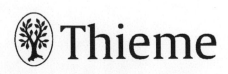

Challenges in the Pandemic

A Multidisciplinary Approach

Chief Editors

Joseph Varon, MD, FACP, FCCP, FCCM, FRSM
Chief of Critical Care Services
United Memorial Medical Center/United General Hospital
Houston, Texas, USA

Paul Marik, MD
Professor of Medicine and Chief of Pulmonary and Critical Care Medicine
Eastern Virginia Medical School
Norfolk, Virginia, USA

Jose Iglesias, DO, FASN
Associate Professor of Medicine
Hackensack Meridian School of Medicine
Nutley, New Jersey, USA
Department of Medicine, Jersey Shore University
Medical Center
Neptune, New Jersey, USA

Christopher de Souza, DORL, MS, DNB, FACS (USA), FRCS (England)
ENT Surgeon
Lilavati Hospital, Holy Family Hospital, Holy Spirit Hospital
Mumbai, Maharashtra, India

Thieme
Delhi • Stuttgart • New York • Rio de Janeiro

Publishing Director: Ritu Sharma
Senior Development Editor: Dr Nidhi Srivastava
Director-Editorial Services: Rachna Sinha
Project Manager: Ronald Dsouza
Vice President, Sales and Marketing: Arun Kumar Majji
Managing Director & CEO: Ajit Kohli

Thieme Medical and Scientific Publishers Private Limited.
A - 12, Second Floor, Sector - 2, Noida - 201 301, Uttar Pradesh, India, +911204556600
Email: customerservice@thieme.in
www.thieme.in

Cover design: Thieme Publishing Group
Cover image source: © Dr Christopher de Souza
Typesetting by RECTO Graphics, India

Printed in India by Replika Press Pvt. Ltd.

5 4 3 2 1

ISBN: 978-93-90553-42-6
eISBN: 978-93-90553-49-5

Important note: Medicine is an ever-changing science undergoing continual development. Research and clinical experience are continually expanding our knowledge, in particular, our knowledge of proper treatment and drug therapy. Insofar as this book mentions any dosage or application, readers may rest assured that the authors, editors, and publishers have made every effort to ensure that such references are in accordance with **the state of knowledge at the time of production of the book.**

Nevertheless, this does not involve, imply, or express any guarantee or responsibility on the part of the publishers in respect to any dosage instructions and forms of applications stated in the book. **Every user is requested to examine carefully** the manufacturers' leaflets accompanying each drug and to check, if necessary, in consultation with a physician or specialist, whether the dosage schedules mentioned therein or the contraindications stated by the manufacturers differ from the statements made in the present book. Such examination is particularly important with drugs that are either rarely used or have been newly released in the market. Every dosage schedule or every form of application used is entirely at the user's own risk and responsibility. The authors and publishers request every user to report to the publishers any discrepancies or inaccuracies noticed. If errors in this work are found after publication, errata will be posted at www.thieme.com on the product description page.

Some of the product names, patents, and registered designs referred to in this book are in fact registered trademarks or proprietary names even though specific reference to this fact is not always made in the text. Therefore, the appearance of a name without designation as proprietary is not to be construed as a representation by the publisher that it is in the public domain.

Thieme addresses people of all gender identities equally. We encourage our authors to use gender-neutral or gender-equal expressions wherever the context allows.

This book is dedicated to Mr Ratan N. Tata
Chairman Emeritus, Tata Trusts
We remain ever grateful to Mr Ratan N. Tata who graciously, generously, and
unselfishly provided for health care workers, during the pandemic.

Contents

Contents

Foreword

I applaud the eminent Editors and contributors for coming out with this timely book *Challenges in the Pandemic: A Multidisciplinary Approach* while we are still in the midst of the pandemic with the looming threat of a 'Third Wave'. They have addressed issues in a very masterful way and shared valuable strategies and solutions that work while we endeavour to get people vaccinated against COVID-19.

It has been a challenging time for me to deal with a very virulent viral infectious disease at Lilavati Hospital which is an extremely well-equipped tertiary care centre in Mumbai, India. With the support of my incredible health care workers, we came up with workable solutions that helped us deal with this challenge very effectively.

Amazingly with the hospital being divided into different zones for safety, we were still able to treat patients with non-COVID related issues safely and effectively without either the patient or the healthcare workers contracting COVID. My Armed Forces background helped me deal with these unprecedented circumstances on a war footing and in a disciplined manner with SOPs being formulated which were rigidly followed by all. All this would not have been possible were it not for our extremely talented, dedicated, and devoted healthcare workers who were committed and saved many lives by putting the lives and concerns of patients ahead of their own.

I foresee that this book will be read by many and will be very popular because of its list of very eminent, widely respected, and deeply influential contributors. It is also likely to serve as a template for other books that address pandemics that might occur in the future.

Lt General (Dr) V Ravishanker, MS, DNB, MCh, FIAC
Lilavati Hospital
Mumbai, India

Preface

We have chosen to write this book during the pandemic in order to provide some clarity on issues that were encountered during the pandemic. It is estimated that approximately 90,000 papers were published in peer-reviewed journals on the pandemic so far. Many of them projected contradictory information. As a result, some high-profile papers were either retracted or withdrawn. Initially, hydroxychloroquinolines (HCQ) were thought to be helpful. These were advocated by many, and their trajectory was propelled by social media leading to enormous misinformation. This was not helped in any way by the presidential elections in the USA where the pandemic was a major issue of debate.

Along the way we learned from our mistakes and some of it through trial and error.

It takes 4 to 5 years for a vaccine to be developed that will be effective and safe, providing immunity from the virus. Vaccines were produced in half that time. This led to vaccine hesitation among the general public. The pandemic has by no means ended. We have gone through the second wave which in many ways was far more devastating than the first. The third wave is now making its presence felt. We still do not know what the long-term consequences are for those who have suffered from COVID-19.

Our book provides insight into dealing with patients and situations in the COVID-19 pandemic. We provide methodologies and treatment strategies that will help health care workers deal effectively with patients who are in various stages of affliction with the coronavirus infection. We also look at how the health care workers while dealing with the pandemic should not suffer from it themselves nor endanger those with whom they come in contact by transmission of the disease.

It will take many years post pandemic to evaluate the effects of the pandemic and to analyze it in an objective, holistic manner.

Until then we do the best we can. Our book attempts to help all who are serving in the pandemic to provide solutions and strategies for those suffering from this terrible malady.

Joseph Varon, MD, FACP, FCCP, FCCM, FRSM
Chief of Critical Care Services
United Memorial Medical Center/United General Hospital, Houston, Texas, USA

Paul Marik, MD
Professor of Medicine and Chief of Pulmonary and Critical Care Medicine
Eastern Virginia Medical School, Norfolk, Virginia, USA

Jose Iglesias, DO, FASN
Associate Professor of Medicine
Hackensack Meridian School of Medicine, Nutley, New Jersey, USA
Department of Medicine, Jersey Shore University
Medical Center, Neptune, New Jersey, USA

Christopher de Souza, DORL, MS, DNB, FACS (USA), FRCS (England)
ENT Surgeon
Lilavati Hospital, Holy Family Hospital, Holy Spirit Hospital
Mumbai, Maharashtra, India

About the Editors

Joseph Varon, MD, FACP, FCCP, FCCM, FRSM
Dr Varon has contributed more than 830 peer-reviewed journal articles, 10 full textbooks, and about 180 book chapters to medical literature. He currently serves as Editor-in-Chief for *Critical Care and Shock* and *Current Respiratory Medicine Reviews*. Dr Varon has won many prestigious awards and is considered one of the top physicians in the United States.

With Dr Carlos Ayus, he co-described the hyponatremia associated with extreme exercise syndrome also known as the "Varon-Ayus syndrome." With Mr James Boston, he co-described the health care provider anxiety syndrome also known as "Boston-Varon syndrome." Along with Professor Luc Montagnier (Nobel Prize winner for Medicine in 2008), Dr Varon founded the Medical Prevention and Research Institute in Houston, Texas, which conducts work on basic sciences projects. During the past 11 months of the COVID-19 pandemic, Dr Varon has become a world leader for his work on COVID-19 and his co-development of the MATH+ protocol to care for these patients. For this he has won multiple awards, including a proclamation by the Mayor of the City of Houston as "Dr. Joseph Varon Day."

Paul Marik, MD
Dr Marik has special knowledge and training in a diverse set of medical fields, with specific training in Internal Medicine, Critical Care, Neurocritical Care, Pharmacology, Anesthesia, Nutrition, and Tropical Medicine and Hygiene. Dr Marik is currently a tenured Professor of Medicine and Chief of the Division of Pulmonary and Critical Care Medicine at Eastern Virginia Medical School in Norfolk, Virginia. Dr Marik has written over 500 peer-reviewed journal articles, 80 book chapters, and authored four critical care books. He has been cited over 43,000 times in peer-reviewed publications and has an H-index of 77.

He is the second most published critical care physician in the world and is a world-renowned expert in the management of sepsis. His contributions to the understanding and management of the hemodynamic, fluid, nutritional, and supportive care practices in sepsis have transformed the care of patients throughout the world. He has already co-authored 10 papers on many therapeutic aspects of COVID-19.

Jose Iglesias, DO, FASN
Dr Iglesias is an Associate Professor of Medicine at the University of Medicine and Dentistry of the N.J. School of Osteopathic Medicine, and Associate Professor of Medicine at Hackensack Meridian School of Medicine. His randomized controlled trial published in the major medical journal *Chest* was the first to demonstrate markedly reduced requirements for vasopressor therapy in septic shock patients treated with intravenous ascorbic acid. He has worked tirelessly at bedsides in ICUs of multiple hospitals in New Jersey throughout the pandemic. His rapidly accumulated clinical insights and expertise helped develop the MATH+ hospital treatment protocol for COVID-19.

Christopher de Souza, DORL, MS, DNB, FACS (USA), FRCS (England)
Dr Christopher de Souza is the Editor-in-Chief of *International Journal of Head and Neck Surgery*. He is presently Consultant ENT - Head Neck Surgeon, Lilavati Hospital and Holy Family Hospital,

Mumbai. He has been on the faculty of State University of New York (SUNY), Brooklyn, New York, USA and Louisiana State University Health Science Center (LSUHSC), Shreveport, USA for 26 years. He is the only Indian and second person in the world to be awarded the Orbit Silver Medal from Europe for work on nose and paranasal sinuses. He is the author and editor of 38 textbooks.

Contributors

Ahmed Ellkhouty, MD
Hospitalist
Department of Internal Medicine
Saint Francis Medical Center
Trenton, New Jersey, USA

Alessandra Chen, MD
Dermatology Resident
Department of Dermatology
Keck USC School of Medicine
Los Angeles, California, USA

Amit Kumar, BS
Graduate student Epidemeology
Harvard School of Public Health
Boston, Massachusetts, USA

Amit Setya, DO
Associate Director
Emergency Medical Services
Community Medical Center RWJ-Barnabas Health
Toms River, New Jersey, USA

Anish Patil, MB, BCh, BAO.SpR (Anesthetics)
SpR in Anesthesia
New Cross Hospital
Wolverhampton, UK

Binh Ngo, MD
Clinical Associate Professor of Dermatology
Keck USC School of Medicine
Department of Dermatology
Los Angeles, California, USA;
The Rose Salter Medical Research Foundation
Newport Coast, California, USA

Carmen Alvarez, PHD
Division of immunology and Virology
UNIR Health Sciences School & Medical Center
Madrid, Spain

Cesar Ivan Patiño-Barrera, MS
Research Coordinator
United Memorial Medical Center
Houston, Texas, USA;
Benemérita Universidad Autónoma de Puebla
Puebla, México

Christine Filippone, DPN
DNP/Adult Nurse Practitioner–Director
Epidemiology/Infection Control
Community Medical Center RWJ–Barnabas Health
Toms River, New Jersey, USA

Christopher de Souza, DORL, MS, DNB, FACS (USA), FRCS (England)
ENT Surgeon
Lilavati Hospital, Holy Family Hospital, Holy Spirit Hospital
Mumbai, Maharashtra, India

Danielle Biggs, MD
Clinical Associate Professor of Emergency Medicine
Robert Wood Johnson Rutgers Medical School
Graduate and Post Graduate Medical Education
New Brunswick, New Jersey, USA

Eric Osgood, MD
Hospitalist
Department of Internal Medicine
Saint Francis Medical Center
Trenton, New Jersey, USA

Jerrold Levine, MD
Professor of Medicine
Department of Medicine Division of Nephrology
University of Illinois at Chicago School of Medicine
Chicago, Illinois, USA

Jill Glasspool Malone, PhD
Consultant
RW Malone MD LLC
Consultancy and Analytics
Madison, Virginia, USA

Jose Iglesias, DO, FASN
Associate Professor of Medicine
Hackensack Meridian School of Medicine Nutley, New Jersey, USA;
Department of Medicine Jersey Shore University Medical Center
Neptune, New Jersey, USA

Joseph Varon, MD, FACP, FCCP, FCCM, FRSM
Chief of Critical Care Services
United Memorial Medical Center/United General
Hospital
Houston, Texas, USA

Joslyn Joseph, MD
Clinical Associate Professor of Emergency
Medicine
Robert Wood Johnson Rutgers Medical School
Graduate and Post Graduate Medical Education
New Brunswick, New Jersey, USA

Kiran Shekade, MD, FNB (Critical Care Medicine)
Intensivist
Lilavati Hospital
Mumbai, Maharashtra, India

Lisa Armstrong, MD
Clinical Associate Professor of Emergency
Medicine
Robert Wood Johnson Rutgers Medical School
Graduate and Post Graduate Medical Education
New Brunswick, New Jersey, USA

Marc Rendell, MD
Medical Director
The Rose Salter Medical Research Foundation
Newport Coast, CA, USA

Marianne M. Holler, MSW, DO, FAAHPM
Director of Palliative Care
Community Medical Center RWJ–Barnabas Health
Toms River, New Jersey, USA

Marie Donaldson, MD
Dermatology Resident
Department of Dermatology
Keck USC School of Medicine
Los Angeles, California, USA

Mariya Mohiuddin, MS
Research Director
United Memorial Medical Center
Houston, Texas, USA

Mika Turkia, MS
Independent Science writer
Helsinki, Finland

Nicole Maguire, DO
Clinical Associate Professor of Emergency
Medicine
Robert Wood Johnson Rutgers Medical School
Graduate and Post Graduate Medical Education
New Brunswick, New Jersey, USA

Paul Marik, MD
Professor of Medicine and Chief of Pulmonary and
Critical Care Medicine
Eastern Virginia Medical School
Norfolk, Virginia, USA

Pierre Kory, MD
President and Chief Medical Officer
Front-Line Covid-19 Critical Care Alliance
Madison, Wisconsin, USA

Prakash Jiandani, MD
Intensivist
Lilavati Hospital
Mumbai, Maharashtra, India

Priyanjan Kata, MD
Research Assistant
Internal Medicine Residency Program Community
Medical Center RWJ–Barnabas Health, Rutgers
Health
Toms River, New Jersey, USA

Rajesh Mohan, MD, MBA, FACC, FSCAI
Interventional Cardiologist;
President North Atlantic Medical Associates;
Former Chief Medical Officer and Chair of Internal
Medicine
Monmouth Medical Center Southern Campus
Lakewood, New Jersey, USA

Robert W. Malone, MD, MS
Consultant
RW Malone MD LLC
Consultancy and Analytics
Madison, Virginia, USA

Rosemarie de Souza, MD
Professor and Head
TN Medica College and MICU, BYL Nair Hospital
Mumbai, Maharashtra, India

Ruchi N. Raval, BS, MPH
Garden State Neurology and Neuro-Oncology PC
100 State Highway 36 East, Suite 1A
West Long branch, New Jersey, USA

Srinivasan Ramnathan, MD
Intensivist
Lilavati Hospital
Mumbai, Maharashtra, India

Steven Hamilton, MD
Hospitalist
Department of Internal Medicine
Saint Francis Medical Center
Trenton, New Jersey, USA

Sumul Raval, MD, DABN
Neurologist and Neuro-oncologist;
Founder and Director
David S. Zocchi Brain Tumor Center at Monmouth
Medical Center
Garden State Neurology and Neuro-Oncology
Toms River, New Jersey, USA

Vicente Soriano, MD, PhD
UNIR Health Sciences School & Medical Center
Madrid, Spain

Vignesh Ravi, BS
Medical Student
Department of Dermatology
Keck USC School of Medicine
Los Angeles, California, USA

Vinod Nookala, MD
Program Director
Internal Medicine Residency Program
Community Medical Center RWJ–Barnabas Health,
Rutgers Health
Toms River, New Jersey, USA

William Dalsey, MD
Attending Physician
Emergency Department Operations
Robert Wood Johnson Rutgers Medical School
Graduate and Post Graduate Medical Education
New Brunswick, New Jersey, USA

**Wouter Jonker, MBChB, DA, FCARCSI, DICM,
FJFICMI**
Consultant Anaesthesiologists Sligo University
Hospital, Ireland

01 Epidemiology of COVID-19

Amit Kumar

Introduction

Coronaviruses—thus named for their unique crownlike spikes visible under microscopy—are a diverse class of viruses that are known to cause intestinal and respiratory infections within both bird and mammal hosts. On a molecular level, they are enveloped, positive-sense viruses that contain single-stranded RNA as their genetic material. Further, coronaviruses belong to the family *Coronaviridae*, which are known to cause respiratory disease in humans.

COVID-19, the infectious disease caused by severe acute respiratory syndrome coronavirus 2 (SARS-CoV-2), has been documented to have a wide range of outcomes. Following infection, certain individuals remain asymptomatic or merely develop mild upper respiratory symptoms, while others present with serious conditions such as pneumonia and/or severe acute respiratory distress syndrome, which could possibly require intubation and lead to complications.

In symptomatic patients, COVID-19 can be modeled by breaking symptoms down into four distinct phases, the first of which is characterized by upper respiratory tract infection accompanied by fever, muscle fatigue, and pain. While most patients experience no further symptoms, individuals that progress further develop pneumonia (which can be either symptomatic or asymptomatic) as well as dyspnea. In the third stage, patients worsen as a result of cytokine release syndrome, also known as "cytokine storm," which floods the bloodstream with inflammatory proteins known as cytokines. This state of hyperinflammation, in turn, can cause renal damage, sepsis, and secondary infection. Finally, in the fourth and final stage, patients either recover or die, the outcome of which is dependent on a myriad of factors including age, race, and past medical history.

Delivering optimal care for SARS-CoV-2 and all future health crises necessitates an understanding of the epidemiological trends of the COVID-19 pandemic; by analyzing and documenting these patterns, we can not only improve our ability to combat future pandemics, but also address current health-related disparities and inform future policy.

Geographic Distribution

Origins of COVID-19 and Global Spread

The origins of SARS-CoV-2 can be traced back to individuals infected within rural locales of the People's Republic of China as early as October 2019. However, the virus appears to have been incapable of efficient human-to-human transmission during this time. In December 2019, a mutation of the virus occurred in Wuhan, a city located in the Hubei Province of China, resulting in improved transmissibility within human hosts.[1,2] Although the Chinese government instituted a quarantine of Wuhan on January 23, 2020, widespread travel among its residents meant the outbreak could no longer be contained, introducing a global pandemic.

The current working theory for the zoonotic basis of SARS-CoV-2 posits that the virus originated in bats before undergoing multiple recombination events as it passed through mammals.[3] Evidence supporting this hypothesis can be found in genomic studies. The genome of SARS-CoV-2 shares a 96% similarity to betacoronavirus isolated from a bat in 2013 (RaTG13).[4] Further, the SARS-CoV-2 receptor binding motif—a portion of the virus instrumental for host infection—is closely related in sequence to the betacoronavirus isolated from a Malayan pangolin, more so than its bat counterpart (98.7 vs. 77.6% similarity).[4]

COVID-19 has since spread exponentially, with greater than 150 million cases having been reported globally spanning every continent. It should be noted that this figure is an underestimate of COVID-19's overall disease burden, as not every case is ultimately reported. This is supported by seroprevalence survey studies conducted in the United States and Europe.[5,6]

Distribution of COVID-19 in the United States

Spread of COVID-19 proceeded rapidly in the United States: community transmission was first identified in February 2020, and by the middle of March, confirmed cases were reported in all 50 states, the District of Columbia, and four U.S. territories. During spring and early summer of 2020—the initial months of the pandemic—case distribution was heavily skewed in favor of densely populated urban centers such as New York, Boston, and New Orleans relative to less populous rural areas. In July 2020, however, this urban–rural disparity began to close, with less densely populated areas beginning to see a rise in case levels.[7]

Risk Factors

Ethnic/Racial Disparities in Disease Outcomes

There exist marked racial/ethnic inequities with respect to age-adjusted COVID-19 disease outcomes. In Chicago, Black individuals make up 30% of the population, yet contributed to 50% of COVID-19 cases and 70% of deaths as of July 2020, most of them concentrated within the city's most vulnerable communities.[8] At the national level, Pacific Islanders, Latinos, Blacks, and Indigenous Americans have a COVID-19 death rate of more than double that of White and Asian Americans after controlling for age (**Fig. 1.1**).[9] Ongoing research seeks to examine the extent to which these observed poorer outcomes among people of color can be attributed to direct effects of the SARS-CoV-2 virus versus indirect consequences of the pandemic such as its effects on the job market, as well as its exacerbation of existing disparities in access to resources and health care.[10] This clear incongruity in outcome measures has shaped the development of targeted economic interventions and vaccine information campaigns.

Social Determinants of Disease Outcome

Existing structural inequities—exacerbated by the brutal socioeconomic effects of the pandemic—likely have contributed to ethnic/racial disparities in COVID-19 outcomes. COVID-19-related mortality rates are also associated with factors such as education and economic status, with U.S. counties comprised of college-educated individuals with high-earning professions suffering fewer deaths on average than counties with a higher poverty prevalence.[11] This observation is linked to risk of exposure, as individuals holding high-earning careers were more likely able to work remotely, allowing for better adherence to social distancing protocols. Persons of color were disproportionately represented among "essential workers" that were exempt from shelter-in-place mandates instituted during heightened waves of COVID-19 spread.[10] Additionally, Blacks make up about roughly a quarter of all public transit users in the United States, further contributing to an increased risk of exposure.[11] Finally, persons of color are more likely to live in crowded conditions such as multigenerational households that not only elevate exposure, but also limit the ability to quarantine.[12]

Ethnic/racial disparities in the incidence of chronic conditions have also been implicated

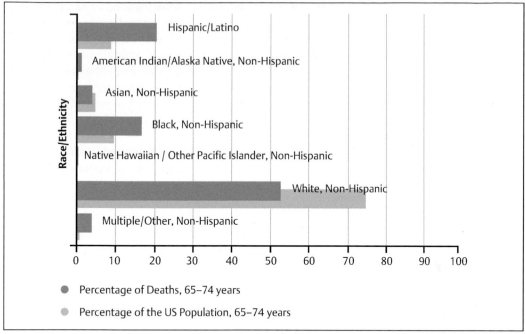

Fig. 1.1 Percentage of COVID-19 deaths among racial and ethnic groups (*blue*) compared to percentage of race and ethnic groups in the United States demonstrating a higher proportion of deaths among minorities compared to non-Hispanic Whites. (Source: https://www.cdc.gov/coronavirus/2019-ncov/community/health-equity/racial-ethnic-disparities/images/atl-disparities-black-patients.)

in COVID-19 outcomes. Previous diagnoses of conditions such as cardiovascular disease, chronic kidney disease, chronic lung diseases (such as chronic obstructive pulmonary disease), diabetes mellitus, hypertension, and obesity have been demonstrated to predispose patients to more severe disease activity, increasing risk of intubation and death[13]: data reported by the Centers for Disease Control and Prevention (CDC) illustrate that over 90% of patients who were hospitalized due to COVID-19 had at least one preexisting condition.[14] Notably, the incidence rates of these chronic diseases are disproportionately high among people of color, partially as a consequence of ethnic/racial disparities within health determinants such as socioeconomic status, education, and availability of health care resources.[15–17] Thus, vulnerability to COVID-19 based on the presence of these comorbidities in part is driven by the convergence of existing structural inequities

along racial lines, further informing the increased mortality rates observed among minorities. Dr. Anthony Fauci, Director of the National Institute of Allergy and Infectious Diseases and Chief Medical Advisor to the President, emphasized these disparities in an April 2020 speech, particularly among Black communities: "Health disparities have always existed for the African American community... [COVID is] shining a bright light on how unacceptable that is because, yet again, when you have a situation like coronavirus, they are suffering disproportionately."[18]

Changes in Racial/Ethnic Distribution of COVID-19 Incidence over Time

Analysis of incidence data reported by the CDC from January through December 2020 indicates that COVID-19 ethnic/racial inequities changed over time in adults aged 25 years or older. Specifically, during the early stages of the pandemic (i.e., January–April), this disparity was more pronounced among ethnic minorities relative to White individuals. Over time, this gap began to close, although as a consequence of increased incidence within White individuals rather than decreases within minority populations. The largest disparities observed were among Native Hawaiian/Pacific Islander, Native American, and Hispanic individuals.[19]

Age-Related Disparities in Disease Outcomes

Among unvaccinated individuals, age is the most significant predictor of poor outcomes and mortality within COVID-19 patients,[20] with the distribution of cases heavily skewed toward older age groups.[21,22] In fact, the SARS-CoV-2 virus has a remarkably low infection rate among children as well as a decreased propensity toward exhibiting symptoms. For instance, it is estimated that the risk of infection in individuals older than 20 years is roughly double that of those younger than 20 years.[23] Further, while individuals between the ages of 18 and 29 years make up the highest percentage of cases in the United States among all age groups, over 94% of COVID-19-related deaths were observed in patients older than 50 years (**Fig. 1.2**).[20]

Factors Driving Increased COVID-19 Mortality among Older Patients

An explanation for this age distribution disparity lies within the presence of chronic health conditions (CHCs), which have been demonstrated to significantly worsen COVID-19 outcomes. Older individuals have a higher prevalence of such CHCs, including hypertension, diabetes, coronary heart disease, and chronic kidney disease: a study conducted on critically ill older patients with SARS-CoV-2 found that 86% had at least one CHC diagnosis.[24] Furthermore, having multiple chronic diseases—the likelihood of which increases with age—has been shown to place

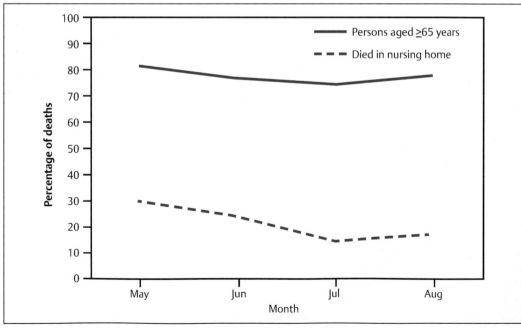

Fig. 1.2   Percentage of deaths from COVID-19 among persons older than 65 years or persons of any age who died in a nursing home. (Reproduced with permission from Gold JAW, Rossen LM, Ahmad FB, et al. Race, ethnicity, and age trends in persons who died from COVID-19—United States, May–August 2020. MMWR Morb Mortal Wkly Rep 2020;69(42):1517–1521.)

patients at even greater risk of mortality from COVID-19.[25]

The use of angiotensin-converting enzyme (ACE) inhibitors—a frequently prescribed type of medication among older patients—has also been thought to worsen outcomes, providing further explanation for the observed distribution of age-related COVID-19 mortality.[25] The foundation of this theory lies in the SARS-CoV-2 viral mechanism of action: external spike proteins anchor the virus to cellular ACE2 receptors, allowing for viral entry. Experimental studies in animal models have found that inhibition of the renin–angiotensin–aldosterone system (RAAS) via ACE inhibitors results in a compensatory increase in tissue expression of these ACE2 receptors, generating speculation as to whether this could adversely affect COVID-19-related outcomes through enhancement of viral binding and cell entry.[26,27] Conversely, other researchers have postulated that RAAS inhibitors could be advantageous in COVID-19 patients by increasing expression of angiotensin 1–7 and 1–9, both of which have vasodilatory and anti-inflammatory effects that could potentially attenuate lung damage. Ultimately, COVID-19 clinical guidelines have cleared ACE inhibitors, stating that there is no evidence of adverse effects as a consequence of continuing these medications.[28-31] To this point, there were no significant differences in the average number of days alive and out of hospital—a composite measure that integrates clinically important outcomes such as death, hospital length of stay, and readmission to hospital—between patients who continued and discontinued ACE inhibitor therapy, lending support to its acceptability within COVID-19 patients.[31]

COVID-19 Infection Rates and Outcomes in Children and Adolescents

By observation, children appear to be less vulnerable to COVID-19 infection than adults: per 2020 data from China, children aged 0 to 15 years make up 17.8% of the population, yet only represent 2.1% of reported cases.[32] However, this does not necessarily indicate that children have a lower rate of infection than adults: a study found that children younger than 10 years who were exposed to COVID-19 were at similar risk of infection compared to all other age groups.[33] Thus, while risk of infection remains the same across age groups, younger patients are less likely to suffer from severe disease activity. Moreover, the number of laboratory-confirmed cases of SARS-CoV-2 infection in children is an underestimate, a consequence of the high proportion of mild and asymptomatic cases within this age group. This assertion is validated by a seroprevalence study that found the reported number of cases within children to be significantly lower than the actual number of infections.[34]

Understanding the factors that drive these clear incongruities in outcomes between children and adults remains an ongoing area of research. One proposed explanation lies in the fact that children have less mature ACE2, potentially disrupting the SARS-CoV-2 virus' ability to anchor onto cells via their spike proteins. Additionally, children—those who are younger, in particular—tend to have frequent viral infections; thus, there is a possibility that this repeated exposure could support the immune system in its response to SARS-CoV-2.[35]

Transmission

Person-to-Person Transmission

Direct Respiratory Transmission: The Dominant Route of Transmission

Direct respiratory transmission is dominant, with proximity and ventilation being key determinants of infection risk. Transmission is thought to occur when two individuals—at least one of whom is infected—come in close contact with each other, specifically within 6 feet distance. When in close proximity, virions suspended on either large droplets or fine aerosol particles are expelled from the respiratory tract of the infected individual via mechanisms such as coughing, sneezing, and/or speaking. When these droplets/aerosols are inhaled or come into contact with a mucous membrane of an uninfected person, SARS-CoV-2 is able to effectively spread from person to person.[36] Therefore, proximity plays a crucial role in SARS-CoV-2 transmission, informing the social distancing and quarantine protocols that have been instituted by public health experts.

Environmental Transmission

Airborne Transmission
In addition to direct person-to-person respiratory transmission, SARS-CoV-2 also has the ability to spread over longer distances via airborne transmission, occurring when individuals inhale viral particles that remain in the air. Recent work has demonstrated that coughs, sneezes, and exhalations produce ejecta that take the form of turbulent clouds composed of hot, humid air and suspended mucosalivary droplets, making them multiphase in nature. This gas-phase component has critical implications toward extending the longevity of these viral droplets: the warm, moist environment within these turbulent clouds allows droplets to evade evaporation for a much greater period of time than if they were isolated. This, in turn, has the ability to increase the lifespan of a droplet from seconds to minutes, allowing for the possibility of infections over time and distance.[37,38] This is validated by studies that analyzed transmission patterns within certain outbreaks (namely, an indoor restaurant, choir practice, and public bus), all of which conclude that airborne spread is plausible, particularly within indoor, poorly ventilated environments.[39–41] Further, a 2020 report from China illustrated that lingering SARS-CoV-2 particles can be found in the hospital rooms of infected patients, underscoring the significance of ventilation in managing transmission.

Overall, however, observational studies utilizing secondary attack rate (SAR) as a means of quantifying spread suggest that this mechanism is not a primary route of transmission. In epidemiology, SAR is defined as the number of cases occurring within the incubation period upon exposure to a primary case divided by the number of susceptible individuals.[42] Overall, only about 5% of close contacts to patients with confirmed COVID-19 become infected, although this rate is dependent upon the duration and intensity of contact.[43] For instance, sharing a meal is associated with a 7% SAR, while passing interactions during shopping has a 0.6% rate. Further, in health care workers unknowingly caring for infected patients, the SAR is roughly 3%.[44] Notably, among these few cases, the providers were found to have performed aerosol-generating procedures and/or underwent prolonged exposure with inconsistent usage of face masks.[45,46]

Fomite Transmission
SARS-CoV-2 also has the capacity to spread indirectly through contaminated intermediates known as fomites, which are defined as objects or materials that are likely to carry infection. These fomites become infected either through direct contact with another fomite or by settling airborne viral particles. Fomite transmission can occur when an individual makes physical contact with a fomite and then touches a facial membrane, although its overall contribution is currently thought to be insignificant.[47] While there are little available data on the environmental stability of SARS-CoV-2, there is evidence to suggest that the virus is able to persist on surfaces such as metal, glass, ceramics, plastic, and rubber to varying degrees of longevity, lasting anywhere from hours to greater than a week.[48]

In general, while this type of transmission necessitates that the virus is able to persist in an area outside of its given host, certain environmental characteristics can influence infectivity retention and speed of spread. Specifically, SARS-CoV-2 transmission is optimized at low temperatures and low humidity, which partially explains the surge of COVID-19 cases observed during colder seasons.[49] Simulated sunlight has also been experimentally determined to inactivate SARS-CoV-2 over the course of 15 to 20 minutes, with higher levels of ultraviolet-B (UVB) linked to more rapid inactivation. These results suggest that persistence and exposure risk, by extension, vary significantly between indoor and outdoor environments, and have contributed to the development of past economic shutdown policies.[50] Taken together, an environment that poses the greatest risk for SARS-CoV-2 fomite transmission are indoor settings with heavy viral contaminations (i.e., an infected patient's hospital room), and it highlights the continued importance of hygiene vigilance and cleaning protocols in public settings.

Transmission within Nonrespiratory Specimens

SARS-CoV-2 has been detected on nonrespiratory specimens including stool, blood, ocular secretions, and semen, although their role in transmission as yet remains unclear. Further, there is no evidence to suggest that transmission can occur through contact with nonmucus sites.

Oral–Fecal Transmission
Given the high expression rate of ACE2 receptors in the small intestine—particularly among proximal and distal enterocytes—infection of the gastrointestinal (GI) tract by SARS-CoV-2 is plausible, and provides an explanation for COVID-19 patients who present with GI symptoms, including diarrhea, nausea, and vomiting. Notably, several studies have demonstrated that viral load within stool samples persists even after SARS-CoV-2 RNA is no longer detected in upper respiratory specimens, illustrating that the duration of virus is longer within this specimen type. Further, peak viral load in stool occurs later relative to upper respiratory specimens, persisting for up to 33 days or more after RNA is no longer detectable in respiratory

specimens.[51,52] In rare cases, replicative SARS-CoV-2 RNA was able to be cultured from stool samples. Despite these findings, an oral–fecal route of transmission has not been documented, although it does remain an area of ongoing research given the presented data.[53,54] Although case studies have implicated transmission via feces, there was insufficient evidence to prove causality in each of these scenarios.[55,56]

Sexual Transmission
SARS-CoV-2 has been detected in the semen of COVID-19 patients, including those who are in the recovery process.[57] Further, ACE2 receptors are located in the testis, introducing discussions on the plausibility of male genital tract infection and viral shedding in semen, as well as implicating sexual intercourse as a potential source of person-to-person transmission.[58–61] The presence of these receptors contributes an explanation for the subset of patients who have reported COVID-19-associated genital symptoms such as testicular/spermatic cord pain.[62,63] Ultimately, while intercourse itself has not been causally linked to SARS-CoV-2 transmission, it can absolutely provide a means for viral spread by virtue of the close proximity between participants required.[64]

Bloodborne Transmission
SARS-CoV-2 can replicate within blood cells, adversely affecting their ability to perform their normal function; therefore, it is unsurprising that low levels have also been detected in serum specimens. Despite this, the likelihood of transmission appears to be low, which is consistent with clinical observations on related respiratory viruses such as the Middle East respiratory syndrome coronavirus (MERS-CoV) and SARS-CoV. In other transfusion-transmitted viral infections such as HIV, the risk of spread is directly related to viral load, indicating that even if bloodborne transmission was possible, its efficacy would be limited.[65]

Period of Infectiousness and Viral Shedding

Infectiousness Timeline

Although the precise time interval during which patients can transmit SARS-CoV-2 to others is unknown, it is well documented that infected individuals are likely at their most contagious in the early stages of the disease. Cultures of upper respiratory specimens validate this, with viral RNA peaks corresponding to this point in the infection timeline as well.[66] Specifically, a study found that infectiousness on average peaks during the following interval: between 2 days prior to the development of symptoms and 1 day after they conclude. Subsequent to this, viral RNA load decreases within a week[67]; specifically, among 28 studies, the pooled median duration of RNA shedding within respiratory specimens was about 18 days after the onset of symptoms.[68] However, it should be noted that positive detection does not necessarily indicate the presence of infectious virus, as studies have illustrated that there is a threshold of viral RNA that must be met to achieve infectiousness.[69] It should be noted that this average duration of RNA shedding refers to immunocompetent patients; within immunocompromised patients, infectious virus have been detected in respiratory specimens that were cultured months after initial diagnosis and onset of symptoms.[70–72]

Transmission among Presymptomatic and Asymptomatic Patients

The potential for transmission can occur in patients who are both presymptomatic (i.e., prior to the development of symptoms) and asymptomatic (patients who do not present with symptoms at all after infection). Although the duration and amount of viral RNA were found to be similar among asymptomatic and symptomatic individuals,[73] it is important to note that the risk of transmission appears to be higher among the latter type of patient. A possible explanation for this lies in the understanding that symptomatic patients are more likely to produce transmissible ejecta as a consequence of increased coughing and sneezing.

Conclusion

The COVID-19 pandemic has posed multiple challenges to global health with a disproportionate increase in mortality among those most vulnerable such as the elderly, the poor, those populations with increasing comorbidities, minorities, and poorer developing countries. Public health measures such as testing, social distancing, wearing masks, aggressive hygiene, and mitigation strategies cannot be underscored.

References

1. Havers FP, Reed C, Lim T, et al. Seroprevalence of antibodies to SARS-CoV-2 in 10 sites in the United States, March 23-May 12, 2020. JAMA Intern Med 2020;180(12):1576–1586
2. Stringhini S, Wisniak A, Piumatti G, et al. Seroprevalence of anti-SARS-CoV-2 IgG antibodies in Geneva, Switzerland (SEROCoV-POP): a population-based study. Lancet 2020;396(10247):313–319
3. Salian VS, Wright JA, Vedell PT, et al. COVID-19 transmission, current treatment, and future therapeutic strategies. Mol Pharm 2021; 18(3):754–771
4. Wong MC, Javornik Cregeen SJ, Ajami NJ, Petrosino JF. Evidence of recombination in coronaviruses implicating pangolin origins of nCoV-2019. bioRxiv 2020 (e-pub ahead of print). doi:10.1101/2020.02.07.939207
5. Jones B, Kiley J. The changing geography of COVID-19 in the U.S. Pew Research Center—U.S. Politics & Policy, Pew Research Center, May 25, 2021. Available at: www.pewresearch.org/politics/2020/12/08/the-changing-geography-of-covid-19-in-the-u-s/
6. Reyes C, Husain N, Gutowski C, St Clair S, Pratt G. Chicago's coronavirus disparity: Black Chicagoans are dying at nearly six times the rate of white residents, data

show. Chicago Tribune. Available at: https://www.chicagotribune.com/coronavirus/ct-coronavirus-chicago-coronavirus-deaths-demographics-lightfoot-20200406-77nlylhiavgjzb2wa4ckivh7mu-story.html. Accessed on June 12, 2021

7. APM Research Lab Staff. The color of coronavirus: COVID-19 deaths by race and ethnicity in the U.S. [Internet]. St. Paul (MN): American Public Media; December 10, 2020 [cited December 18, 2020]. Available at: https://www.apmresearchlab.org/covid/deaths-by-race

8. Polyakova M, Udalova V, Kocks G, Genadek K, Finlay K, Finkelstein AN. Racial disparities in excess all-cause mortality during the early COVID-19 pandemic varied substantially across states. Health Aff (Millwood) 2021; 40(2):307–316

9. Choi YJ, Lee HY, An S, Yoon YJ, Oh J. Predictors of cervical cancer screening awareness and literacy among Korean-American women. J Racial Ethn Health Disparities 2020;7(1): 1–9

10. BLS Reports. Labor force characteristics by race and ethnicity. 2018. Available at: https://www.bls.gov/opub/reports/race-and-ethnicity/2018/home.htm. Accessed June 13, 2021

11. American Public Transportation Association. Who rides public transportation. April 27, 2020. Available at: www.apta.com/research-technical-resources/research-reports/who-rides-public-transportation/

12. Gallo Marin B, Aghagoli G, Lavine K, et al. Predictors of COVID-19 severity: a literature review. Rev Med Virol 2021;31(1):1–10

13. Centers for Disease Control and Prevention. Coronavirus disease 2019 (COVID-19). June 25, 2020. Available at: https://www.cdc.gov/coronavirus/2019-ncov/need-extra-precautions/people-with-medical-conditions.html?CDC_AA_refVal=https%3A%2F%2Fwww.cdc.gov%2Fcoronavirus%2F2019-ncov%2Fneed-extra-precautions%2Fgroups-at-higher-risk.html. Accessed June 27, 2020

14. Centers for Disease Control and Prevention. COVID-19 laboratory-confirmed hospitalization. Preliminary data as of June 6, 2020. Available at: https://gis.cdc.gov/grasp/COVIDNet/COVID19_5.html

15. Tanner RM, Gutiérrez OM, Judd S, et al. Geographic variation in CKD prevalence and ESRD incidence in the United States: results from the reasons for geographic and racial differences in stroke (REGARDS) study. Am J Kidney Dis 2013;61(3):395–403

16. Barker LE, Kirtland KA, Gregg EW, Geiss LS, Thompson TJ. Geographic distribution of diagnosed diabetes in the U.S.: a diabetes belt. Am J Prev Med 2011;40(4):434–439

17. Piccolo RS, Yang M, Bliwise DL, Yaggi HK, Araujo AB. Racial and socioeconomic disparities in sleep and chronic disease: results of a longitudinal investigation. Ethn Dis 2013;23(4):499–507

18. Nelson S. Anthony Fauci compares race disparities of coronavirus to AIDS epidemic. New York Post. April 8, 2020. Available at: nypost.com/2020/04/07/anthony-fauci-compares-race-disparities-of-coronavirus-to-aids-epidemic/

19. Price-Haywood EG, Burton J, Fort D, Seoane L. Hospitalization and mortality among black patients and white patients with Covid-19. N Engl J Med 2020;382(26):2534–2543

20. Pollard CA, Morran MP, Nestor-Kalinoski AL. The COVID-19 pandemic: a global health crisis. Physiol Genomics 2020;52(11): 549–557 10.1152/physiolgenomics.00089. 2020

21. Epidemiology Working Group for NCIP Epidemic Response, Chinese Center for Disease Control and Prevention. The epidemiological characteristics of an outbreak of 2019 novel coronavirus diseases (COVID-19) in China [in Chinese]. Zhonghua Liu Xing Bing Xue Za Zhi 2020;41(2):145–151

22. Sun K, Chen J, Viboud C. Early epidemiological analysis of the coronavirus disease 2019 outbreak based on crowdsourced data: a population-level observational study. Lancet Digit Health 2020;2(4):e201–e208

23. Davies NG, Klepac P, Liu Y, Prem K, Jit M, Eggo RM; CMMID COVID-19 working group. Age-dependent effects in the transmission and control of COVID-19 epidemics. Nat Med 2020;26(8):1205–1211

24. Arentz M, Yim E, Klaff L, et al. Characteristics and outcomes of 21 critically ill patients with COVID-19 in Washington state. JAMA 2020;323(16):1612–1614

25. Shahid Z, Kalayanamitra R, McClafferty B, et al. COVID-19 and older adults: what we know. J Am Geriatr Soc 2020;68(5):926–929

26. Ferrario CM, Jessup J, Chappell MC, et al. Effect of angiotensin-converting enzyme inhibition and angiotensin II receptor blockers on cardiac angiotensin-converting enzyme 2. Circulation 2005;111(20):2605–2610

27. Soler MJ, Barrios C, Oliva R, Batlle D. Pharmacologic modulation of ACE2 expression. Curr Hypertens Rep 2008;10(5):410–414

28. Vaduganathan M, Vardeny O, Michel T, McMurray JJV, Pfeffer MA, Solomon SD. Renin-angiotensin-aldosterone system inhibitors in patients with Covid-19. N Engl J Med 2020;382(17):1653–1659

29. Zheng YY, Ma YT, Zhang JY, Xie X. COVID-19 and the cardiovascular system. Nat Rev Cardiol 2020;17(5):259–260

30. Grewal E, Sutarjono B, Mohammed I. Angioedema, ACE inhibitor and COVID-19. BMJ Case Rep 2020;13(9):237888

31. Lopes RD, Macedo AVS, de Barros E Silva PGM, et al; BRACE CORONA Investigators. Effect of discontinuing vs continuing angiotensin-converting enzyme inhibitors and angiotensin II receptor blockers on days alive and out of the hospital in patients admitted with COVID-19: a randomized clinical trial. JAMA 2021;325(3):254–264

32. Statista Research Department. Population distribution in China in 2019, by broad age group. March 5, 2020. Available at: https://www.statista.com/statistics/251524/population-distribution-by-age-group-in-china/. Accessed June 28, 2021

33. Bi Q, Wu Y, Mei S, et al. Epidemiology and transmission of COVID-19 in 391 cases and 1286 of their close contacts in Shenzhen, China: a retrospective cohort study. Lancet Infect Dis 2020;20(8):911–919. Erratum in: Lancet Infect Dis 2020;20(7):e148

34. Hobbs CV, Drobeniuc J, Kittle T, et al; CDC COVID-19 Response Team. Estimated SARS-CoV-2 seroprevalence among persons aged <18 years—Mississippi, May-September 2020. MMWR Morb Mortal Wkly Rep 2021; 70(9):312–315

35. Ludvigsson JF. Systematic review of COVID-19 in children shows milder cases and a better prognosis than adults. Acta Paediatr 2020;109(6):1088–1095

36. Meyerowitz EA, Richterman A, Gandhi RT, Sax PE. Transmission of SARS-CoV-2: a review of viral, host, and environmental factors. Ann Intern Med 2021;174(1):69–79

37. Bourouiba L. Turbulent gas clouds and respiratory pathogen emissions: potential implications for reducing transmission of COVID-19. JAMA 2020;323(18):1837–1838

38. Scharfman BE, Techet AH, Bush JWM, Bourouiba L. Visualization of sneeze ejecta: steps of fluid fragmentation leading to respiratory droplets. Exp Fluids 2016;57(2):24

39. Lu J, Gu J, Li K, et al. COVID-19 outbreak associated with air conditioning in restaurant, Guangzhou, China, 2020. Emerg Infect Dis 2020;26(7):1628–1631

40. Hamner L, Dubbel P, Capron I, et al. High SARS-CoV-2 attack rate following exposure at a choir practice - Skagit County, Washington, March 2020. MMWR Morb Mortal Wkly Rep 2020;69(19):606–610

41. Shen Y, Li C, Dong H, et al. Community outbreak investigation of SARS-CoV-2 transmission among bus riders in eastern China. JAMA Intern Med 2020;180(12):1665–1671. Erratum in: JAMA Intern Med 2021;181(5): 727

42. Shah K, Saxena D, Mavalankar D. Secondary attack rate of COVID-19 in household contacts: a systematic review. QJM 2020; 113(12):841–850

43. Klompas M, Baker MA, Rhee C. Airborne transmission of SARS-CoV-2: theoretical considerations and available evidence. JAMA 2020;324(5):441–442

44. Chen Y, Wang AH, Yi B, et al. Epidemiological characteristics of infection in COVID-19 close contacts in Ningbo city [in Chinese]. Zhonghua Liu Xing Bing Xue Za Zhi 2020; 41(5):667–671

45. Heinzerling A, Stuckey MJ, Scheuer T, et al. Transmission of COVID-19 to health care personnel during exposures to a hospitalized patient - Solano County, California, February 2020. MMWR Morb Mortal Wkly Rep 2020;69(15):472–476

46. Ng K, Poon BH, Kiat Puar TH, et al. COVID-19 and the risk to health care workers: a case report. Ann Intern Med 2020;172(11): 766–767

47. Castaño N, Cordts SC, Kurosu Jalil M, et al. Fomite transmission, physicochemical

origin of virus-surface interactions, and disinfection strategies for enveloped viruses with applications to SARS-CoV-2. ACS Omega 2021;6(10):6509–6527

48. Aboubakr HA, Sharafeldin TA, Goyal SM. Stability of SARS-CoV-2 and other coronaviruses in the environment and on common touch surfaces and the influence of climatic conditions: a review. Transbound Emerg Dis 2021;68(2):296–312

49. Ficetola GF, Rubolini D. Containment measures limit environmental effects on COVID-19 early outbreak dynamics. Sci Total Environ. 2021;761:144432. doi:10.1016/j.scitotenv.2020.144432

50. Ratnesar-Shumate S, Williams G, Green B, et al. Simulated sunlight rapidly inactivates SARS-CoV-2 on surfaces. J Infect Dis 2020;222(2):214–222

51. Cheung KS, Hung IFN, Chan PPY, et al. Gastrointestinal manifestations of SARS-CoV-2 infection and virus load in fecal samples from a Hong Kong cohort: systematic review and meta-analysis. Gastroenterology 2020;159(1):81–95

52. Zheng S, Fan J, Yu F, et al. Viral load dynamics and disease severity in patients infected with SARS-CoV-2 in Zhejiang province, China, January-March 2020: retrospective cohort study. BMJ 2020;369:m1443

53. Wang W, Xu Y, Gao R, et al. Detection of SARS-CoV-2 in different types of clinical specimens. JAMA 2020;323(18):1843–1844

54. Xiao F, Sun J, Xu Y, et al. Infectious SARS-CoV-2 in feces of patient with severe COVID-19. Emerg Infect Dis 2020;26(8):1920–1922

55. Hong Kong Government. WHO Environmental Health Team reports on Amoy Gardens. 2003. Available at: https://www.info.gov.hk/gia/general/200305/16/0516114.htm

56. Kang M, Wei J, Yuan J, et al. Probable evidence of fecal aerosol transmission of SARS-CoV-2 in a high-rise building. Ann Intern Med 2020;173(12):974–980

57. Li D, Jin M, Bao P, Zhao W, Zhang S. Clinical characteristics and results of semen tests among men with coronavirus disease 2019. JAMA Netw Open 2020;3(5):e208292

58. Douglas GC, O'Bryan MK, Hedger MP, et al. The novel angiotensin-converting enzyme (ACE) homolog, ACE2, is selectively expressed by adult Leydig cells of the testis. Endocrinology 2004;145(10):4703–4711

59. Chen Y, Guo Y, Pan Y, Zhao ZJ. Structure analysis of the receptor binding of 2019-nCoV. Biochem Biophys Res Commun 2020;525(1):135–140

60. Abobaker A, Raba AA. Does COVID-19 affect male fertility? World J Urol 2021;39(3):975–976

61. Massarotti C, Garolla A, Maccarini E, et al. SARS-CoV-2 in the semen: where does it come from? Andrology 2021;9(1):39–41

62. Özveri H, Eren MT, Kırışoğlu CE, Sarıgüzel N. Atypical presentation of SARS-CoV-2 infection in male genitalia. Urol Case Rep 2020;33:101349

63. Pan F, Xiao X, Guo J, et al. No evidence of severe acute respiratory syndrome-coronavirus 2 in semen of males recovering from coronavirus disease 2019. Fertil Steril 2020;113(6):1135–1139

64. Naik BS. Can a health care worker have sex in the time of COVID-19? Eur J Obstet Gynecol Reprod Biol 2020;252:622–623

65. Pham TD, Huang C, Wirz OF, et al. SARS-CoV-2 RNAemia in a healthy blood donor 40 days after respiratory illness resolution. Ann Intern Med 2020;173(10):853–854

66. To KK, Tsang OT, Leung WS, et al. Temporal profiles of viral load in posterior oropharyngeal saliva samples and serum antibody responses during infection by SARS-CoV-2: an observational cohort study. Lancet Infect Dis 2020;20(5):565–574

67. He X, Lau EHY, Wu P, et al. Temporal dynamics in viral shedding and transmissibility of COVID-19. Nat Med 2020;26(5):672–675. Erratum in: Nat Med 2020;26(9):1491–1493

68. Fontana LM, Villamagna AH, Sikka MK, McGregor JC. Understanding viral shedding of severe acute respiratory coronavirus virus 2 (SARS-CoV-2): review of current literature. Infect Control Hosp Epidemiol 2021;42(6):659–668

69. Wölfel R, Corman VM, Guggemos W, et al. Virological assessment of hospitalized patients with COVID-2019. Nature 2020;581(7809):465–469. Erratum in: Nature 2020;588(7839):E35

70. Avanzato VA, Matson MJ, Seifert SN, et al. Case study: prolonged infectious SARS-CoV-2

shedding from an asymptomatic immuno-compromised individual with cancer. Cell 2020;183(7):1901–1912.e9

71. Tarhini H, Recoing A, Bridier-Nahmias A, et al. Long-term severe acute respiratory syndrome coronavirus 2 (SARS-CoV-2) infectiousness among three immuno-compromised patients: from prolonged viral shedding to SARS-CoV-2 superinfection. J Infect Dis 2021;223(9):1522–1527

72. Baang JH, Smith C, Mirabelli C, et al. Prolonged severe acute respiratory syndrome corona-virus 2 replication in an immunocomprom-ised patient. J Infect Dis 2021;223(1):23–27

73. Lee S, Kim T, Lee E, et al. Clinical course and molecular viral shedding among asympto-matic and symptomatic patients with SARS-CoV-2 infection in a community treatment center in the Republic of Korea. JAMA Intern Med 2020;180(11):1447–1452

02 Paradigm Shifts in Understanding SARS-CoV-2 Virology and Disease

Robert W. Malone and Jill Glasspool Malone

Introduction

Severe acute respiratory syndrome coronavirus 2 (SARS-CoV-2) is the species of coronavirus responsible for the ongoing outbreak. This virus was named by a consensus scientific committee assembled by the World Health Organization, with classification based on genetic and structural analysis similarities relating to the general family of coronaviruses, genus *Betacoronavirus* and subgenus *Sarbecovirus*, and specifically relating to another *Sarbecovirus* responsible for a prior outbreak.[1,2] It has been designated SARS because it is genetically related to the SARS-CoV *Sarbecovirus* and causes a similar clinical disease. In contrast, the *Sarbecovirus* named Middle East respiratory syndrome coronavirus (MERS-CoV) is less closely related based on genetic analyses.[2]

Pretty much everyone reading this has been infected by milder forms of coronaviruses without knowing it. Four different strains of human coronaviruses cause about one-fifth of all common colds. Until 2003, coronaviruses were generally thought to only cause mild disease in humans. Then SARS came along and changed that assumption forever. SARS-CoV-2 is the seventh recognized coronavirus with human hosts.[1-3] The four human adapted "common cold" coronaviruses are 229E, NL63, OC43, and HKU1. The more recently discovered sarbe-coronavirus, known as SARS-CoV, MERS-CoV, and SARS-CoV-2, are able to cause severe morbidity and mortality, with mortality rates of 10, 37, and 1.04 to 3.09% worldwide (0.7–2.3% in the United States), respectively.[1,2,4] Other feline enteric coronavirus (FECV) types of coronaviruses are pathogenic and endemic in certain animal populations, and some readers may have heard of coronaviruses infecting cats, dogs, or cattle (FECV, canine respiratory coronavirus [CRCoV], and bovine coronavirus [BCV], which are different from SARS-CoV-2 virus and COVID-19 disease).[5]

Coronaviruses: The Transition from Zoonotic Nuisance to Human Pandemic

The SARS-CoV-2 epidemic, which started in China during 2003, abruptly shifted the paradigm that human coronaviruses only cause mild disease. Susan Weiss of the University of Pennsylvania has stated that "Everybody in the field was shocked," and then added: "People started really caring about this group of viruses."[6] It is thought that the epidemic began when a coronavirus spread from other mammals to humans. Infectious diseases that pass from animals to humans are called zoonotic diseases or zoonosis. SARS, MERS, and SARS-CoV-2 are all zoonotic diseases. To illustrate the importance of SARS, the government of the People's Republic of China is estimated to spend well over the equivalent of over a billion U.S. dollars per year every year since the initial SARS outbreak to monitor and protect its citizens from SARS and to eliminate the disease.[3] There is no vaccine for SARS; numerous, well-funded vaccine development efforts have all failed. The propensity of this family of coronaviruses to demonstrate the ability to transition from animal species to humans was again highlighted in 2012, when the MERS-CoV adapted from camels to humans.[7] As of the end of December 2020, there have been a total of 2,566 laboratory-confirmed cases of MERS, including 882 associated deaths.[8] As with SARS, all efforts to date to develop a MERS vaccine have failed. MERS is a good reason to not quit your day job to join the circus and become a camel trainer or handler.

SARS and SARS-CoV-2 most likely originated in bats (SARS-CoV-2 *may* have been a product of gain-of-function research) and probably had an intermediate animal host.[3,4] The sequence of SARS-CoV-2 as isolated from humans is genetically closely related to coronaviruses isolated from bats of the genus *Rhinolophus* ("horseshoe bats"), and SARS is also related to coronaviruses found in bats.[2,9] Similar viruses also exist in pangolins and civet cats.[10–12] These close genetic relations suggest that all of these sarbecoviruses have their ecological origin in bat populations. Bats of the genus *Rhinolophus* are found across Asia, Africa, the Middle East, and Europe. Analysis of genomic sequences of SARS-CoV-2 also shows that it is very adapted to human cell receptors.[13] This enables it to invade human cells and easily infect people. Bats have similar immune systems to humans, but it is sort of like the volume is turned down on how bats respond to viral infections. One interesting thing about bats is that their body temperature spikes as they fly, which may inhibit virus replication. This and other factors appear to make it easier for bats to live with certain types of viral infections, including some coronaviruses. However, when a bat coronavirus evolves to be able to infect a human, everything changes. The immune system of humans is generally turned up toward stronger immediate responses ("inflammation") relative to bats. SARS-CoV-2 in a bat is not very pathogenic to the bat, due to the bat's higher immunologic level of tolerance of viruses compared to humans. However, when this virus infects a human, it can result in the human immune system reacting in new, different, and unusual ways. SARS-CoV-2 in humans causes immune upregulation of mast cells, which control the release of histamine. The very high histamine release then causes damage to the human body. This is one new important aspect of the severe COVID-19

disease threat that we are now facing.[14] How the SARS-CoV-2 first came to productively infect humans (apparently during October–November 2019) remains a mystery, but there are many theories ranging from natural zoonotic transmission to escape from a research laboratory.

Initial reports from Chinese scientists theorized that the virus originated from snakes because of similarities in fragments of both genomes, but that theory was quickly debunked. Then, based on bat biology and an analysis of sequence data from various strains of coronavirus, the primary animal host species was determined most likely to be the horseshoe bat. According to local officials in Wuhan, China, where the outbreak is thought to have started, there were no bats being sold at the live animal market in Wuhan city. However, 66% of the original cases had contact with the animal market. However, after tracing down the earliest cases of disease caused by this virus, epidemiologists have not been able to establish a clear link between early human cases of disease and any exposure to the live animal food market in Wuhan, China. However, the World Health Organization believes that this is the probable cause.[15] This report suggests that an intermediate host species may have been involved but then goes on to disclose that although 188 animals spanning 18 species were tested, none were positive for COVID-19.[15] The Wuhan Institute of Virology and the live animal market are in close proximity, so another theory is that the virus is an escaped mutation from the institute. This theory is supported by many in the U.S. government, although the World Health Organization investigated this thoroughly and no data have ever been found by western investigators linking the virus to the institute.

Having an intermediate animal host other than bat seems to be a common feature of zoonotic coronaviruses.[1,2,9,11] This is what happened with MERS and its intermediary host, the camel. These intermediate animal hosts may increase the viruses' genetic diversity and mammalian host range by facilitating development of more or different mutations via cross-species virus transmission. Viruses infrequently develop the potential to spread efficiently within a new host that has never been exposed to or sensitive to them. Devastating epidemics can occur when there is increasing exposure or viruses acquire mutations that permit them to overcome limits to infect new hosts.[16]

In the case of SARS-CoV-2, the intermediary host probably served as a sort of bridge between bat and human. The pangolin, an endangered animal that some Chinese use for traditional Chinese medicine (sold for as much as $350 per kilo), supports replication of a coronavirus that shares about 90% homology with SARS-CoV-2.[9,16–18] Early on in the outbreak, it was hypothesized to be the animal intermediate. As the horseshoe bat range does not overlap with Wuhan, the most likely mammalian host of SARS-CoV-2 may reside far outside of the Wuhan province. Based on this logic, the original crossover from bat to human may have happened elsewhere in China and then transported to Wuhan by either an intermediary animal or human host. Members of the cat family (felids) as well as civets (there are a dozen members of the "civet cat" family) share an angiotensin-converting enzyme 2 (ACE2) receptor similar to the human version.[5,9,11] These and other species that can be infected by this virus have also been considered as an intermediate host. In the end, the origins of how this virus cross into humans remain shrouded in mystery and clouded by conspiracy theories. As the science on the evolution of the virus progresses into how it made the leap from an animal host to human, that data will influence how humans interact with and treat other species. This, in of itself, could influence culture beyond the current crisis and could change how humans view and interact with the natural world. For example, the high transmissibility rate of this virus has permanently impacted global tourism, travel, and commerce.

There are many vulnerable species, such as those in the great ape family, that can be infected by this virus. The transmissibility and disease severity in most of these is not known. How this may affect other species found in domestic or wild populations including those found in urban zoos is not yet determined. For example, during January 2021, two gorillas at the San Diego Zoo tested positive for SARS-CoV-2 and developed COVID-19 disease, exhibiting mild respiratory symptoms. Since then, zoos have begun to vaccinate animal species that may be in danger of contracting this virus.[19–21] But how this virus may impact other mammalian and even avian species is still unknown. Many animals do have cell surface receptors (such as ACE2) that will support SARS-CoV-2 infection. Studies have shown that critically endangered nonhuman primate species are predicted to be at very high risk of infection by SARS-CoV-2 via their ACE2 receptors. Other animals that are at high risk include other nonhuman primates and marine mammals. Domestic animals demonstrate a medium risk for getting infected with this virus. However, dogs, horses, and pigs were found to have low risk for ACE2 binding. Documented SARS-COV-2 infection of mink, cats, dogs, hamsters, lions, and tigers may rely on ACE2 receptors or may employ alternate pathways to acquire entry to host cells.[22] Furthermore, as the virus continues to mutate and become more transmissible, there is the potential that future virus mutations may support infection in additional animal populations.

About the Virus

Coronaviruses are about 120 nm in diameter, which is fairly large for a virus. Just for comparison, the thickness of a single human hair is more than 1,000 times wider than a single coronavirus. Coronaviruses are spherical in shape, and under high-powered microscopes they look like they have a ring or halo around a central sphere, like the corona around the sun. And no, coronaviruses have nothing to do with the famous Mexican Corona brand beer! These viruses use a single strand of RNA, rather than a double strand of DNA, to carry their genetic code. RNA is not as stable as DNA, and so even a simple dish soap can do a lot of damage to a coronavirus.[23]

Coronaviruses are known to cause pulmonary and gastrointestinal diseases in various animals with coughing, pneumonia, and diarrhea all being typic symptoms.[24] Examples of animals that get infected by different coronaviruses include camels, cattle, chickens, bats, mice, alpacas, swine, dogs, horses, and cats as well as other mammals and (of course) human and nonhuman primates.[24] There are many different types of coronaviruses, and different coronaviruses tend to specialize in infecting different animals. For example (as discussed previously), SARS-CoV-2 is in the same coronavirus family (group 3) as MERS and SARS, but is different from cat (feline) coronavirus and also different from the human coronaviruses that cause the common cold. MERS, SARS, and the novel coronavirus demonstrate genetic homology and each has its genesis in bats, although the MERS virus also infects camels and is primarily transmitted to humans from camels. Genetic analysis demonstrate that SARS-CoV-2 is more closely related to SARS than to MERS, but is even most closely related to a subset of group 3 coronaviruses that virologists refer to as the bat SARS-like coronaviruses.[2,5,9,11] SARS, SARS-CoV-2, and closely related pangolin, civet cat, and horseshoe bat coronaviruses all show significant levels of conserved nucleocapsid 2 protein COX-2 promoter transactivation domains and nuclear localization regions.[25]

Coronaviruses and other single-stranded RNA viruses are classified as positive- or negative-stranded depending on the polarity of the RNA.[26,27] One can think of RNA polarity as sort of like reading a sentence from left to right (positive polarity) or right to left (negative polarity). The machinery in cells that makes proteins from RNA reads the RNA (message) from left to right. Therefore, getting really technical, coronaviruses are a type of positive-polarity single-stranded enveloped RNA virus, which is to say that virus proteins can be produced directly from the RNA

genome by reading it from left to right.[26,27] The RNA does not have to go through another round of replication (as is required for negative-polarity RNA viral genomes) to get back to a form that can be read from left to right to produce proteins after infecting a cell. At a practical level, this also means that the RNA genome of a coronavirus can be infectious; the RNA alone, if transferred into a cell, can cause that cell to produce complete and infectious new coronaviruses. This is why mRNA vaccines only use a fragment of the mRNA genome, so that the mRNA cannot reproduce virus. The life cycle of SARS coronavirus and cellular disruption induced by viral invasion are demonstrated in **Fig. 2.1**.

Using RNA as the genetic material is very efficient (a single strand is easier and cheaper to make than two!), but it is also very likely to develop errors during replication relative to using double-stranded DNA (like human beings use). Among other problems with this viral strategy is that this means that viruses that use RNA often mutate very fast. Good thing that human beings use DNA to store their genetic information! For humans, lots of mutations would generally be very bad. However, RNA viruses make this high mutation rate work for them. The high mutation rate of RNA viruses is one reason why it is difficult to make effective vaccines against many of these types of viruses. Influenza virus is an RNA virus, and often mutates from one year to the next, requiring new and slightly different influenza vaccines to be produced every year. Positive-sense RNA viruses account for a significant proportion of all known human viruses, including many pathogenic viruses such as HIV (the AIDS virus), hepatitis C virus (liver cancer), rhinoviruses (common cold), West Nile virus, dengue virus, Zika virus, SARS and MERS coronaviruses, and COVID-19. Even though the single-stranded RNA strategy comes with the problem of high mutation rate, these viruses replicate so efficiently and produce so many viruses so fast that it does not slow them down. In fact, the high mutation rate is sort of an advantage for viruses—it

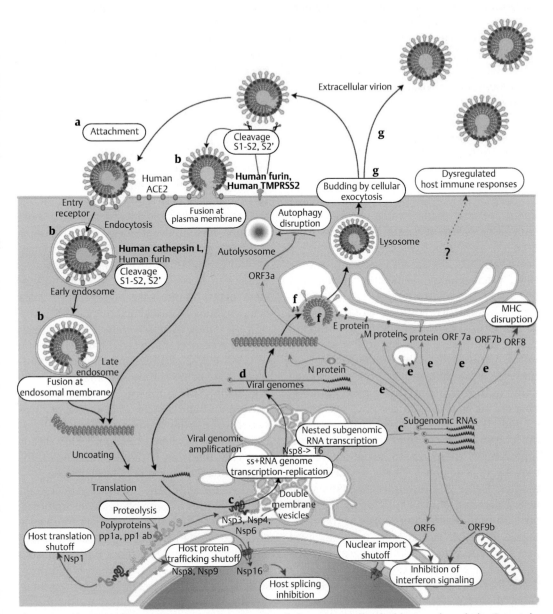

Fig. 2.1 Life cycle of SARS-CoV-2. (**a**) Attachment of virus occurs via viral interaction via its S protein and ACE2 and TMPRSS2, resulting in endocytosis of virion. (**b**) S2-mediated fusion of virus membrane with endosomal membrane with resultant release of genome +ssRNA into cell cytoplasm. (**c**) Synthesis of replicase polyprotein products of subgenomic mRNA, inducing disruption of cellular processes. (**d**) Transcription of new viral genomes. (**e**) Structural proteins encoded by subgenomic mRNA. (**f**) Assembly and budding at membranes of the endoplasmic reticulum Golgi body complex. (**g**) Exocytotic release. (Source: ViralZone, SIB Swiss Institute of Bioinformatics; http://creativecommons.org/licenses/by/4.0/.)

makes it easy for them to evolve and adapt to a new host (you and me) very rapidly, and to adapt to escape immunity in the animals that they infect (including us). The SARS-CoV-2 virus that is currently circulating in humans is a group of closely related quasi-species; in other words, there is still significant diversity in the genetic sequences of all SARS-CoV-2 viral genomes when different samples of the novel coronavirus are sequenced.[28]

Variants

There are now many strains of SARS-CoV-2 circulating, with new strains being discovered on a regular basis. The occurrence of new variants affects viral transmissibility (R0), pathogenicity, reinfection rates, and SARS-CoV-2 vaccine effectiveness. These factors will influence how the world responds to the virus. Travel, commerce, government policy, health care systems, and other social infrastructure will all be influenced by how these new variants impact on the human body differently than the current strain(s) now circulating.

Mutations within the virus genome are clustered, and it appears that the most important of these genetic variation clusters may be in a region defined as ORF8 (open reading frame 8). Mutations in ORF8 were also associated with adaptation of the SARS virus to human infection. ORF8 (or the alternative form ORF8ab) appears to be involved in viral replication and/or disease, but the way that it works has not been completely defined at this point. What is known is that ORF8 disrupts IFN-I signaling when exogenously overexpressed in cells.[29] Also known is that ORF8 of SARS-CoV-2 downregulates MHC-I in cells, but that the ORF8 in SARS does not.[30] These data imply that the SARS-CoV-2 is still evolving to adapt to a new host (humans), and has not settled in on a predominant final strain. Therefore, any current assessments or predictions of future behavior (infectivity, incidence of disease, and death) may change as the virus settles down into a dominant viral strain and sequence, if it does

settle. It is also important to know that this is a single-stranded RNA virus and these viruses mutate very fast. There have been reports of the virus' genome being different at various time points within an individual. Another RNA virus with this capability that we are all familiar with is HIV.

Mode of Action

Viral infections can cause multiple different pathophysiologic patterns. One example of this is damage caused by direct virus injury and another example involves reactive host immune-mediated pathology in response to the pathogen. These could also be described as a hyperinflammatory immune response, which can cause significant clinical injury or even death. In the case of COVID-19, mast cell activation releases histamine and is a significant cause of organ damage.[14] Although there are reports that a significant proportion of SARS-CoV-2-positive individuals demonstrate little or no symptoms, a large systematic review of literature documented that between 20 and 31% of SARS-CoV-2-positive patients are truly asymptomatic throughout the entirety of their infection.[31] This means that viral infection is required but not sufficient for development of clinical disease.

The predominant pathophysiology in COVID-19 disease involves hyperimmune-mediated responses that are most frequently observed in high-risk patients, such as those with advanced age and those with comorbid medical conditions such as high blood pressure, obesity, diabetes, and cardiac, vascular, neurologic, renal, chronic lung, and asthmatic diseases. In particular, metabolic syndrome, caused by insulin resistance, hyperglycemia, high blood pressure, and subclinical inflammation are linked with a high risk of severe disease.[32] All of these risk factors are associated with chronic proinflammatory states, which may predispose the patient to the hyperinflammatory responses typical of COVID-19 disease.

Viral spike protein and nucleocapsid N protein induce overexpression of COX-2.

COX-2 is an enzyme that is the inducible form of cyclo-oxygenase.[14,25] This enzyme catalyzes the conversion of arachidonic acid to prostaglandins. Prostaglandins are a class of lipids that are produced at locations of tissue damage or infection and modulate the disease process.

They control processes such as inflammation, thrombosis, and circulation at an injury site. COX-2 is expressed by inflammatory cells, such as macrophages, and can be induced by tumor necrosis factor (TNF) and epidermal growth factor.

COX-2 is most likely the dominant source of prostaglandin formation in inflammation. Patients with COVID-19 disease frequently have abnormally high amounts of prostaglandin E2 (PGE2). PGE2 and histamine are two of the inflammatory signaling molecules likely involved in mediating COVID-19 hyperinflammatory responses to viral infection as well as the superimposed coagulopathy.[14,25] Coagulopathy results in thromboembolic events, leading to significant morbidity and mortality. The increased hyperinflammatory responses and coagulopathy correlate with a parallel rise in markers of inflammation. Many of these inflammatory processes are mediated by the COX-2 isoenzyme system. Pharmaceutical inhibition of COX-2 can provide reduce inflammation and hence modulate the hyperimmune-mediated responses associated with severe COVID-19.[14,25]

COX-2 is expressed in many different types of cells, including lung fibroblasts, vascular endothelial cells, type II alveolar pneumocytes, and alveolar macrophages. These cell types are all found in compromised pulmonary gas exchange tissue during the early stages of COVID-19 disease.[33] Vascular endothelial cells and type II alveolar pneumocytes are primary targets for viral infection and replication, and alveolar macrophages are permissive to infection.[34]

SARS-CoV can transactivate the inducible COX-2 gene promoter in infected cells. SARS transcriptional upregulation of COX-2 is mediated by the nucleocapsid protein (N, directly via specific N2 protein sequences) and spike glycoprotein (S, via indirect transactivation cascade), promoting upregulation of COX-2 in a dose-dependent manner in infected cells.[35,36] The ability of SARS-CoV-2 to similarly transactivate COX-2 expression is untested, but nonclinical studies reveal viral infection does upregulate COX-2 expression.[37] Homology analysis of the analogous N2 sequences of SARS-CoV-2 and other betacoronaviruses relative to SARS has not been reported. Based on urinary levels of PGE2, viral infection is associated with high levels of PGE2 production, which were several fold higher than levels observed in normal uninfected individuals (17,040 vs. 18,138 ng/mL, $p = 0.01$), and in some cases increased to 150 times the normal level in one study of hospitalized patients.[38] These investigators postulated that increases in PGE2 potentially play a pivotal role in the pathophysiology of COVID-19 by binding to EP2, EP3, and EP4 receptors.[38] EP2 receptor binding is associated with pyrexia, pain, acute inflammation, and enhanced capillary leak. EP3 receptor binding via a mast cell activation–dependent pathway leads to edema, inflammatory mucus secretion, and increased viscosity of alveolar exudate, resulting in mucous plugging of alveolar and respiratory bronchioles.[39] EP4 receptor binding causes bronchial contractions and spasms, resulting in increased airway resistance, and is associated with pulmonary and circulatory disorders, acute respiratory distress syndrome (ARDS), and multiorgan failure.[40] Excessive PGE2 binding to EP4 is also associated with inhibition of T lymphocyte functionality by promoting amplification, differentiation, and proliferation of Th1 and Th17 subtypes.[41] In addition, PGE2 and thromboxane A2 activation can cause platelet aggregation and thrombosis.[42] All of these signs and symptoms of excessive signaling by the products of arachidonic acid metabolism resulting from COX-2 activation are features of COVID-19 disease.

Researchers have attempted to elucidate COVID-19 clinical and pathologic data using just traditional models of antiviral innate and adaptive immune responses, which overlook the contribution of mast cell activation and degranulation. Other investigators highlight the inflammatory cell response cascade related with monocytes, macrophages, and adaptive T and B lymphocyte helper and effector responses.[43,44] These immune responses have also been suggested as a possible explanation for the unique microvascular and macrovascular pulmonary and systemic coagulopathy linked to COVID-19.[45] All of these reviews are flawed because they do not show the entire landscape of the virus–host immunologic interactions and cascading immunologic events.

Clinically, the most serious effects of COVID-19 disease are the pathologic hyperinflammatory host responses described in the subset of critically ill symptomatic SARS-CoV-2-infected patients. These responses manifest as exuberant immunological and paracrine pathway alterations. While COVID-19 symptoms are systemic in nature, ARDS is the most common cause of morbidity and mortality. Evaluation of RNA transcriptomic profiles of the cells that contribute to pulmonary anatomy and function reveals the existence of multiple ACE2/transmembrane protease serine 2 (TMPRSS2)-positive cell types susceptible to viral infection in the lung. Furthermore, these and other associated lung cells that express histamine receptors H1 and H2 may react to local histamine release following mast cell degranulation.[46]

Mast cell activation caused by SARS-CoV-2 infection is responsible for a portion of the central pathophysiological cascade and much of the unique manifestations linked with COVID-19.[14,25,47] A fair number of the unique symptoms observed in the early stages of COVID-19 are compatible with established histamine-related consequences.[48] Histamine may function in an autocrine fashion regulating mast cell cytokine and TNF-α release mediated by a PGE2-dependent mechanism. In vitro studies demonstrate the autocrine feedback appears to be mediated by H2 and H3.[14,49] This model is consistent with the histopathologic findings observed during surgery and postmortem studies, and is substantiated by clinical pharmacologic findings suggesting potential benefits of histamine H2 receptor blockade, such as famotidine for treatment of COVID-19 disease. Substantial overlap exists between the clinical manifestations of the early phase of COVID-19 and those of mast cell activation syndrome[14,25,50,51]

There are also many resemblances to dengue hemorrhagic fever and shock syndrome (including T cell depletion) during the later stages of COVID-19.[50-52] The cardiovascular complications, cerebrovascular accidents, and related complications linked with COVID-19 are similar to the Kounis syndrome.[53-55] This theory is substantiated by the discovery of increased amount of mast cells in the alveolar septal walls and lung tissues of SARS-CoV-2-infected African green monkeys and in the alveolar septa of COVID-19 patients.[56]

If COVID-19 is partially driven by dysfunctional mast cells, then a variety of treatments employing FDA-approved therapeutic agents useful in the management of mast cell–associated diseases may lead to a reduction in morbidity and mortality in patients suffering from COVID-19.[14] These include mast cell stabilizers such as beta-2 adrenoceptor antagonists or cromolyn sodium, other histamine antagonists (for example H1 and H4 types), leukotriene antagonists and leukotriene receptor antagonists, anti-inflammatory agents such as those developed for inflammatory bowel diseases, and mast cell activation inhibitors.[57-65] If such repurposed drugs are used in combination with pharmaceuticals that directly inhibit SARS-CoV-2 infection or replication, it may be possible to rapidly develop potent, safe, and effective outpatient treatments for preventing or treating COVID-19. The emergence of new variants can affect viral transmissibility, disease severity, reinfection rates, and SARS-CoV-2 vaccine effectiveness. The need for antiviral and therapeutic drugs to treat COVID-19 disease and long hauler syndrome has not diminished with the advent of emergency-use authorized vaccines. Breakthrough disease, undervaccinated populations, and new variants that continue to evolved mean that this disease needs more effective treatments. By understanding the link between COVID-19, mast cells, and histamine release, combined with the structural elements of this virus, new therapeutics can be developed.

ACE2 is a transmembrane protein that was first discovered in 2000.[66,67] This protein is found on epithelial and endothelial cells of the upper and lower respiratory tract, heart and vasculature, kidneys, and portions of the gastrointestinal tract.[68] ACE2 is an ectoenzyme. An ectoenzyme means that its actions occur outside of the cell. ACE2 is found in many different organs that can be affected by SARS-CoV-2.[68] The primary role of the ACE2 protein is to counterbalance the effects of the first angiotensin-converting enzyme, commonly referred to as ACE.[68] The primary role of ACE2 relates to the renin–angiotensin system (RAS)—the hormone system that regulates blood pressure: volume and tone, electrolyte balance, and systemic vascular resistance. RAS is regulated by the action of angiotensin II, which is a peptide hormone.[68]

In SARS-CoV-2 infection, the viral S (spike) protein receptor-binding domain binds to ACE2. This allows the virus to enter the host cell. ACE2 expression in the lungs is relatively low, but it is present in type II pneumocytes, which are the surface epithelial cells of the alveoli that are adapted to carry out gas exchange. This cell type is also endowed with TMPRSS2.[68] This protease binds the SARS-CoV-2 S protein to ACE2. That is the key that allows entry into the cells. Blocking TMPRSS2 could potentially be an effective clinical therapy for COVID-19, as it would effectively not allow the viruses spike protein to bind and enter the cell.[69]

SARS-CoV-2 include four major structural proteins. These proteins are the spike (S), nucleocapsid (N), membrane (M), and envelope (E) proteins. The S, M, and E proteins are all embedded in the viral surface envelope. The other structural protein (N) forms the viral ribonucleoprotein core.[68-70] S proteins are involved in recognition of the host cellular receptor to initiate virus entry. The M proteins are in and shape the virion envelope.[70] E proteins are small polypeptides that are responsible for coronavirus infectivity. N proteins are the building blocks of the helical nucleocapsid and they bind along the viral RNA genome. As well as these four structural proteins, SARS-CoV-2 encodes at least 16 nonstructural proteins and nine accessory proteins.[70] Several of these viral proteins could potentially serve as targets of vaccine-induced immune responses.[70]

For the development of vaccine against SARS-CoV-2, the spike (S) protein is most often chosen.[70] The spike (S) protein of SARS-CoV-2 is an important element in the receptor recognition and cell membrane fusion process. The spike protein is composed of two subunits, named S1 and S2. The S1 subunit contains a receptor-binding domain that recognizes and binds to the host receptor ACE2.[70] The S2 subunit is responsible for viral cell membrane fusion. It does this by forming a six-helical bundle via the two-heptad repeat domain.[71] The spike protein is essential for viral entry into cells, and it is present on the outer layer of the virus. This makes it an ideal target for vaccination strategies against SARS-CoV-2, as antibodies and cytotoxic T lymphocyte (in the case of mRNA vaccines) targeting the S protein prevent the virus from entering the host cell. If the virus does not enter the cell, it cannot replicate inside the host cell.[72] The Moderna, Pfizer, and AstraZeneca vaccines all target the spike (S) protein. The fundamental role of the S protein in viral infection indicates that it is a potential target not just for vaccines, but also for antibody-blocking therapies and small molecule inhibitors (antiviral drugs).

Conclusion

The cost of this disease in mortalities, disabilities, and economic loss is enormous. This disease has the potential to not only continue to devastate human populations but also ravage critical animal populations. Understanding the molecular virology of

SARS-CoV-2 is important to help allevi-
ate these individual and macroeconomic
hardships. First, it will allow new therapeutics and vaccines to be developed. It will also
help in the understanding of the biology of
the disease, which will impact strategies for
infection control. SARS-CoV-2 mutates very
rapidly, and there are many strains of SARS-
CoV-2 circulating. The emergence of new
variants affects viral transmissibility, disease
severity, reinfection rates, and SARS-CoV-2
vaccine effectiveness. In the future, these
new variants will impact travel, infection
control, and vaccination strategies as well
as new therapeutics. As three new human-
adapted and closely related betacoronaviruses have emerged in the last two decades, it
is likely that more will emerge in the future.
Understanding the molecular virology of
these viruses will help combat the next betacoronavirus that jumps into humans from an
animal host.

The mechanism of action for this virus is
different from other viruses in that it elicits
an hyperimmune response/mast cell activation that in of itself can cause severe disease
and even death. Some of the basic pathophysiologic cascade and the peculiar manifestations linked with COVID-19 are attributed
to viral-initiated mast cell activation.[14,25,47]A
large number of the clinical symptoms seen
during the early stages of COVID-19 are
consistent with histamine-related consequences.[48] This knowledge will contribute to
the discovery of new therapeutics.

References

1. Zheng J. SARS-CoV-2: an emerging corona-virus that causes a global threat. Int J Biol Sci 2020;16(10):1678–1685
2. Petrosillo N, Viceconte G, Ergonul O, Ippolito G, Petersen E. COVID-19, SARS and MERS: are they closely related? Clin Microbiol Infect 2020;26(6):729–734
3. Bouey J. From SARS to 2019-coronavirus (nCoV): U.S.-China collaborations on pande-mic response. RAND Corporation; 2020. Available at: https://www.rand.org/pubs/testimonies/CT523.html
4. Petersen E, Koopmans M, Go U, et al. Comparing SARS-CoV-2 with SARS-CoV and influenza pandemics. Lancet Infect Dis 2020; 20(9):e238–e244
5. Colina SE, Serena MS, Echeverría MG, Metz GE. Clinical and molecular aspects of veterinary coronaviruses. Virus Res 2021;297:198382
6. Makin S. How coronaviruses cause infection–from colds to deadly pneumonia. Scientific American. February 5, 2020. Available at: www.scientificamerican.com/article/how-coronaviruses-cause-infection-from-colds-to-deadly-pneumonia1/
7. Azhar EI, El-Kafrawy SA, Farraj SA, et al. Evidence for camel-to-human transmission of MERS coronavirus. N Engl J Med 2014; 370(26):2499–2505
8. WHO. MERS situation update, January 2020. January 1, 2020. Available at: http://www.emro.who.int/pandemic-epidemic-diseases/mers-cov/mers-situation-update-january-2020.html
9. Latinne A, Hu B, Olival KJ, et al. Origin and cross-species transmission of bat corona-viruses in China. Nat Commun 2020;11(1): 4235
10. Liu P, Chen W, Chen J-P. Viral metagenomics revealed Sendai virus and coronavirus infection of Malayan pangolins (*Manis javanica*). Viruses 2019;11(11):E979
11. Wang L-F, Shi Z, Zhang S, Field H, Daszak P, Eaton BT. Review of bats and SARS. Emerg Infect Dis 2006;12(12):1834–1840
12. Cyranoski D. Did pangolins spread the China coronavirus to people? Nature 2020 (e-pub ahead of print). doi:10.1038/d41586-020-00364-2
13. Boni MF, Lemey P, Jiang X, et al. Evolutionary origins of the SARS-CoV-2 sarbecovirus lineage responsible for the COVID-19 pandemic. Nat Microbiol 2020;5(11): 1408–1417
14. Malone RW, Tisdall P, Fremont-Smith P, et al. COVID-19: famotidine, histamine, mast cells, and mechanisms. Front Pharmacol 2021;12:633680
15. Maxmen A. WHO report into COVID pandemic origins zeroes in on animal markets, not labs. Nature 2021;592(7853):173–174
16. Parrish CR, Holmes EC, Morens DM, et al. Cross-species virus transmission and the emergence of new epidemic diseases. Microbiol Mol Biol Rev 2008;72(3):457–470

17. Sharma S, Sharma HP, Katuwal HB, Chaulagain C, Belant JL. People's knowledge of illegal Chinese pangolin trade routes in central Nepal. Sustainability 2020;12(12):4900

18. Wang Y, Turvey ST, Leader-Williams N. Knowledge and attitudes about the use of pangolin scale products in Traditional Chinese Medicine (TCM) within China. People Nat 2020;2(4):903–912

19. Machemer T. Gorillas at California zoo test positive for covid-19. Smithsonian Magazine. January 31, 2021. Available at: https://www.smithsonianmag.com/smart-news/gorillas-california-zoo-test-positive-covid-19-180976740/

20. Tizard IR. Vaccination against coronaviruses in domestic animals. Vaccine 2020;38(33):5123–5130

21. Sharun K, Dhama K, Pawde AM, et al. SARS-CoV-2 in animals: potential for unknown reservoir hosts and public health implications. Vet Q 2021;41(1):181–201

22. Damas J, Hughes GM, Keough KC, et al. Broad host range of SARS-CoV-2 predicted by comparative and structural analysis of ACE2 in vertebrates. Proc Natl Acad Sci U S A 2020;117(36):22311–22322

23. Jahromi R, Mogharab V, Jahromi H, Avazpour A. Synergistic effects of anionic surfactants on coronavirus (SARS-CoV-2) virucidal efficiency of sanitizing fluids to fight COVID-19. Food Chem Toxicol 2020;145:111702

24. Mahdy MAA, Younis W, Ewaida Z. An overview of SARS-CoV-2 and animal infection. Front Vet Sci 2020;7:596391

25. Malone R, Tomera K, Kittah J. Hospitalized COVID-19 patients treated with celecoxib and high dose famotidine adjuvant therapy show significant clinical responses. SSRN 2020 (e-pub ahead of print). http://dx.doi.org/10.2139/ssrn.3646583

26. Payne S. Introduction to RNA Viruses. Viruses. 2017:97–105. doi: 10.1016/B978-0-12-803109-4.00010-6. Epub 2017 Sep 1. PMCID: PMC7173417.

27. Pal M, Berhanu G, Desalegn C, Kandi V. Severe acute respiratory syndrome coronavirus-2 (SARS-CoV-2): an update. Cureus 2020;12(3):e7423

28. Ceraolo C, Giorgi FM. Genomic variance of the 2019-nCoV coronavirus. J Med Virol 2020;92(5):522–528

29. Li J-Y, Liao C-H, Wang Q, et al. The ORF6, ORF8 and nucleocapsid proteins of SARS-CoV-2 inhibit type I interferon signaling pathway. Virus Res 2020;286:198074

30. Zhang Y, Chen Y, Li Y, et al. The ORF8 protein of SARS-CoV-2 mediates immune evasion through down-regulating MHC-I. Proc Natl Acad Sci U S A 2021;118(23):e2024202118

31. Buitrago-Garcia D, Egli-Gany D, Counotte MJ, et al. Occurrence and transmission potential of asymptomatic and presymptomatic SARS-CoV-2 infections: a living systematic review and meta-analysis. PLoS Med 2020;17(9):e1003346

32. Stefan N, Birkenfeld AL, Schulze MB. Global pandemics interconnected — obesity, impaired metabolic health and COVID-19. Nat Rev Endocrinol 2021;17(3):135–149

33. Çınar HNU, İnce Ö, Çelik B, Saltabaş F, Özbek M. Clinical course of COVID-19 pneumonia in a patient undergoing pneumonectomy and pathology findings during the incubation period. Swiss Med Wkly 2020;150:w20302

34. Yang D, Chu H, Hou Y, et al. Attenuated interferon and proinflammatory response in SARS-CoV-2-infected human dendritic cells is associated with viral antagonism of STAT1 phosphorylation. J Infect Dis 2020;222(5):734–745

35. Yan X, Hao Q, Mu Y, et al. Nucleocapsid protein of SARS-CoV activates the expression of cyclooxygenase-2 by binding directly to regulatory elements for nuclear factor-kappa B and CCAAT/enhancer binding protein. Int J Biochem Cell Biol 2006;38(8):1417–1428

36. Liu M, Yang Y, Gu C, et al. Spike protein of SARS-CoV stimulates cyclooxygenase-2 expression via both calcium-dependent and calcium-independent protein kinase C pathways. FASEB J 2007;21(7):1586–1596

37. Chen JS, Alfajaro MM, Chow RD, et al. Non-steroidal anti-inflammatory drugs dampen the cytokine and antibody response to SARS-CoV-2 infection. J Virol 2021;95(7):JVI.00014-21

38. Hong W, Chen Y, You K, et al. Celebrex adjuvant therapy on coronavirus disease 2019: an experimental study. Front Pharmacol 2020;11:561674

39. Morimoto K, Shirata N, Taketomi Y, et al. Prostaglandin E2-EP3 signaling induces inflammatory swelling by mast cell activation. J Immunol 2014;192(3):1130–1137

40. Säfholm J, Dahlén S-E, Delin I, et al. PGE2 maintains the tone of the guinea pig trachea through a balance between activation of contractile EP1 receptors and relaxant EP2 receptors. Br J Pharmacol 2013;168(4): 794–806

41. Niwa H, Satoh T, Matsushima Y, et al. Stable form of galectin-9, a Tim-3 ligand, inhibits contact hypersensitivity and psoriatic reactions: a potent therapeutic tool for Th1- and/or Th17-mediated skin inflammation. Clin Immunol 2009;132(2):184–194

42. Zamora CA, Baron DA, Heffner JE. Thromboxane contributes to pulmonary hypertension in ischemia-reperfusion lung injury. J Appl Physiol (1985) 1993;74(1):224–229

43. Merad M, Martin JC. Pathological inflammation in patients with COVID-19: a key role for monocytes and macrophages. Nat Rev Immunol 2020;20(6):355–362

44. Vabret N, Britton GJ, Gruber C, et al; Sinai Immunology Review Project. Immunology of COVID-19: current state of the science. Immunity 2020;52(6):910–941

45. McGonagle D, Bridgewood C, Ramanan AV, Meaney JFM, Watad A. COVID-19 vasculitis and novel vasculitis mimics. Lancet Rheumatol 2021;3(3):e224–e233

46. Krystel-Whittemore M, Dileepan KN, Wood JG. Mast cell: a multi-functional master cell. Front Immunol 2016;6:620

47. Kritas SK, Ronconi G, Caraffa A, Gallenga CE, Ross R, Conti P. Mast cells contribute to coronavirus-induced inflammation: new anti-inflammatory strategy. J Biol Regul Homeost Agents 2020;34(1):9–14

48. Conti P, Caraffa A, Tetè G, et al. Mast cells activated by SARS-CoV-2 release histamine which increases IL-1 levels causing cytokine storm and inflammatory reaction in COVID-19. J Biol Regul Homeost Agents 2020; 34(5):1629–1632

49. Bissonnette EY. Histamine inhibits tumor necrosis factor alpha release by mast cells through H2 and H3 receptors. Am J Respir Cell Mol Biol 1996;14(6):620–626

50. Mongkolsapaya J, Dejnirattisai W, Xu XN, et al. Original antigenic sin and apoptosis in the pathogenesis of dengue hemorrhagic fever. Nat Med 2003;9(7):921–927

51. Guzman MG, Harris E. Dengue. Lancet 2015;385(9966):453–465

52. Redoni M, Yacoub S, Rivino L, Giacobbe DR, Luzzati R, Di Bella S. Dengue: status of current and under-development vaccines. Rev Med Virol 2020;30(4):e2101

53. González-de-Olano D, Alvarez-Twose I, Matito A, Sánchez-Muñoz L, Kounis NG, Escribano L. Mast cell activation disorders presenting with cerebral vasospasm-related symptoms: a "Kounis-like" syndrome? Int J Cardiol 2011;150(2):210–211

54. Kounis NG. Kounis syndrome: an update on epidemiology, pathogenesis, diagnosis and therapeutic management. Clin Chem Lab Med 2016;54(10):1545–1559

55. Kounis NG, Koniari I, Tzanis G, Soufras GD, Velissaris D, Hahalis G. Anaphylaxis-induced atrial fibrillation and anesthesia: pathophysiologic and therapeutic considerations. Ann Card Anaesth 2020;23(1):1–6

56. Motta Junior JDS, Miggiolaro AFRDS, Nagashima S, et al. Mast cells in alveolar septa of COVID-19 patients: a pathogenic pathway that may link interstitial edema to immunothrombosis. Front Immunol 2020; 11:574862

57. Han Y-S, Chang G-G, Juo C-G, et al. Papain-like protease 2 (PLP2) from severe acute respiratory syndrome coronavirus (SARS-CoV): expression, purification, characterization, and inhibition. Biochemistry 2005;44(30): 10349–10359

58. Zhang T, Finn DF, Barlow JW, Walsh JJ. Mast cell stabilisers. Eur J Pharmacol 2016; 778:158–168

59. Okayama Y, Benyon RC, Lowman MA, Church MK. In vitro effects of H1-antihistamines on histamine and PGD2 release from mast cells of human lung, tonsil, and skin. Allergy 1994;49(4):246–253

60. Marone G, Granata F, Spadaro G, Genovese A, Triggiani M. The histamine-cytokine network in allergic inflammation. J Allergy Clin Immunol 2003;112(4, Suppl):S83–S88

61. Hogan Ii RB, Hogan Iii RB, Cannon T, et al. Dual-histamine receptor blockade with cetirizine–famotidine reduces pulmonary symptoms in COVID-19 patients. Pulm Pharmacol Ther 2020;63:101942

62. Fidan C, Aydoğdu A. As a potential treatment of COVID-19: montelukast. Med Hypotheses 2020;142:109828

63. Castells M, Butterfield J. Mast cell activation syndrome and mastocytosis: initial treatment options and long-term management. J Allergy Clin Immunol Pract 2019;7(4):1097–1106

64. Theoharides TC. Potential association of mast cells with coronavirus disease 2019. Ann Allergy Asthma Immunol 2021;126(3): 217–218

65. Scola A-M, Chong LK, Suvarna SK, Chess-Williams R, Peachell PT. Desensitisation of mast cell beta2-adrenoceptor-mediated responses by salmeterol and formoterol. Br J Pharmacol 2004;141(1):163–171

66. Tipnis SR, Hooper NM, Hyde R, Karran E, Christie G, Turner AJ. A human homolog of angiotensin-converting enzyme. Cloning and functional expression as a captopril-insensitive carboxypeptidase. J Biol Chem 2000;275(43):33238–33243

67. Donoghue M, Hsieh F, Baronas E, et al. A novel angiotensin-converting enzyme-related carboxypeptidase (ACE2) converts angiotensin I to angiotensin 1-9. Circ Res 2000;87(5):E1–E9

68. Samavati L, Uhal BD. ACE2, much more than just a receptor for SARS-COV-2. Front Cell Infect Microbiol 2020;10:317

69. Hoffmann M, Kleine-Weber H, Schroeder S, et al. SARS-CoV-2 cell entry depends on ACE2 and TMPRSS2 and is blocked by a clinically proven protease inhibitor. Cell 2020;181(2):271–280.e8

70. Dai L, Gao GF. Viral targets for vaccines against COVID-19. Nat Rev Immunol 2021; 21(2):73–82

71. Huang Y, Yang C, Xu XF, Xu W, Liu SW. Structural and functional properties of SARS-CoV-2 spike protein: potential anti-virus drug development for COVID-19. Acta Pharmacol Sin 2020;41(9):1141–1149

72. Walls AC, Park Y-J, Tortorici MA, Wall A, McGuire AT, Veesler D. Structure, function, and antigenicity of the SARS-CoV-2 spike glycoprotein. Cell 2020;181(2):281–292.e6

03
COVID-19 Testing

Cesar Ivan Patiño-Barrera, Mariya Mohiuddin, and Joseph Varon

Introduction

As the world recognized that this new virus was rapidly spreading, the need for rapid identification aired, and COVID-19 testing rapidly began. Unfortunately, the logistical issues with massive testing also evolved. To start massive testing efforts, a coordinated scientific and logistic approach must occur. An essential aspect of a containment strategy is employment of extensive testing, which allows health organizations to identify the individuals currently or previously infected by severe acute respiratory syndrome coronavirus 2 (SARS-CoV-2). Accurate diagnostic testing is crucial to identify symptomatic and asymptomatic individuals to ensure adequate treatment and isolation measures, thus preventing further disease transmission.

This chapter describes the importance of testing, the refinement of different diagnostic tests, the differences between them, and the challenges faced while undergoing massive diagnostic testing.

Background

COVID-19 was first publicly announced in December 2019 to the world, following the outbreak in Wuhan, China. The virus, now recognized as SARS-CoV-2, was identified and sequenced in early January 2020.[1–3] It consisted of a positive-sense single-stranded RNA β-family coronavirus that shares significant genetic homology with the SARS coronavirus and bat SARS-like coronaviruses, with a genomic size of 29.9 kb. Each intact virus consists of four structural proteins. The N protein holds the RNA genome of the virus, and S, E, and M proteins create the virus envelope together.[4–6]

Isolation and identification of the virus paved the way to the prompt development of diagnostic testing based on real-time reverse transcription polymerase chain reaction (RT-PCR) technology. Currently, this is one of the most extensively employed diagnostic tests for COVID-19.[7,8]

As testing evolved, the World Health Organization (WHO) and the Centers for Disease Control and Prevention (CDC) stressed massive widespread testing, tracking infected people, and tracing those exposed, as an effective strategy to decrease viral transmission.[9]

Emergency Development of COVID-19 Testing

During the beginning of the pandemic in Wuhan, China, where the first cases were reported, the primary scientific task was to identify why this atypical pneumonia was causing so many critical care admissions due to acute hypoxemic respiratory failure. The first step was an attempt to culture the pathogenic agent that was causing the disease. After identifying the single-stranded virus, the second step was to start the task to decode its genome, which was accomplished in a very short time thanks to the efforts of the scientific community.[10] After that was achieved, the new goal was to develop accurate tests to help in the early diagnosis and identification of patients and begin containing measures. Immediately, the scientific community started the task of developing those tests, and soon three principal types of diagnostic tests for COVID-19 were developed: nucleic acid amplification tests (NAATs), antibody tests, and antigen tests.[11,12] NAATs identify viral genetic material. Antibody tests examine the presence of antibodies generated from the human immune response to the viral infection. Antigen tests identify the presence of viral antigens.[13]

Early in the pandemic, the CDC developed real-time RT-PCR diagnostic panels for viral detection.[14] The CDC's Real-Time RT-PCR Diagnostic Panel is a test formulated to qualitatively detect two different regions of the N gene, N1 and N2, and the RNase P (RP) gene from specimens obtained from the upper and lower respiratory tract.[14] The RP gene test performs as an internal control to confirm that the RT-PCR was performed properly.[15] Because the virus is found in the upper and lower respiratory tract, specimens from the nasopharynx will represent the presence of viral RNA in the upper and lower respiratory tract.

The CDC's Real-Time RT-PCR Diagnostic Panel was the first to obtain approval on February 4, 2020, and employs the N1 and N2 genomic segments.[16] The CDC developed the primers and probes and made the materials obtainable for other diagnostic labs that wanted to employ the same test.[16]

Most of the antigen tests focus on the four viral structural proteins. The spike (S) and nucleocapsid (N) proteins are the main immunogens.[17] The S1 subunit shares less homology with other coronaviruses and is very specific to SARS-CoV-2.[18] Furthermore, the receptor-binding domain (RBD) of the S protein demonstrates a reduced amount of cross-reactivity between SARS-CoV-2 and other coronavirus strains.[19]

The serological test came into play to try to detect rapidly and inexpensively the immune response of a suspected patient for COVID-19, mainly focusing on the presence of immunoglobulin M (IgM) in the blood to diagnose an acute infection and the presence of immunoglobulin G (IgG) to address acquired immunity, as well as diagnose people who had the infection without noticing.

Although all of these tests were getting developed as fast as possible, limitations in sample collection, transportation, and kit performance during the beginning of the

pandemic led regulatory agencies to decide to grant emergency and special approval to try to face the challenge of massive testing (**Table 3.1**).

FDA Emergency Approval

In the United States, transmission of the virus outpaced the ability to test for it, with more patients developing the symptoms and no available test to obtain a certain diagnostic test. It was one of the main reasons why the Food and Drug Administration (FDA) eventually used its Emergency Use Authorizations (EUAs) on February 4, 2020, to permit for prompt and widespread development and deployment of in vitro testing.[14]

Any laboratory or commercial company developing molecular tests to detect SARS-CoV-2 that wanted to obtain this approval had to submit an application to the FDA and obtain EUA status to offer the test for diagnostic purposes to release it to the market.[20] However, all these tests had to contain the legend "Emergency Use Authorization," either in the boxes of the testing supplies or in the reports given to the patients.[21]

Several more tests were added in early March 12, 2020, under a different permission by a Presidential directive, enabling laboratories with Clinical Laboratory Improvement Amendment accreditation to add tests without regulatory clearance.[22] This produced an unprecedented scenario in which the medical profession and the general public were unaware about the new COVID-19 tests that were being given to patients and health care facilities. However, the objective of all of these measures was to provide as many feasible testing resources available for all levels of care.

Screening for Testing

The determination to test ought to be predicated on clinical, epidemiological circumstances and linked to appraising the probability of infection.[23] At the beginning of the pandemic, testing of asymptomatic or

Table 3.1 Test type overview

Test type	Sample	Summary	Results time	Limitations
Viral culture	Respiratory tract	The gold standard to identify an emerging virus	3–7 d	Very specific laboratory capabilities as well as skilled personal. Not useful in the clinical setting
NAAT whole-genome sequencing	Respiratory tract and blood	Detects every pathogen present in the sample obtained and can identify mutations as well	20 h	High cost, time-consuming. Requires a high complexity laboratory. Not available in all the clinics
NAAT, real-time RT-PCR	Respiratory tract, stool, urine, rectal, vaginal, and blood	Most widely approved and preferred test for the diagnosis of SARS-CoV-2 infection. Gold standard	1.5–3 h	High cost. Requires a high complexity laboratory and skilled personal. Not available in all hospitals
Antigen test	Respiratory tract	Provides the fastest results, and therefore they are widely use point-of-care diagnoses	5–30 min	Possible cross-reaction with other coronaviruses. NAAT must confirm the result
Antibody test	Serum, plasma, and blood	Simple to use cassettes, useful to evaluate immunity and epidemiology surveillance	15–45 min	Timing specific. Possible cross-reaction with other coronaviruses

Abbreviations: NAAT, nucleic acid amplification test; RT-PCR, reverse transcription polymerase chain reaction; SARS-CoV-2, severe acute respiratory syndrome coronavirus 2.

presymptomatic individuals who have had contact with COVID-19-positive patients was contemplated and screening protocols were then adapted to different locals and laws.[24]

The clinical manifestations of infection are often nonspecific, including pyrexia, fatigue, cough, anosmia, and dyspnea. Also, a large proportion of individuals demonstrate no symptoms throughout their disease course, and this poses difficulty in determining who should be tested.[25]

Only a few studies have matched the timing of detection of the viral RNA, and the timing of the detection of antibodies, with

the course of the disease beginning with the incubation phase ending with recovery.[26-28] However, the available information at this point suggests that a patient can be carrying the virus for 2 to 14 days and can be a "negative" patient in a first test but become "positive" in a test done in 6 to 8 days after the first day.[29]

Both the WHO and CDC advise testing individuals exhibiting symptoms and close contacts of individuals with identified infections.[9] Furthermore, both advise testing for a wide range of respiratory pathogens on patients' samples suspected for COVID-19 to reduce the risk of untreated coinfection.[30] The same guidelines advise testing asymptomatic or presymptomatic patients only if they have had contact with a COVID-19-positive patient.[9,30]

In the United States and most countries, the decision to test a person had to be precise, as there was a lack of resources and materials to test everyone. This brought to importance the clinical diagnosis of COVID-19, which was solely grounded on epidemiological history and clinical manifestations.[23] However, this process had several flaws, such as patients not recalling a complete history of present illness or lying to be tested.

Due to the uncertainty and different presentations of COVID-19, it comes only as an intelligent decision to treat every patient as a possible COVID-19 until a PCR negative is obtained.[30] Moreover, even though a negative result comes back if the patient is still displaying symptoms or the clinical presentation changes, it is a good clinical practice to retest the patient.[30]

Mutations

The mutation of this virus is of great concern for the scientific community, primarily because of the velocity that these mutations are taking place.[31] In the context of COVID-19, this poses an unprecedented threat to the efforts to contain the virus because most of these variants are also more transmissible or the infection the patients develop is worst.[32]

An unexpectedly increased quantity of mutations may occur involving all locations of the viral genome and will have substantial effects on diagnostic kits, vaccines, and the development of therapeutic agents.[32] That is why every test that has been developed in COVID-19 will have to be rechecked in a short period of time. For example, the nucleocapsid gene may not be an optimum target for diagnostic kits, and the existing test kits targeting the nucleocapsid gene should be appropriately modified for testing accuracy.

Types of Tests

The three main types of tests available to detect SARS-CoV-2 and accurately diagnose COVID-19 include NAATs, serological tests, and antigen tests (**Table 3.2**).

It is critical that clinicians understand the difference between all the available tests, the correct diagnostic test, and, more importantly, interpret the results (**Fig. 3.1**). One should always remember that all of these tests are aiding the diagnosis.

As a rule, all tests have main and dependent variables, accuracy, and cost. When we select to lower the price, the accuracy of the test reduces. Therefore, it is crucial to understand that even though a test might seem accessible, this does not guarantee that it will be accurate.

Nucleic Acid Amplification Test

Because viremia is frequently detected early in the course of an illness, NAATs are the most sensitive assays and widely recommended diagnostics for detecting early viral infections,[9] For a quick and reliable diagnosis of COVID-19, many NAATs have been developed. Most assays have a detection limit of between 3.4 and 4.5 log10 copies/mL of virus.[9]

All methods based on nucleic acid are complex (and expensive), involving sophisticated equipment and testing reagents and requiring highly trained technicians. As a consequence, it is not feasible to employ this type of testing as point-of-care diagnostic or bedside tests in resource-limited settings. Furthermore, the tests take 4 to 6 hours to complete on average, but the necessity to transport clinical samples takes time, thus delaying reporting of results.

These types of tests have three main processes that can influence their results. These are the collection of the specimen, handling of the specimen, and processing of the specimen.[33] Proper technique and

Table 3.2 Test types: significant points to remember

Important points and characteristics	Type		
	NAATs	Antigen	Antibody
How does it work?	By detecting viral genome, most commonly using a polymerase chain reaction	By detecting specific proteins located on the surface of the virus	By detecting IgG and IgM antibodies
Sample	Respiratory tract specimen	Respiratory tract specimen	Blood
Pros	This is the most accurate kind of test available. Ideal when a tracing strategy is being implemented	Faster and less expensive than a NAAT Turnaround time makes them ideal for screening patients	It can help identify which patients have acquired immunity. It can orient us to analyze if the patient's immune system is responding.
Cons	NAATs do not quantify the viral load; they are primarily qualitative. They do not tell us if there was a prior infection.	Less sensitive than a NAAT. A negative or positive result has to be confirmed by a NAAT.	This test fails to detect an acute infection due to its nature. FDA does not recommend it for diagnosis.
Risk of false-positive test	If a false-positive is obtained, all resources for contact tracing would be wasted.	Unnecessary initiation of treatment if not confirmed using a NAAT	Patients would believe they are immune and put themselves and others at risk.
Risk of false-negative test	The patient would infect other people by not self-isolating	Same as a false-positive NAAT	Patients would not know that they have had the infection in the past.

Abbreviations: NAATs, nucleic acid amplification tests; FDA, Food and Drug Administration; IgG, immunoglobulin G; IgM, immunoglobulin M; NAATs, nucleic acid amplification tests.

well-trained medical staff reduce the chances of erroneous results from a deficient collection of a sample. When it comes to handling the specimens, the manufacturer of each collection kit specifies different temperatures at which the samples must be stored; the last part is processing the sample.[34]

Real-Time Reverse Transcription Polymerase Chain Reaction Test

The RT-PCR test was one of the first tests to be developed and the first one that the CDC approved for the diagnosis of COVID-19.[9] To this day, it retains its position as the gold standard at diagnosing suspected cases of COVID-19.[35] RT-PCR has been deemed the "gold standard" for diagnosis as it has been demonstrated to be highly sensitive for accurately identifying viral genomes present, down to just one molecule of RNA.[36]

RT-PCR is an example of molecular testing. RT-PCR is a NAAT that detects unique sequences of SARS-CoV-2 (**Fig. 3.2**).

The first RT-PCR assays were intended to identify viral RNA from upper or lower

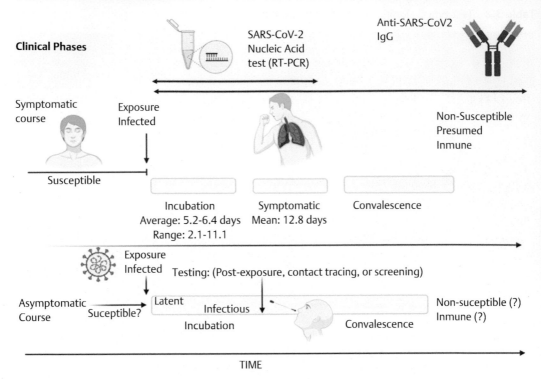

Fig. 3.1   Test comparison to disease presentation in time.

respiratory tract samples.[9] However, later development and curiosity from researchers allowed obtaining specimens to test from vaginal and anal swabs and even urine samples.[37]

Apart from nasopharyngeal (NP) and oropharyngeal sample, sputum samples can be collected to diagnose infection by expectorating deep cough into a sterile container.[37] In contrast to oropharyngeal samples, increased positive rates are observed with NP swabs performed by trained medical personnel.[38]

When it comes to the results of this test, clinicians must be cautious; different panels available can vary drastically from one laboratory to another. For example, some tests detect two or more viral genes.[37] Test results are interpreted differently in various assays. Some assays require that both viral genes be identified for the test result to be interpreted as positive, while others require detecting one of two viral genes for a positive

interpretation.[37] Furthermore, it is important to recall that due to the small amount of RNA that can be identified, these test results can be positive during the incubation period, which occurs several days prior to the development of disease symptoms, and remain positive for the duration of symptoms.[9] That is why it has been an ideal test to detect patients who report themselves as asymptomatic. Indeed, in our practice, we have seen patients remain "positive" for weeks after they had no more symptoms of the illness. This has been specially observed to be true in specimens obtained from anal swabs.[39]

In general, a positive result in an RT-PCR test indicates the presence of viral nucleic acid in the specimen obtained. However, testing in conjunction with the clinical evaluation, clinical history, doctors' perception, and further diagnostic techniques should be used to establish the patient's infection

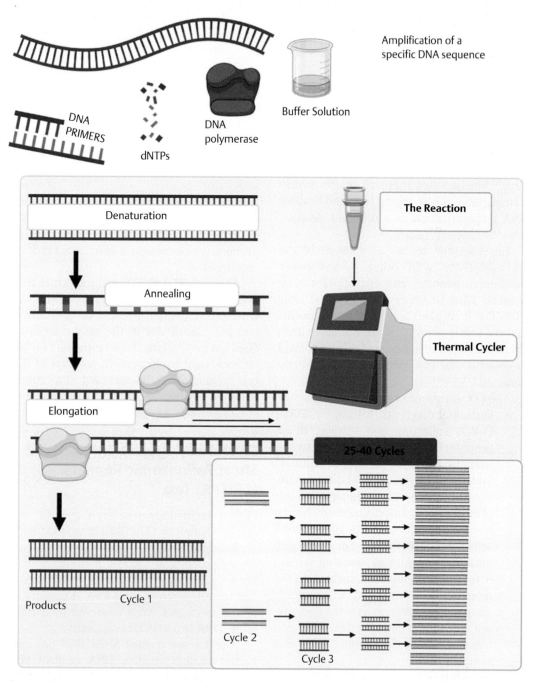

Fig. 3.2 Illustration of the RT-PCR process. PCR, Polymerase Chain Reaction

status.[9,23,29,37,40] Negative results should not mislead to rule out SARS-CoV-2 infection and must be used in combination with other clinical features and testing to determine patient management.[9,23,29,37,40]

The results of the RT-PCR tests might take anywhere from a few hours to a few days, depending on the PCR version and the panel.[37] This test can be done in a one-step or two-step process. The one-step method, which combines RT and DNA polymerase to carry out their reactions in the same tube, is the recommended method for identifying the virus.[41] The two-step approach entails reverse transcription of RNA in one tube and ensuing DNA polymerization in a different reaction tube.[42]

False-positive results as a result of the cross-reactivity with other coronaviruses, the human genome, and microflora can be reduced with sequence fidelity.[9] A reliable RT-PCR test contains a control, which means that the test is also looking for human epithelial cells as a safety measure of quality control to confirm that the specimen was correctly obtained.[9,23,29,37,40]

The CDC recommends the following:

- For initial diagnostic testing for SARS-CoV-2, collecting and testing NP or oropharyngeal samples, sterile swabs must be employed to collect samples. Swabs must be transferred directly into a sterile transport containing 2 to 3 mL of either viral transport medium, Amies transport medium, phosphate-buffered saline, or sterile saline. For personnel obtaining samples or working within 6 feet of individuals suspected to be infected, it is essential to maintain appropriate infection control and use the recommended personal protective equipment (PPE) while obtaining samples.[43]
- Providers handling sampling but not involved in the collection (e.g., self-collection) and not working within 6 feet of the patient should follow standard precautions. Providers are recommended to wear a face mask at all times while in the facility.[43]
- Samples should be stored at 2 to 8°C for up to 72 hours after collection. If a delay is anticipated, store samples at −70°C or below.

Reverse Transcription Loop-Mediated Isothermal Amplification

Loop-mediated isothermal amplification (LAMP) is a qualitative PCR-based nucleic acid amplification, which can precisely amplify the target sequence very efficiently, rapidly under isothermal conditions (usually 60–65°C).[44] The method employs multiple primers, which recognize specific areas of the target gene.[45]

Although RT-LAMP-based molecular technologies are available, they have not met with widespread use as a result cross-reactivity and poor sensitivity of the assays. RT-LAMP does not necessitate skilled providers or high technological equipment. In contrast to PCR, this technique can be executed in a limited-resource setting by heating the specimens and reagents in a single reaction tube.[46]

Clustered Regularly Interspaced Short Palindromic Repeats (CRISPR) Test

CRISPR technology has been applied as a diagnostic tool by COVID-19 iinvestigators.[47]

Recently, assays combining isothermal amplification and CRISPR technology have been developed as diagnostic tools for the fast identification of viral RNA. A distinct set of *Cas* nucleases were observed to demonstrate DNA and RNA cleavage activity.[48–50]

A technique termed SHERLOCK has been harnessed for sensitive DNA or RNA viral identification. Employing this technology requires very little laboratory resources and facilitates amplification of target RNA, and this technique is able to detect viral RNA in under 1 hour.[48–51]

There are many adaptations of CRISPR platform technology and amplification techniques in development that will be valuable in assisting the diagnosis of COVID-19; however, they are beyond the scope of this chapter.[47]

Antigen Tests

Rapid antigen tests are rapid diagnostic methods (point-of-care tests) due to the practicality of testing the patient at the bedside and with fast turnaround time of results.[52] Most of these tests are based on lateral immunochromatography; they are already in use for other respiratory viruses (e.g., influenza virus, syncytial virus) and do not require specific and expensive equipment or supplies, which makes them very accessible for clinics or places where a high complexity laboratory is not in the near vicinity.[53]

Most of these tests do rapid qualitative viral identification. They detect viral antigen, which is usually a protein, by the immobilized coated viral antibody on the apparatus. They usually come in immunofluorescence-based lateral flow technology.[5] These tests do not employ amplification technology and are more likely to produce a false-negative results than NAATs. Their main advantage is that they are fast to deliver results, with the fastest turnaround times for all tests.

It is necessary that a negative antigen test be confirmed by further molecular testing before infection is ruled out in a COVID-19-suspected individual.[54]

Trusting just an antigen result would be a big mistake by the clinician. In the authors' experience, a false-negative rate of 30% is commonly encountered with some of these tests.

Three different main types of antigens are commonly used: (1) the recombinant nucleocapsid protein, from SARS-CoV-2, which is highly conserved among all seven members of coronaviruses and led to poor specificity in tests in the general population; (2) the Spike1 protein from SARS-CoV, which has very different antigenicity from its counterpart in

SARS-CoV-2; and (3) the RBD of SARS-CoV-2 Spike1. Among these antigens, the nucleocapsid shares significant homology with other coronaviruses, leading to low specificity of the test.[55]

Most of the antigen tests' specimens have to be collected from an NP or nasal sample. This means the existence of same limitations as noted in the PCR tests about requiring well-trained health care workers.

Serological Tests (Antibody)

Currently, several antibody tests are available for clinical use, some of which initially appeared on the market as point-of-care test. These tests are mainly directed at immunogenic proteins: spike protein, the most vulnerable viral protein, and nucleocapsid proteins, which are abundantly expressed during infection.[56] In addition, the RBDs along the spike protein are viable targets for detecting the presence of SARS-CoV-2-specific antibodies.[57] There are two types of antibody tests: binding antibody and neutralizing antibody identification.[58] Antibody testing offers data on the serologic status of individuals during their clinical course of infection and convalescence. Furthermore, antibody testing provides evidence on the serologic status of undiagnosed asymptomatic patients. Although SARS-CoV-2 is a novel virus, the process of antibody formation raised against it is not dissimilar to that of other diseases. Initially, there is a rise in IgM production, with IgG following thereafter. The interesting or complex situation about this test is the window in which it becomes ideal for testing; this is mainly dependent on the immune system of the individual to be tested.[59] So far, we have a theoretical timeline that seems to be the window in which it would be good to test a patient.

Antibody testing can identify current and previous infections. Testing for IgM or IgG does not detect the SARS-CoV-2 virus per se, but the immune response if the antibodies are identified during a reasonable timeline after the onset of the disease. In general, antibody production and rise begin 1 to 3 weeks after the initiation of the infection.[60]

Serologic analysis for neutralizing IgG may be a superior marker of sustained immunity.

Several tests to identify individuals' antibodies include rapid diagnostic tests (RDTs), enzyme-linked immunosorbent assay (ELISA) tests, and chemiluminescence immunoassay tests.[54,61] Interestingly, the RDT employs lateral flow nanoparticle immunologic technology and only requires a minimal amount of blood acquired from finger prick.[54,61]

Compared with RNA detection–based testing, antibody-based tests have lower clinical sensitivity and specificity.[62] This is due to several factors, which include but are not limited to: the patient's IgG and IgM antibody production, which in other terms means the immune response of the patient to the infection, also named seroconversion, which depends on the onset of symptoms, but on average occurs 5 to 10 days after the onset of initial symptoms. Another limitation is the number of circulating immunoglobulins for the test to detect, which translates to less analytical sensitivity. Of importance, the day on which the analysis is conducted may impact the identification and quantification of antibodies. Furthermore, methodologies may result in false-positive results from acute infection with a different coronavirus resulting in antibody cross-reactivity.

It is important in clinical practice not to rely on serologic testing for diagnosis. Molecular testing that detects the presence of viral RNA is the current diagnostic gold standard.[63]

The supplementation of antibody testing with molecular testing provides a higher sensitivity than PCR alone in the diagnosis of infection. When employing serologic testing in the diagnostic evaluation of individuals, it is important to remember that according to the information available, the amount of IgG produced after infection starts declining after an average of 3 months.[64,65] Therefore, serological tests should not be used as a single diagnostic tool but should be employed in conjunction with molecular

testing with PCR-based technology the patients' clinical history, and evaluation from other laboratory tests.

Enzyme-Linked Immunosorbent Assay

An ELISA test has been developed for measuring presence of antibody directed against the recombinant RBD of the spike protein or entire spike protein.[66]

Lateral Flow Immunoassays

Lateral flow immunoassays employ a point-of-care testing for the rapid identification of an antibody response to infection. It utilizes the sandwich immunodetection method. This point-of care testing methodology provides the advantage of being able to perform assays without requiring an operational clinical laboratory,[67] i.e., the fluorescent conjugates in the detection buffers are bound to the antibodies present in the sample, forming antigen–antibody complexes, and migrate to the nitrocellulose matrix.[67]

Chemiluminescence Immunoassay

The identification of antibodies is predicated by the enzymatic reaction of enzyme and substrate, which is converted to chemiluminescent substrate and can then be measured. The assay has a high sensitivity and is automated, allowing the processing of a large number of samples.[68]

Immunoassays employed to detect the antibodies to the virus may produce false-negative results during the early stage of the infection or in asymptomatic or presymptomatic individuals who may be producing low-titer antibodies. ELISA and chemiluminescence assays based on the antibodies have shown a sensitivity of 70 to 95% and 82 to 97%, respectively. The sensitivity may be low when tested in asymptomatic or mildly symptomatic individuals who may generate only low-titer antibodies.

Sensitivity and Specificity

Testing during a pandemic poses many challenges and relies on the performance of the test in terms of assisting in containment of disease spread and the management of infected individuals.

In regards to testing it is important to have an understanding that there are two types of specificity and sensitivity, clinical and analytical. Both are not dependent, meaning that a test can have a high analytical sensitivity and low clinical sensitivity.[69,70] When dealing with a test to help us diagnose infected individuals during a pandemic, clinical specificity and sensitivity are essential for mitigation, containment, and quarantining. However, many patients are asymptomatic at the time of testing and the turnaround time for PCR testing poses some limitation on its effectiveness in surveillance, containment, and early treatment of infected individuals. Ideally, for these tests to be effective in surveillance, they should have a rapid turnaround time, be inexpensive, and be feasibly deployed for rapid testing. Clinical sensitivity refers to the accuracy of a test in identifying infected individuals.[69,70] A test with 95% sensitivity will identify 95% of patients who have the disease and produces false-negatives in 5% of infected individuals. Tests with a high sensitivity are necessary in order to identify the greatest number of patients with infection and would be important for containment and mitigation purposes. Thus, a lower sensitivity test will not identify patients who truly have infection and would be a poor screening test to be employed during a pandemic. Clinical specificity determines how accurately a test identifies negative patients who do not have SARS-COV-2. A test with 95% specificity will identify 95% of individuals who do not have the infection and incorrectly identify 5% of patients who test positive but are not infected; a lower specificity test means higher false-positives. Furthermore, it is important to note that the prevalence of the disease will impact the performance of the test.[69,70] For example, a rapid test with a high specificity employed in an area where prevalence of the disease is low will result in a substantially high percentage of false-positive tests.[70]

The SARS-CoV-2 shares significant genetic homology with human SARS-CoV. Thus, in order to develop a highly specific and sensitive test, it is of high interest to select or avoid certain regions of interest that share genetic homology with other viruses when designing primers and probes.

Many pretest variables and the individual's clinical status impact the clinical sensitivity and test performance. This means that timing is a critical part of this topic; as we explained before, the complexity and variability of the presentation of COVID-19 lead to multiple windows for the best time to test for a determined test depending on the disease state. The dynamic changes that occur during the immune response and the impact of viral clearance on test sensitivity may present a particular challenge in the interpretation of the test.

Ideally, specimens should undergo processing and tests should be performed in a rapid and timely matter. Specimens can be or stored (2–8°C) for up to 72 hours.

In order to ensure accuracy of the results, it is essential that appropriate sample collection, appropriate procedure, proper storage, and reliable transportation are available.

Drive-Thru Testing

In order to understand the transmissibility and impact of the virus, public health measures that increase testing and enable testing of large percentages of the population are important. In addition, increases in testing improve predictive modeling and bioepidemiological analysis.[71] Furthermore, an insufficient and inaccurate evaluation on the prevalence of viral infection and transmission in communities could lead to the premature discontinuation of public health measures such as wearing of masks, social distancing orders, opening of indoor areas, and relaxing other mitigation strategies, resulting in increased transmission rates.

Drive-thru testing became the answer to deploy massive efforts for COVID-19 testing. It was initially started in Asia and was rapidly followed by the United States. The authors of this chapter have participated in drive-thru testing of more than half a million individuals over 15 months.

Drive-thru testing centers must have particular characteristics and components for them to be a successful way to accomplish the goal of rapidly and efficiently processing a large number of individuals. As noted, we have been fortunate to have the experience to start a drive-thru testing operation (**Fig. 3.3**).

Drive-thru testing centers must be remote from populated zones or in locations isolated from nearby bystanders or houses. For example, a large school or store parking lot provides sufficient space. However, small areas and lots can be used efficiently with scheduling appointments. In fact, many small community clinics and urgent care centers employing a scheduling system have efficiently used small spaces. When using a parking lot, the entrance and exit should be strictly marked and delimited to avoid accidents and people entering the wrong way. When implementing signs or information handed at the drive-thru, it is imperative to have these signs in multiple languages (in Texas, English and Spanish due to the high population of individuals speaking only Spanish).

When using a parking lot as the space of a drive-thru center, it must be considered to protect the personnel performing the tests.

One structure that is easy to obtain is an open tent, which is inexpensive and provides adequate aeration. However, open tents and outdoor testing are susceptible to inclement weather and outdoor conditions. Although it requires a higher startup cost, a provisional structure/edifice provides better security for providers and equipment against inclement weather and outdoor conditions. Areas in a provisional edifice can be designated as either a clean or contaminated zone, subject to the design of the process.

The main components of a drive-thru testing center are as follows: entrance–screening–registration–specimen collection–instructions–exit (**Fig. 3.3**). This whole process must be completed to avoid the patient's necessity to get out of the car and minimize the time of direct contact.

At the beginning of the pandemic, screening of patients was critical, and this was because of the significant shortages of testing supplies that were experienced throughout the whole United States, leading the CDC to establish a criterion of patients who could get tested that was mainly focused on their exposure to a known COVID-19 patient, symptoms, and recent traveling. Health care personnel in charge of performing the tests should be well instructed to perform the test and avoid cross-contamination and self-contamination. We recommend the use of RT-PCR as the method for testing. However, not all of the testing centers perform an NP swab.

Some advantages of drive-thru testing are that it provides an efficient, convenient, and safe option to carry out massive testing for a large population in a quick time while at the same time allowing for social distancing and preventing or potentially minimizing exposure and infected individuals from transmitting the disease in closed environments.

Some of the disadvantages of drive-thru reported at the start of this pandemic included prolonged waiting times, language barriers, and, depending on the location, heat exhaustion inside the vehicles.

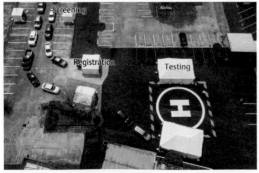

Fig. 3.3 United Memorial Medical Center COVID-19 drive-thru.

Sampling Areas

Nasopharyngeal Swab

Molecular diagnostics need an NP swabbed specimen, an invasive technique that is painful for the patient when done correctly, and those conducting the test require training. NP swabs are now the preferred specimen for COVID-19 diagnoses; however, they must be collected by skilled providers (**Fig. 3.4**).

NP swabs can induce coughing and thus have the potential to generate aerosols, and providers are at risk of exposure to large viral loads from aerosols and droplets.[72] In addition, providers require PPE to perform this testing safely. The reliability of high viral loads in NP specimens as a prognostic indicator of mortality has been previously characterized in SARS with or without a high viral load in serum.[73]

To perform a correct NP swab, the person who will test should at least know the basics of the nose anatomy, remembering that the passage from the nostril to the choanae is straight; thus, making an angle aiming upward would result in a different trajectory of the swab (**Fig. 3.4**).

Obtaining the NP specimen is uncomfortable for the patient. One of the risks faced is involuntary aggression of the person being tested to the health care provider carrying out the test. In addition, voluntary or involuntary head movements may break the swab used to collect the sample, creating the risk of losing the tip of the swab inside the nose.

So far, NP swab remains the most reliable method to obtain specimen for COVID-19 testing. This is mainly due to the easy accessibility, the large cohorts that have been analyzed, and the majority of centers employing RT-PCR prefer this method of sampling over the others.

Nasal Swab

This alternative arose due to the evident shortage of health care workers adequately trained to collect NP swabs.[74] Moreover, the CDC approved this type of collection and later authorized onsite individual self-swab-collected specimens from nasal midturbinates and anterior nares (nasal) swabs under the supervision of a health care professional (**Fig. 3.5**).

The consensus to this day keeps favoring the NP swabbing because of the virus preference of the NP cavity over the nasal.

Saliva Sampling

Another kind of collection method is saliva samples, where the patient has to fill a cup or a sampling tube with a certain amount of saliva for it to be processed. This simple and noninvasive self-collection procedure eliminates the necessity for invasive NP swabbing,

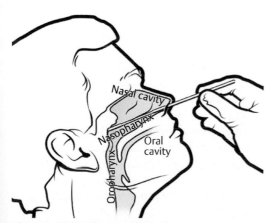

Fig. 3.4 Nasopharyngeal swab.

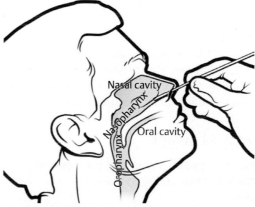

Fig. 3.5 Nasal swab.

eliminates exposure risk to providers, and can be obtained by the individual in any setting.[75]

One of the limitations of this collection methodology is that some patients do not collect enough saliva, thinking that they have provided enough when they have not, leading to the need for recollection and delays in the results. This type of testing is less consistent when compared to an NP swab.[76]

Anal Swab

The existence of viral shedding in fecal or anal samples seems to be independent of the patient's symptoms. Even though patients might not present any gastrointestinal symptoms, the virus can be detected.

It has been observed that positive tests can be obtained on patients with COVID-19 up to 5 days before the patient starts developing any symptoms.[77] In addition, it has been shown that this is a significant way of shedding. Asymptomatic, presymptomatic, or convalescing individuals may continue to shed the virus at detectable levels. However, asymptomatic individuals may not shed it for shorter periods of time or lesser amounts compared to severely infected individuals required to be hospitalized.[39]

The behavior of virus shedding is very similar to the one observed in SARS-CoV-1, in which there is an increasing viral load that peaks at approximately 12 days after the patient's first 5 days of being ill but then starts decreasing but can still be detected up to 30 days or 2 weeks after the patient's symptoms stop.[77]

A particular challenge is the presence of PCR inhibitors in fecal material (e.g., bile salts, lipids) that can lead to underestimating viral abundance or the reporting of false-negatives, thus leading to poor sensitivity of the test.[78]

Vaginal Swabs

Vaginal swabs came to the spotlight of obstetricians and gynecologists who were interested to know if it was possible to detect SARS-CoV-2 from patients who had been previously diagnosed or patients who have not been diagnosed but were going to deliver soon.[79]

The primary purpose of most of the studies investigating this form of specimen collection was to confirm or deny the possibility of vertical transmission.[80]

Urine Samples

This type of specimen was noted when SARS-CoV-1 was being studied in order to best understand virus shedding and the possibility of environmental transmission. Few studies pertinent to SARS-CoV-2 have been published so far and confirm that urine is a way in which the virus is shed.[81] Thus, it can be used to evaluate the patient's status; most of the studies suggest that the length of virus shedding is around 14 days.[81]

Similar to the anal swabs or fecal samples, the virus has been isolated successfully, suggesting the possibility of a possible infection route, but more studies are underway to confirm this possibility.

Blood Samples

Blood has also been tested to evaluate the disease of the patients, which has yielded different results.[82] The central concept is that blood samples are used to evaluate the severity of illness and understand if the infection has become systemic. Not all laboratories are equipped to manage these samples as other blood-borne pathologies can be found as coinfections.[83] Some tests have avoided blood-borne diseases using a dry spot method.

There are two main ways to obtain a sample to do a test of COVID-19; the easiest one preferred by the public is the finger prick because it does not cause the discomfort that getting blood drawn causes, which is the other method to obtain a venous sample.

Gold Standard

Confirmatory testing is generally by molecular testing usually by employing RT-PCR, which can identify unique nucleotide sequences of viral RNA.[35,36] Molecular (RT-PCR panels) testing can identify genomic sequences that code for the spike (S) protein, the nucleocapsid (N) proteins 1 and 2, the membrane protein, and the envelope (E) protein, in addition to different open reading frame segments, 1a and 1b. RNA extraction should be done in a biosafety cabinet in a Biosafety Level 2 or equivalent facility.[9]

The CDC's 2019-nCoV Real-Time RT-PCR Diagnostic Panel has a clinical sensitivity of 100% (13/13; 95% confidence interval [CI]: 77.2–100) and a clinical specificity of 100% (104/104; 95% CI: 96.4–100).[9]

False-Negative Results

Almost all the tests will, unfortunately, provide false-negative results. This can be due to multiple reasons, but even if the other variables are adequately controlled for, tests will have by design the chance of giving false-negatives.

We would like to emphasize that one or more negative results do not rule out the possibility of COVID-19 virus infection. Clinicians must always trust their assessment and use other diagnostic tools available if there is a reason to believe that the test result is incorrect.

Several factors could lead to a negative result in an infected individual, including but not limited to the following:

- Poor quality of the specimen, containing little patient material (most of the NAATs available include a human target control in the primers that their test contains enough sample material).[9,23,29,37,40]
- The specimen was collected late or very early in the infection; as we discussed before, every test has a window in which it can be the most effective to detect the target; hence, if we try to

test the patient in a nonrecommended period, the results might end up being false-negatives.[9,23,29,37,40]

- Most of all, the test kits have a specific temperature or time to be used.
- The specimen was not handled and shipped appropriately. If we used expired tests or let them be in an environment harmful to the specimen, it will modify the result.

Technical reasons inherent in the test, such as virus mutation, cause the test to miss the target designed to identify. In addition samples may contain natural inhibitors like fecal samples where PCR inhibition naturally occurs.

False-negative tests become problematic as public health authorities and governmental institutions move forward with relaxing lockdown restrictions.

When to Test?

One of the most recurrent questions is when to get a person tested for COVID-19. The CDC has developed guidelines for this, which states the following[9,23,29,37,40]:

- Symptomatic patients consistent with COVID-19.
- Individuals who have had close contact with an individual with confirmed COVID-19 (within 6 feet for an aggregate total of 15 minutes or more over 24 hours).
- People who are at higher risk for COVID-19 because they cannot socially distance as needed, such as travel, attending large social or mass gatherings, or being in congested indoor settings.
- Individuals who have been requested to get tested or referred to get testing by their health care provider or state health department.

However, this does not include the hospital setting. In the middle of a pandemic, every person admitted to a hospital should be tested for COVID-19 even if this patient is not displaying symptoms or denies any exposure.

Because, as we have shown before, the risk of a patient being an asymptomatic COVID-19 patient is high, this would help decrease the number of patients admitted, which later produce an outbreak due to the failure to have the preventive and isolation techniques.

Please note that testing for COVID-19 always requires the patient's consent, and the patient should understand the risk of not being tested affects the health care worker staff and other patients who could already be in critical condition.

The other situation is the outpatient setting. What would be the best advice to give to a patient exposed to many people due to work, not being able to confirm if one of them was a COVID-19-positive patient? We should refer to the guidelines, which allow these patients to be tested. The question that we would face is: How often should they be tested if they are asymptomatic? This is not an easy question to answer because we have to consider the possibility of getting tested, but a good time to test in general would be every 10 to 15 days.

Conclusion

During the pandemic, testing has been an important role in mitigation and containment strategies, providing local, state, and federal governments with important data to assist them in making public health decisions. In addition, testing plays an essential role in patient management. Understanding the dynamics and the advantages and disadvantages of different types of testing will allow researchers, clinicians, and scientists to properly deploy and utilize the appropriate testing technique for the particular situation at hand.

References

1. Wu F, Zhao S, Yu B, et al. Author Correction: A new coronavirus associated with human respiratory disease in China. Nature 2020; 580(7803):E7

2. Kuiken T, Fouchier RA, Schutten M, et al. Newly discovered coronavirus as the primary cause of severe acute respiratory syndrome. Lancet 2003;362(9380):263–270

3. Zhou P, Yang X-L, Wang X-G, et al. A pneumonia outbreak associated with a new coronavirus of probable bat origin. Nature 2020;579(7798):270–273

4. Wang Y, Grunewald M, Perlman S. Coronaviruses: an updated overview of their replication and pathogenesis. Methods Mol Biol 2020;2203:1–29

5. Naqvi AAT, Fatima K, Mohammad T, et al. Insights into SARS-CoV-2 genome, structure, evolution, pathogenesis and therapies: structural genomics approach. Biochim Biophys Acta Mol Basis Dis 2020; 1866(10):165878

6. Pal M, Berhanu G, Desalegn C, Kandi V. Severe acute respiratory syndrome coronavirus-2 (SARS-CoV-2): an update. Cureus 2020; 12(3):e7423

7. Corman VM, Landt O, Kaiser M, et al. Detection of 2019 novel coronavirus (2019-nCoV) by real-time RT-PCR. Euro Surveill 2020;25(3)

8. Vandenberg O, Martiny D, Rochas O, van Belkum A, Kozlakidis Z. Considerations for diagnostic COVID-19 tests. Nat Rev Microbiol 2021;19(3):171–183

9. Centers for Disease Control and Prevention. CDC 2019-Novel Coronavirus (2019-nCoV) Real-Time RT-PCR Diagnostic Panel for Emergency Use Only Instructions for Use. Atlanta, GA: CDC.; 2020

10. Rastogi M, Pandey N, Shukla A, Singh SK. SARS coronavirus 2: from genome to infectome. Respir Res 2020;21(1):318

11. Carter LJ, Garner LV, Smoot JW, et al. Assay techniques and test development for COVID-19 diagnosis. ACS Cent Sci 2020; 6(5):591–605

12. Cheng MP, Papenburg J, Desjardins M, et al. Diagnostic testing for severe acute respiratory syndrome-related coronavirus 2: a narrative review. Ann Intern Med 2020;172(11):726–734

13. Nguyen NNT, McCarthy C, Lantigua D, Camci-Unal G. Development of diagnostic tests for detection of SARS-CoV-2. Diagnostics (Basel) 2020;10(11):905

14. U.S. Food and Drug Administration. New York SARS-CoV-2 Real-Time Reverse Transcriptase (RT)-PCR Diagnostic Panel. Albany, NY: Wadsworth Center, New York State Department of Health; 2020. Available at: https://www.fda.gov/media/135847/download

15. Ravi N, Cortade DL, Ng E, Wang SX. Diagnostics for SARS-CoV-2 detection: a comprehensive review of the FDA-EUA COVID-19 testing landscape. Biosens Bioelectron 2020; 165:112454

16. U.S. Food and Drug Administration. FDA takes significant step in coronavirus response efforts, issues emergency use authorization for the first 2019 novel coronavirus diagnostic. February 4, 2020. Available at: https://www.fda.gov/news-events/press-announcements/fda-takes-significant-step-coronavirus-response-efforts-issues-emergency-use-authorization-first

17. Nguyen T, Duong Bang D, Wolff A. 2019 novel coronavirus disease (COVID-19): paving the road for rapid detection and point-of-care diagnostics. Micromachines (Basel) 2020; 11(3):E306

18. Tian Y, Lian C, Chen Y, et al. Sensitivity and specificity of SARS-CoV-2 S1 subunit in COVID-19 serology assays. Cell Discov 2020; 6:75

19. Ou X, Liu Y, Lei X, et al. Characterization of spike glycoprotein of SARS-CoV-2 on virus entry and its immune cross-reactivity with SARS-CoV. Nat Commun 2020;11(1):1620

20. U.S. Food and Drug Administration. Coronavirus (COVID-19) update: serological tests. April 7, 2020. Available at: https://www.fda.gov/news-events/press-announcements/coronavirus-covid-19-update-serological-tests. Accessed January 27, 2021

21. U.S. Food and Drug Administration. Emergency use authorizations for medical devices. Available at: https://www.fda.gov/medical-devices/emergency-situations-medical-devices/emergency-use-authorizations-medical-devices#covid19ivd. Accessed January 27, 2020

22. FEMA. COVID-19 emergency declaration. March 14, 2020. Available at: https://www.fema.gov/press-release/20210318/covid-19-emergency-declaration

23. Patel R, Babady E, Theel ES, et al. Report from the American Society for Microbiology COVID-19 International Summit, 23 March 2020: value of diagnostic testing for SARS-CoV-2/COVID-19. MBio 2020; 11(2):e00722-e20

24. Pulia MS, O'Brien TP, Hou PC, Schuman A, Sambursky R. Multi-tiered screening and diagnosis strategy for COVID-19: a model for sustainable testing capacity in response to pandemic. Ann Med 2020;52(5):207-214

25. Zhu CQ, Gao SD, Xu Y, et al. A COVID-19 case report from asymptomatic contact: implication for contact isolation and incubation management. Infect Dis Poverty 2020; 9(1):70

26. Jiang H, Li Y, Zhang H, et al. SARS-CoV-2 proteome microarray for global profiling of COVID-19 specific IgG and IgM responses. Nature Communications. 2020;11(1):3581. doi:10.1038/s41467-020-17488-8

27. Amanat F, Stadlbauer D, Strohmeier S, et al. A serological assay to detect SARS-CoV-2 seroconversion in humans. Nat Med 2020; 26(7):1033-1036

28. Xu Y, Xiao M, Liu X, et al. Significance of serology testing to assist timely diagnosis of SARS-CoV-2 infections: implication from a family cluster. Emerg Microbes Infect 2020;9(1):924-927

29. Sethuraman N, Jeremiah SS, Ryo A. Interpreting diagnostic tests for SARS-CoV-2. JAMA 2020;323(22):2249-2251

30. World Health Organization. Global Surveillance for Human Infection with Coronavirus Disease (COVID-2019): Interim Guidance. Geneva: World Health Organization; 2020. Available at: https://www.who.int/publications/i/item/who-2019-nCoV-surveillanceguidance-2020.8

31. Kupferschmidt K. Viral mutations may cause another 'very, very bad' COVID-19 wave, scientists warn. Science January 5, 2021. doi:10.1126/science.abg4312

32. Centers for Disease Control and Prevention. What you need to know about variants. Available at: https://www.cdc.gov/coronavirus/2019-ncov/transmission/variant.html

33. Chan JF, Yip CC, To KK, et al. Improved molecular diagnosis of COVID-19 by

the novel, highly sensitive and specific COVID-19-RdRp/Hel real-time reverse transcription-PCR assay validated *in vitro* and with clinical specimens. J Clin Microbiol 2020;58(5):e00310-20

34. American Society for Microbiology. ASM expresses concern about coronavirus test reagent shortages. March 10, 2020. Available at: https://asm.org/Articles/Policy/2020/March/ASM-ExpressesConcern-about-Test-Reagent-Shortages

35. Jung Y, Park GS, Moon JH, et al. Comparative analysis of primer-probe sets for RT-qPCR of COVID-19 causative virus (SARS-CoV-2). ACS Infect Dis 2020;6(9):2513–2523

36. Wang Y, Kang H, Liu X, Tong Z. Combination of RT-qPCR testing and clinical features for diagnosis of COVID-19 facilitates management of SARS-CoV-2 outbreak. J Med Virol 2020;92(6):538–539

37. Tsang NNY, So HC, Ng KY, Cowling BJ, Leung GM, Ip DKM. Diagnostic performance of different sampling approaches for SARS-CoV-2 RT-PCR testing: a systematic review and meta-analysis. Lancet Infect Dis 2021;21(9):1233–1245

38. Tan SY, Tey HL, Lim ETH, et al. The accuracy of healthcare worker versus self collected (2-in-1) Oropharyngeal and Bilateral Mid-Turbinate (OPMT) swabs and saliva samples for SARS-CoV-2. PLoS One 2020;15(12):e0244417

39. Kipkorir V, Cheruiyot I, Ngure B, Misiani M, Munguti J. Prolonged SARS-CoV-2 RNA detection in anal/rectal swabs and stool specimens in COVID-19 patients after negative conversion in nasopharyngeal RT-PCR test. J Med Virol 2020;92(11):2328–2331

40. Ai T, Yang Z, Hou H, et al. Correlation of chest CT and RT-PCR testing for coronavirus disease 2019 (COVID-19) in China: a report of 1014 cases. Radiology 2020;296(2):E32–E40

41. Vogels CBF, Brito AF, Wyllie AL, et al. Analytical sensitivity and efficiency comparisons of SARS-CoV-2 RT-qPCR primer-probe sets. Nat Microbiol 2020;5(10):1299–1305

42. Tahamtan A, Ardebili A. Real-time RT-PCR in COVID-19 detection: issues affecting the results. Expert Rev Mol Diagn 2020;20(5):453–454

43. McFee DRB. COVID-19 laboratory testing/CDC guidelines. Dis Mon 2020;66(9):101067

44. González-González E, Lara-Mayorga IM, Rodríguez-Sánchez IP, et al. Scaling diagnostics in times of COVID-19: Colorimetric Loop-mediated Isothermal Amplification (LAMP) assisted by a 3D-printed incubator for cost-effective and scalable detection of SARS-CoV-2. medRxiv. Published online January 1, 2020:2020.04.09.20058651. doi:10.1101/2020.04.09.2005865

45. Kim JH, Kang M, Park E, Chung DR, Kim J, Hwang ES. A simple and multiplex loop-mediated isothermal amplification (LAMP) assay for rapid detection of SARS-CoV. Biochip J 2019;13(4):341–351

46. Butt AM, Siddique S, An X, Tong Y. Development of a dual-gene loop-mediated isothermal amplification (LAMP) detection assay for SARS-CoV-2: a preliminary study. medRxiv 2020 (e-pub ahead of print). doi:https://doi.org/10.1101/2020.04.08.20056986

47. Broughton JP, Deng X, Yu G, et al. CRISPR-Cas12-based detection of SARS-CoV-2. Nat Biotechnol 2020;38(7):870–874

48. Ding X, Yin K, Li Z, Liu C. All-in-One Dual CRISPR-Cas12a (AIOD-CRISPR) Assay: A Case for Rapid, Ultrasensitive and Visual Detection of Novel Coronavirus SARS-CoV-2 and HIV virus. bioRxiv. Published online March 21, 2020. doi:10.1101/2020.03.19.998724

49. Hou T, Zeng W, Yang M, et al. Development and evaluation of a rapid CRISPR-based diagnostic for COVID-19. PLoS Pathog. 2020; 16(8):e1008705. doi:10.1371/journal.ppat.1008705

50. Chen JS, Ma E, Harrington LB, et al. CRISPR-Cas12a target binding unleashes indiscriminate single-stranded DNase activity. Science 2018;360(6387):436–439

51. Joung J, Ladha A, Saito M, et al. Point-of-care testing for COVID-19 using SHERLOCK diagnostics. medRxiv 2020 (e-pub ahead of print). doi:10.1101/2020.05.04.20091231

52. Riccò M, Ferraro P, Gualerzi G, et al. Point-of-care diagnostic tests for detecting SARS-CoV-2 antibodies: a systematic review and meta-analysis of real-world data. J Clin Med 2020;9(5):1515

53. Stevens B, Hogan CA, Sahoo MK, et al. Comparison of a point-of-care assay and a high-complexity assay for detection of

SARS-CoV-2 RNA. J Appl Lab Med 2020;5(6): 1307–1312

54. Michel M, Bouam A, Edouard S, et al. Evaluating ELISA, immunofluorescence, and lateral flow assay for SARS-CoV-2 serologic assays. Front Microbiol 2020;11:597529

55. Zhao P, Praissman JL, Grant OC, et al. Virus-receptor interactions of glycosylated SARS-CoV-2 spike and human ACE2 receptor. Cell Host Microbe 2020;28(4):586–601.e6

56. Lee CY-P, Lin RTP, Renia L, Ng LFP. Serological approaches for COVID-19: epidemiologic perspective on surveillance and control. Front Immunol 2020;11:879

57. Theel ES, Slev P, Wheeler S, Couturier MR, Wong SJ, Kadkhoda K. The role of antibody testing for SARS-CoV-2: is there one? J Clin Microbiol 2020;58(8):e00797-20

58. Okba NMA, Muller MA, Li W, et al. Severe acute respiratory syndrome coronavirus 2-specific antibody responses in coronavirus disease patients. Emerg Infect Dis 2020;26(7):1478–1488

59. Wang P. Combination of serological total antibody and RT-PCR test for detection of SARS-COV-2 infections. J Virol Methods 2020;283:113919

60. Maxmen A. The researchers taking a gamble with antibody tests for coronavirus. Nature 2020 (e-pub ahead of print). doi:10.1038/d41586-020-01163-5

61. Meyer B, Drosten C, Müller MA. Serological assays for emerging coronaviruses: challenges and pitfalls. Virus Res 2014;194: 175–183

62. Yongchen Z, Shen H, Wang X, et al. Different longitudinal patterns of nucleic acid and serology testing results based on disease severity of COVID-19 patients. Emerg Microbes Infect 2020;9(1):833–836

63. Zhang W, Du RH, Li B, et al. Molecular and serological investigation of 2019-nCoV infected patients: implication of multiple shedding routes. Emerg Microbes Infect 2020;9(1):386–389

64. Krammer F, Simon V. Serology assays to manage COVID-19. Science 2020; 368(6495):1060–1061

65. Bermingham WH, Wilding T, Beck S, Huissoon A. SARS-CoV-2 serology: Test, test, test, but interpret with caution! Clin Med (Lond) 2020;20(4):365–368

66. Kubina R, Dziedzic A. Molecular and serological tests for COVID-19 a comparative review of SARS-CoV-2 coronavirus laboratory and point-of-care diagnostics. Diagnostics (Basel) 2020;10(6):434

67. Torres R, Rinder HM. Double-edged spike. Am J Clin Pathol 2020;153(6):709–711

68. Paradiso AV, De Summa S, Loconsole D, et al. Rapid Serological Assays and SARS-CoV-2 Real-Time Polymerase Chain Reaction Assays for the Detection of SARS-CoV-2: Comparative Study. J Med Internet Res. 2020;22(10):e19152. doi:10.2196/19152

69. Chau CH, Strope JD, Figg WD. COVID-19 clinical diagnostics and testing technology. Pharmacotherapy 2020;40(8):857–868

70. Mina MJ, Parker R, Larremore DB. Rethinking Covid-19 test sensitivity—a strategy for containment. N Engl J Med 2020;383(22): e120

71. Ton AN, Jethwa T, Waters K, Speicher LL, Francis D. COVID-19 drive through testing: an effective strategy for conserving personal protective equipment. Am J Infect Control 2020;48(6):731–732

72. Jayaweera M, Perera H, Gunawardana B, Manatunge J. Transmission of COVID-19 virus by droplets and aerosols: a critical review on the unresolved dichotomy. Environ Res 2020;188:109819

73. Fajnzylber J, Regan J, Coxen K, et al; Massachusetts Consortium for Pathogen Readiness. SARS-CoV-2 viral load is associated with increased disease severity and mortality. Nat Commun 2020;11(1):5493

74. Wang X, Tan L, Wang X, et al. Comparison of nasopharyngeal and oropharyngeal swabs for SARS-CoV-2 detection in 353 patients received tests with both specimens simultaneously. Int J Infect Dis 2020;94: 107–109

75. Becker D, Sandoval E, Amin A, et al. Saliva is less sensitive than nasopharyngeal swabs for COVID-19 detection in the community setting. medRxiv 2020 (e-pub ahead of print). doi: https://doi.org/10.1101/2020.05.11.20092338

76. Williams E, Bond K, Zhang B, Putland M, Williamson DA. Saliva as a noninvasive specimen for detection of SARS-CoV-2. J Clin Microbiol 2020;58(8):e00776–e20

77. Sun M, Guo D, Zhang J, et al. Anal swab as a potentially optimal specimen for

SARS-CoV-2 detection to evaluate hospital discharge of COVID-19 patients. Future Microbiol 2020;15:1101–1107. Erratum in: Future Microbiol 2021;16(6):453

78. Udugama B, Kadhiresan P, Kozlowski HN, et al. Diagnosing COVID-19: the disease and tools for detection. ACS Nano 2020; 14(4):3822–3835

79. Narang K, Enninga EAL, Gunaratne MDSK, et al. SARS-CoV-2 infection and COVID-19 during pregnancy: a multidisciplinary review. Mayo Clin Proc 2020;95(8):1750–1765

80. Kotlyar AM, Grechukhina O, Chen A, et al. Vertical transmission of coronavirus disease 2019: a systematic review and meta-analysis. Am J Obstet Gynecol 2021;224(1):35–53.e3

81. Kashi AH, De la Rosette J, Amini E, Abdi H, Fallah-Karkan M, Vaezjalali M. Urinary viral shedding of COVID-19 and its clinical associations: a systematic review and meta-analysis of observational studies. Urol J 2020;17(5):433–441

82. Woo PC, Lau SK, Wong BH, et al. Differential sensitivities of severe acute respiratory syndrome (SARS) coronavirus spike poly-peptide enzyme-linked immunosorbent assay (ELISA) and SARS coronavirus nucleo-capsid protein ELISA for serodiagnosis of SARS coronavirus pneumonia. J Clin Microbiol 2005;43(7):3054–3058

83. Woo PCY, Lau SKP, Wong BHL, et al. Detection of specific antibodies to severe acute respiratory syndrome (SARS) coronavirus nucleo-capsid protein for serodiagnosis of SARS coronavirus pneumonia. J Clin Microbiol 2004;42(5):2306–2309

04   COVID-19 Prevention and Vaccines

Carmen Alvarez and Vicente Soriano

SARS-CoV-2 Transmission

From the beginning, the major role of airborne transmission was highlighted for severe acute respiratory syndrome coronavirus 2 (SARS-CoV-2) infection.[1] In addition, contact with contaminated surfaces was considered a potential source of contagion. Indeed, studies reporting the different times of viral particle survival as infectious on distinct materials were published.[2] However, over time, it became clear that inhalation of infectious particles through aerosols is by far the major route of infection.

Resembling what is well established for other respiratory viral infections, such as influenza, the size of the inoculum determines in SARS-CoV-2 infection both the risk of contagion and the chances of developing severe disease.[3] This observation was made during the first wave of COVID-19 comparing outbreaks in different settings (e.g., chorus singers in close spaces). In Madrid, Spain, we reported several clusters of infected people, some of them developing severe pneumonia and others mostly remaining asymptomatic or developing mild disease.[3] The estimated airborne viral inoculum was the major determinant of this discordant outcome, with an indoor meeting associated with severe disease and living in a large home with a garden linked to mild infection, as shown in **Fig. 4.1**.[3]

A unique feature of SARS-CoV-2 compared to other life-threatening coronaviruses such as severe acute respiratory syndrome (SARS) or Middle East respiratory syndrome (MERS)

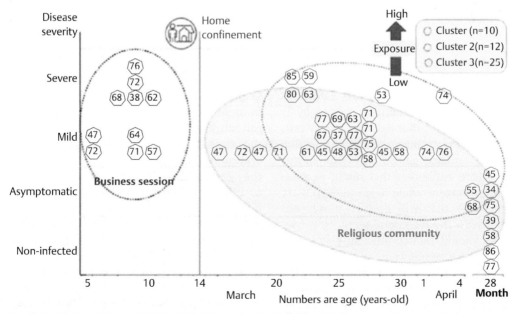

Fig. 4.1 Three clusters of SARS-CoV-2 infection in Madrid with divergent clinical outcomes according to estimated inoculum at infection.

is that infected persons may transmit the virus before they begin symptoms, during the incubation period. In this way, preventive strategies such as isolation are often implemented too late, when contacts already have been exposed unnoticed.[4]

Vaccines

Vaccines are very effective biologic agents that prevent infections, save lives, and reduce global mortality. The incidence of vaccine-preventable diseases among children has decreased enormously during the last five decades in developed countries. Four vaccine-preventable diseases were eradicated by 2015: smallpox, poliomyelitis, rubella, and congenital rubella syndrome.[5] Other important achievements regarding vaccination during this period involved at least three major advances. First, the administration of the first recombinant vaccine, the hepatitis B vaccine, was found to reduce the infection rates and the liver cancer risk.[5] Second, the license of the first polysaccharide-protein conjugate vaccine decreased the incidence of invasive *Haemophilus influenzae* type B in children.[5] Third, the first vaccine was designed for people in low-income countries as the vaccine for *Neisseria meningitides* group A.[6]

Effective vaccines should stimulate the immune system and elicit adaptive and long-lasting immunity to a particular infectious disease. Adaptive immunity is exerted by T- and B-lymphocytes that induce memory cells and amplify the response to a later infection with the microorganism. B-lymphocytes will produce antibodies that might neutralize the pathogen, while T-lymphocytes are effector cells that will destroy those cells infected with the infectious agent. However, vaccines should induce efficiently not only adaptive but also innate immune responses. In the past, innate immunity was considered to induce nonspecific immune responses throughout phagocytic cells such as monocytes, macrophages, or dendritic cells, which recognize pathogens throughout pattern

recognition receptors and lack immunologic memory. However, more recently, it was discovered that innate immune cells presented a heterologous memory of past infections, a process known as trained immunity that involves specificity.[7]

There are two main requirements to design prophylactic vaccines. First, a target antigen that elicits a strong immune response and correlates with protection is needed. Classical antigens used in vaccine designs are either main virulence factors or relevant factors involved in the entry of a pathogen into cells. The second requirement implies a vaccine platform that allows the antigen expression and allows a safe and convenient administration while generating an adequate prophylactic immune response. While the target antigen differs in each pathogen, vaccine platforms might be common to a great variety of pathogens. In this regard, vaccine platforms prepared with small molecules such as DNA, mRNA, recombinant proteins, peptides, polysaccharides, nanoparticles, or cellular vaccines as dendritic cells loaded with small molecules, filled into the category of flexible vaccine platforms. In this regard, we would like to stress the pioneering work of Robert Malone in the late 1980s.[8,9]

Vaccine formulations based on small molecules, except cellular dendritic-based vaccines, require adjuvants to help to amplify the immune response, improve the immunogenicity of the antigens or elicit a preferred immune response. For instance, adjuvants can attract the antigen-presenting cells to the site of vaccination, increase the generation of memory immune cells or improve the generation of neutralizing antibodies or effector T cells. Very few adjuvants are licensed for human use since the approval of aluminum salts in 1920 that induce Th2-immune responses.[10,11] Live attenuated or inactivated microorganisms are other types of vaccines composed of whole pathogens and do not require adjuvants. Vaccine formulations that do not include whole microorganisms in their design should also include adjuvants.[12] Finally, vaccine formulations also include preservatives in their compositions such as formaldehyde, thimerosal, phenol, polyethilenglycol, and stabilizers such as sugars, gelatin, proteins as human albumin, and hydrolyzed collagen.[10,11]

Once the vaccine formulation is ready, several parameters are explored before the approval of a vaccine for commercialization, such as toxicity, immunogenicity, and efficacy. These parameters are examined first in pre-clinical trials using experimental animals and in vitro human testing and second in human trials after authorization by the Food and Drug regulatory agencies. Human trials for vaccine approval involve three phases.[13]

Phase 1

It examines the induction of fatal toxicities or severe pathologies. It is performed in 20 to 100 recruited healthy volunteers. This phase usually takes around three months.

Phase 2

It explores the immune response against the infectious agent, the vaccine doses, and the vaccine protocol. For this phase, rand-omized 200 to 500 volunteers are recruited. Volunteers should be adults, between 18 and 55 years, healthy, that they have not had the infection. The election of the groups depends on the risk groups for each infectious disease. Half of the volunteers are inoculated with the complete vaccine and half of them with placebo, a vaccine formulation without the target antigen of the pathogen. Volunteers should live together with the pathogen to evaluate if the vaccine can protect against the infection. Phase 2 can last at least 6 months.

Phase 3

It has the purpose of evaluating long-lasting immune responses. In this stage, thousands of volunteers are recruited, usually between 30,000 and 50,000 persons, with the same features and groups as the previous phase. That is healthy individuals that did not have

the infection. Since this phase includes a high number of volunteers, the results of this phase have a great statistical value to detect secondary adverse effects that were not detected in previous phases. These toxicities are always mild and not severe. This phase also measures vaccine efficacy. A normal vaccine efficiency is at least 60%. This phase usually lasts between 9 and 12 months.

Which Clinical Effects are Explored with the Analysis of Toxicity, Immunogenicity, and Efficacy?

The toxicity explores any severe or fatal adverse effects of the vaccine design. The most common severe adverse effects associated with vaccines are caused by an inflammation elicited that is accompanied by the release of proinflammatory cytokines that evokes an acute-phase response involving the production of IL-6, C-reactive protein (CRP), fibrinogen, or TNF.[14] The entry of these acute-phase cytokines into the bloodstream might trigger fever or malaise. Since vaccines are administrated by intramuscular injection, they might also cause some local trauma and small pain that does not last longer than a week but, in some cases, might be longer. Another type of severe adverse effects is the induction of autoimmune diseases in rare cases as the cases of systemic lupus erythematosus detected in some adolescent girls after HPV vaccination or the Guillain-Barré syndrome, a neurological complication immune-mediated, a rare event observed six weeks after a dose of tetanus, oral polio, rabies or influenza containing vaccines.[15,16] In fact, autoimmune diseases can be explained by the molecular mimicry of the antigen and the production of autoantibodies. Some viruses such as Epstein-Barr (EBV), cytomegalovirus (CMV), human immunodeficiency virus (HIV), influenza (HIN1) or human T lymphotropic virus (HTLV-1) are examples that might induce autoimmune diseases, and SARS-CoV-2 infection can also trigger autoantibodies.[17] Also, some components of the vaccine formulation such as adjuvants that induce innate immunity and are required to augment the immune response or other ingredients such as preservatives or stabilizers might cause some toxicities or some autoimmune associated reactions.[18]

The immunogenicity is based on the ability of an antigen or antigens to induce the adaptive immune system, formed by T-lymphocytes, both CD4[+] and CD8[+] T cells, as well as B-lymphocytes.[19] To measure the vaccine immunogenicity specific antibodies in the blood are measured. If vaccines induced a good immune memory, a large increase in the antibody levels occurs after the application of a booster dose of the vaccine. But not only do antibodies measure the immunogenicity of a vaccine, but vaccines also induce the expansion of CD4[+] and CD8[+] T cells specific for the vaccine antigen, and therefore, antigen-specific T cells are examined to determine if a vaccine induces a strong cellular immune response.

The efficacy is measured as a percentage of the reduction in disease between individuals vaccinated and control participants, known as the placebo group, and performed in optimal conditions. Therefore, it is a measurement of the protection attributable to a vaccine. However, vaccine efficacy does not always predict their effectiveness, known as the protection attributable to a vaccine administered under field conditions. For instance, vaccines for older age groups may implement methods to improve their immunogenicity, including the use of adjuvants. Therefore, prospective studies of vaccine effectiveness in real scenarios are needed for adjustments.[20]

Vaccines for Coronaviruses

Coronaviruses are a group of viruses of the *Coronaviridae* family that demonstrate spike glycoproteins on the nucleocapsid envelope, which are necessary to attach to host cells.[21] Coronavirus has a positive-sense single-stranded RNA genome and a nucleocapsid with helicoid symmetry. They infect mammals and birds and caused respiratory tract and diarrhea symptoms. Coronavirus infections in humans can be lethal as the cases of SARS or MERS.

After the SARS epidemic in 2002–2003, several laboratories performed vaccine developments to prevent this lethal disease whose symptoms are high fever, shortness of breath, and pneumonia. The origin was southern China, with more than 8096 cases and 774 deaths that involved 26 countries. No vaccines were commercially available, and SARS cases ceased from 2004. Most subunit vaccines targeted the spike (S) glycoprotein as the main virulence factor used by the virus to bind and enter host cells. Vaccines inducing strong immune responses against S protein would affect the entry of the virus to host cells. Vaccines prepared for SARS used different technologies, mainly live-attenuated or inactivated virus, recombinant viral vectors, DNA, virus-like particles (VLPs), and soluble proteins, but all of them were studied in preclinical studies, none of these vaccines passed to clinical trials.[22]

Live attenuated or inactivated viral vaccines imply first to transform the virus into a non-replicating virus, and therefore, the virus infectivity is reduced either deleting components of the virus genome or using physical-chemical methods such as heat or formaldehyde. Recombinant viral vectors prepared as SARS vaccines used a different virus able of host cell infection that has been genetically engineered to express components of SARS virus. VLPs are non-infectious multiprotein structures from other virus proteins that self-assemble into virus-like particles (**Table 4.1**).[22] Human clinical trials of phase I were only performed with vaccines that used inactivated SARS, DNA, or soluble proteins based on S glycoprotein.[22] To be able to examine protection with these vaccines from virus infection and clinical signs, vaccinated individuals should be exposed to the virus. However, it should be noted that SARS has high virulence, and challenge studies were not performed in humans, and

Table 4.1 Vaccines platforms for SARS: description in humans, side effects, and status

Vaccine	Target	Description	Side effects	Status
Inactivated	All structural proteins	Induce neutralizing antibodies and showed no severe adverse effects **(in humans)**	Local pain, erythema, abdominal pain, diarrhea	Preclinical and Phase 1 clinical trial
Live attenuated (E-deleted)	All genome except the envelope protein	Induction of neutralizing antibodies and CD4/CD8 T cell responses in mice **(not in human)**	Not reported	Preclinical
Live attenuated recombinant virus (parainfluenza virus, VSV, Newcastle disease virus)	S glycoprotein, nucleocapsid (N) protein	Induction of protection from viral replication in lungs (African green monkeys) Long-term protection in mice **(not in human)**	Enhanced lung immunopathology after challenge when using N protein.	Preclinical
Recombinant modified vaccinia Ankara (MVA) virus	Spike (S) glycoprotein or nucleocapsid (N) protein	Induction of neutralizing antibodies and protection from viral replication in lungs in mice, rabbits, rhesus monkeys, and macaques **(not in human)**	High levels of ALT indicating hepatic lesion when expressing S protein, hepatitis in ferrets after viral challenge	Preclinical
Recombinant non-replicating adenovirus (E-deleted)	S glycoprotein or nucleocapsid (N) protein	Incomplete protection but a reduction of viral replication in mice and ferrets. Great immune responses in lungs after intranasal Immunization **(not in human)**	Redirection of vector to olfactory bulbs by intranasal administration in mice	Preclinical
DNA-based vaccines	Full spike (S) glycoprotein or fragments	Induction of neutralizing antibodies and T cell responses after 2–3 doses **(in human)** Neutralizing antibodies and CD4/CD8 T cells and viral protection in lungs **(in mice)**	Lung immunopathology (in mice)	Preclinical and Phase 1 clinical trial
Soluble proteins/adjuvant	Full spike (S) glycoprotein or fragments	Protection from lung viral replication and pneumonia in mice and hamsters. Induction of neutralizing antibodies in rabbits	Enhancement of virus entry in B cells	Preclinical and Phase 1 clinical trial

(Continued)

Table 4.1 *(Continued)* Vaccines platforms for SARS: description in humans, side effects and status

Vaccine	Target	Description	Side effects	Status
VLP/adjuvant	Spike (S) glycoprotein	Induction of neutralizing antibodies and protection from lung viral replication in mice	Lung immunopathology	Preclinical
Combination vaccines (DNA/ peptides, DNA/ recombinant viral vector, viral vector/peptides)	Spike (S) glycoprotein or fragments	Induction of neutralizing antibodies and T cell responses	Not reported	Preclinical

Adapted from Padron-Regalado (2020).

consequently, protection efficacy was not assessed.

MERS coronavirus emerged in 2012. Similar to SARS vaccines, most of the subunit vaccines were targeted to S glycoprotein. Vaccines based on live attenuated viruses, recombinant viral vectors, nanoparticles, DNA, and soluble proteins were tested in experimental animal models (**Table 4.2**).[22] Only a DNA-based vaccine went into a clinical trial at phase I and viral replication vaccines using modified Ankara virus MVA.[23]

Current COVID-19 Vaccine Overview

Since the formal declaration by WHO of a global pandemic on 11 March 2020 due to a SARS-CoV-2 that caused the coronavirus disease (COVID-19), a year later, over 3 million deaths had been reported in the world. There has been a race to develop safe and effective vaccines in a scale and manner never reported before. More than 200 potential vaccines are using different approaches and platforms. Genome sequencing and structural analyses revealed that this positive-sense single-stranded RNA encodes for structural proteins spike (S), envelope (E), membrane (M), and nucleocapsid (N), as well as several accessory and non-structural proteins. The virion shape is giving by M and N proteins,

while the spikes on the viral surface that confers a solar corona appearance are provided by the S protein.[24] S protein forms a homotrimeric glycoprotein that binds to the functional receptor human for angiotensin-converting enzyme 2 (ACE2). Spike protein binding to ACE2 is responsible for the virus entry into target cells via the receptor binding domain (RBD).[25] The S protein exists in a prefusion conformation that undergoes major structural rearrangements to fuse the viral membrane with the host cell membrane. The RBD performs conformational movements that hide or expose receptor binding determinants, implying two states, the down and inaccessible state and the up and receptor-accessible state. These studies also revealed key epitopes, amino acids A475 and F486, as the binding sites for neutralizing antibodies.[26,27] Therefore, S protein and the RBD appeared as the primary targets to block viral entry and the focus of most vaccine developments, therapeutic antibodies, and diagnostics.

Immune responses to SARS-CoV-2 is characterized by the following issues that condition the designs of vaccines:

Induction of Innate Immunity

Innate immunity is triggered via pattern associated molecular patterns (PAMPS) expressed

Table 4.2 Vaccines platforms for MERS

Vaccine	Target	Description	Side effects	Status
Live attenuated (E-deleted)	All genome except the envelope protein	Not tested in vivo	Not reported	In vitro
Inactivated	S protein and S1 subunit	Induce neutralizing antibodies and protection from viral lung loads and pathologic damage **(in humanized mice)**	Enhanced lung eosinophil infiltrations after challenge	Preclinical
Replication-deficient viral vaccines (poxvirus, adenovirus, measles, rabies)	S glycoprotein, S1 subdomain (containing the RBD)	Induction of neutralizing antibodies and T cell responses and protection from lung replication and lethal viral dose **(in humanized mice)**	Use of S1 in an adenovirus-based vaccine-induced lung pathology after challenge	Phase 1
Soluble proteins/ adjuvant	S glycoprotein and fragments	Induction of neutralizing antibodies and protection from lethal doses **(in humanized mice),** partial protection in rhesus macaques (do not prevent pneumonia)	Not reported	Pre-clinical
Nanoparticles	S glycoprotein	Induction of neutralizing antibodies and reduction of virus replication **(in mice)**	Not reported	Preclinical
DNA-based vaccines	S glycoprotein and subunits	Induction of neutralizing antibodies and T cell responses after three doses **(in humans)**	Moderate to mild symptoms	Phase 1/2a (South Korea) and 2 (Middle East)
Combination vaccines (protein/ DNA	S glycoprotein and subunits	Induction of long-life neutralizing antibodies and protection from pneumonia **(in non-human primates)**	Not reported	Preclinical

Adapted from Padron-Regalado (2020).

by the virus, such as RNA that stimulates multiple immune pathways such as Toll-like receptors (TLR) 3 and 7, cytosolic retinoic acid-inducible gene 1 (RIG-1), and melanoma differentiation associated protein 5 (MDA5).[28] Local tissue damage in the lungs released damage molecular patterns (DAMPS) that induce local inflammation. These inflammatory responses provide anti-viral immunity after activating type I and III IFN-1 pathways that upregulate certain acute phase cytokines such as IL-6 or IL-1βa nd recruit neutrophils and other innate immune cells that elicit anti-SARS-CoV-2 adaptive memory T and B cells.[29] Uncontrolled inflammation in COVID-19 patients described as the "cytokine storm" causes tissue damage with inflammatory cell infiltration. Acute respiratory distress syndrome is characteristic of the severe manifestations of COVID-19.[30] Patients with severe disease demonstrate high levels of IL-6, IL-2R, IL-10, and TNF-α while having low levels of IFN.[29] Patients requiring ICU admission show high levels of IL-2, IL-7, IL-10, G-CSF, MCP-1, TNF-α.[30,31] Vaccine design should avoid the production of this cytokine storm while inducing IFN regulatory cytokines.

Production of SARS-CoV-2 Specific Neutralizing Antibodies

Activated B cells produce antibodies that play several roles as anti-viral immunity, viral neutralization, antibody-dependent cellular cytotoxicity (ADCC), and antibody-dependent cellular phagocytosis, and antibody-dependent complement activation.[32] While the generation of high levels of neutralizing antibodies would be important for a successful human vaccine; COVID-19 patients can recover without producing high levels of neutralizing antibodies.[33] In this regard, the IgG memory B cells to S protein and RBD observed in COVID-19 patients are essential for a rapid recall response to further contact with the virus. Some COVID-19 patients lose neutralizing antibodies rapidly; however, other patients maintained high levels even 3–4 months post-infection.[32]

Adaptive Immunity

Processing and presentation of SARS-CoV-2 epitopes by antigen presenting cells (APC) and binding to histocompatibility class I molecules activate CD8+ T cells to become cytolytic effectors that destroy infected cells.[29] SARS-CoV-2 epitope binding to histocompatibility class II molecules activates CD4+ T cells. Activation of Th1 CD4+ T cells enhances the CD8+ T cell response, and activation of Th2 CD4+ T cells increases virus-specific antibody production.[34] Effective viral clearance requires the combination of CD8+ and CD4+ T cells enhancement of B cells and CD8+ effector cells. While some activated T cells apoptose and die, some persist and induce long-lasting virus-specific T cell immunity. Severe COVID-19 patients showed T cell energy or exhaustion, especially in lungs; they contained high levels of CD8+ T cells expressing exhaustion markers.[35] While patients recovered from moderated or severe COVID-19 appeared to have robust memory T cells with high levels of markers of activation and cytotoxicity. Therefore, vaccines should induce CD4+ and CD8+ T cells involved in SARS-CoV-2 clearance.

Coronavirus Vaccine Designs

During the last 10–20 years have involved modified or killed whole microorganisms. Vaccine development usually took several years. The fastest vaccine that was constructed, developed, and approved for use was the mumps vaccine, which took five years.[13] Therefore, it is a challenge to develop a vaccine for COVID-19 in less than 24 months. The advances with vaccines for last viral epidemics such as SARS, MERS, Ebola, or Zika have developed new technologies that can be applied to the design of vaccines for SARS-CoV-2. In this regard, besides the classical whole microorganism vaccines, four types of vaccine technology have been used for COVID-19 vaccines: viral vector, subunit protein/ peptide-based vaccines, nucleic acid vaccines with DNA or mRNA.[13,24,36,37]

Author describes all the putative vaccine designs used for coronavirus and available up to date for vaccination after Phase 3 clinical trials (**Table 4.3**).

Inactivated Virus

Inactivated vaccines result from growing virus and killing or deactivating it to block viral replication. Heat or formaldehyde inactivation of whole virus formulated with alum as an adjuvant is a strategy followed by Sinovac-Sinopharm (China) that was immunogenic in experimental animals, mice, rats, and non-human primates.[36,37] These vaccine-induced neutralizing antibodies to the vaccine and non-vaccine SARS-CoV-2 virus and provide partial or complete protection of primates in challenge studies. The vaccine went to phase 3 trial already and was approved by China and under study at the European regulatory agency (EMA). Currently, this vaccine has been used in China, Indonesia, Pakistan, Brazil, and Turkey. The efficacy reported varies from 50 to 74%, and the trials have included the elderly above 60 years of age.[38]

Viral Vector Vaccines

These vaccines are bases inserted in a non-replicative virus different than coronaviruses that have been genetically modified to reduce their virulence and made them non-replicative. They are engineered to carry the gene encoding S protein. Their advantage is that the immunogen expressed in a heterologous viral infection is able to induce innate and adaptive immune responses. However, the downside effect implies the possibility to induce prior immunity to the viral vector, that is, Ad5 or Ad26 pre-existing immunity that conditions its efficacy. The most common ones are monkey adenoviruses as ChAdOx1 (AstraZeneca/Oxford vaccine) or human adenoviruses Ad5 or Ad26 (Janssen, Sputnik V or Cansino). The efficacy of the different viral vector vaccines is 65,7% for Cansino (Ad5), 59-86% for AstraZeneca/Oxford (ChAdOx1), 85% for Janssen (Ad26) or 97.6% for Sputnik V (Ad26-Ad5).[39] Adverse effects reported with these adenovirus vaccines for COVID-19 are mainly two types, either small fever and local pain and or a severe thrombocytopenia auto-immune similar to those observed with heparin described in 1–4 out of 1,000,000 cases.[40]

Subunit Protein/Peptide-Based Vaccines

Subunit vaccines of viral proteins inoculated into the host might have the potential to protect humans from viral infection. Since only a few viral components can be included, their protective efficacy might be limited. Some subunit vaccines in the case of COVID-19 were constructed using the residues 319–545 of SARS-CoV-2 RBD produced through a baculovirus expression system and including an adjuvant in the formulation.[41] The preclinical study in non-human primates indicated that it could protect from SARS-CoV-2 infection with little toxicity (Anhui Zhifei Longcom Biopharmaceutical/Institute of Microbiol, Chinese Academy of Sciences).[42] Recombinant Spike protein formulated with AdvaxTM adjuvant (Vaxine Ltd, Adelaide, Australia).[43] Virus-like particles (VLPs) are another type of subunit protein vaccine that includes the full-length trimeric S protein and Matrix M™ adjuvant (Novavax, USA).[44] Clinical trials finished with Novavax vaccine indicated efficacy of 96,4%.[44] The other two subunit vaccines from the Chinese Microbiology Institute or Vaxine company are still in Phase 3 trials, and efficacy is not known. One of the advances of these vaccines is the easy scale up in production and the conservation as lyophilized vaccines at room temperature, being possible to be transported easily to developing countries.

Nucleic Acid Vaccines (mRNA or DNA)

Nucleic acid vaccines, either mRNA or DNA once inoculated into humans, can be transcribed into viral proteins. mRNA vaccines are a promising vaccine platform since they have high potency, rapid development, and cost-efficient production. However, the physiochemical properties influence their cellular delivery and organ distribution. In this regard, three mRNA vaccines finished the clinical trials, (i) BNT162b1 (Pfizer/Biontech, USA-Germany) targeted to the RBD of S protein

Table 4.3 COVID-19 vaccines

Vaccine	Company/ Organization	Country	No. of doses	Immunization	Results
Inactivated (formaldehyde & alum)	Sinovac Biotech	China	2	Intramuscular	Doses: 12 and 6 µg/ mL, produce antibodies after 14 days
Inactivated (alum)	Wuhan Institute & SinoPharm	China	2	Intramuscular	6% of vaccinated group had adverse reactions
Non-replicative adenovirus (Ad5-nCoV)	Cansino	China	1	Intramuscular	Produce antibodies after 14 días (efficacy: 65,7%)
Non-replicative adenovirus (ChAdOx1-proteina S)	Oxford University & AstraZeneca	UK	1	Intramuscular	Produce antibodies and cytotoxic T cells, adverse effects (local systemic reaction, neurological effect, and thrombocytopenia with thrombosis induction; efficacy: 59–86%)
Non-replicative adenovirus-Sputnik V (rAd26-S/rAd5-S)	Gamaleya Institute	Russia	1	Intramuscular	Produce antibodies and cytotoxic T cells (efficacy: 97,6%)
Non-replicative adenovirus (Ad26COVS1)	Janssen-Johnson & Johnson)	USA-Belgium	1	Intramuscular	Produce antibodies (adverse effects: thrombocytopenia with thrombosis induction; efficacy: 85%)
ARNm-1273 (encapsulated with nanolipids-LNP)	Moderna & NIAID	USA	2	Intramuscular	Produce antibodies and cytotoxic T cells (adverse effects: local pain, efficacy: 93,6%)
ARN-BNT162 (encapsulated with nanolipids-LNP)	Pfizer & BioNtech & Fosum Pharma	USA Germany	2	Intramuscular	Produce antibodies and cytotoxic T cells (efficacy: 93,8%)
ARN-CnVCoV (encapsulate delivery with nanolipids- LNP)	CureVac	Germany	2	Intramuscular	Finishing Phase 3 (data not liberated yet)
Recombinante proteína S-VLPs	Novavax	USA	2	Intramuscular	Produce antibodies and cytotoxic T cells (efficacy: 96,4%)

Adapted from Dong et al. (2020) and Chung et al. (2020).

and encapsulated within nanolipids (LNP) mainly ionizable cationic lipids.[24] This vaccine caused mild to moderate local and systematic symptoms (local pain, some fever, muscular pain, vomits), eliciting the vaccine higher neutralizing titers of antibodies after the second dose and compared to the COVID-19 convalescent sera as well as CD4 and CD8 T cell responses. Phase 3 clinical trials indicated an efficacy of 93.8% and require two doses. (ii) mRNA-1273 (Moderna/NIAID, USA) encodes the prefusion form of the S antigen and encapsulated within nanolipids (LNP) composed of four lipids.[45] The vaccine produces neutralizing antibodies and cytotoxic T cells as T cell responses. This vaccine has an efficacy of 93.8% and also requires two doses. (iii) mRNA CVnCoV (CureVac, Germany) encodes the S antigen and is also encapsulated within nanolipds. This vaccine has entered Phase 3, and results will be soon released regarding immune response and efficacy (Flanagan et al, 2020).[24] DNA vaccines

These are plasmids that produce the S protein as the Inovio Farmaceuticals vaccine (Pennsylvania, USA) with a new vaccination system without needles using electroporation (INO-4800 CELLECTRA), inducing humoral and cellular immune responses or the Osaka University/Anges-Takara (Japan) vaccine including an adjuvant (AG0301-COVID-19). The efficacy of DNA vaccines is unknown as they are in clinical trials. India currently has three approved vaccines, Covaxin (Bharat Biotech) which is a whole inactivated SARs-COV-2 vaccine, two adenovirus delivered viral DNA vaccines Covishield (Serum Institute of India) and Sputnik(Gamaleya institute Russia). Interestingly, Covaxin uses a Toll like receptor(TLR) 7/8 agonist as an adjuvant and the Sputnik Vaccine employs a series of two injection each employing a different adenovirus delivery system rAd26 for the first and rAd 5 for the second injection. None of India's approved vaccines require sub zero refrigeration.

With a vaccination rate worldwide of 7–50% in most cases, it can be assumed that these available vaccines seemed to stop COVID-19 severity but also community transmission of the virus. Some questions are remaining regarding these vaccines: the long-lasting of the immune protection, the possibility to combinate the vaccines, and the ability of these vaccines to block the infection.

COVID-19 Vaccine Prospects

There are some vaccines that are in the different stages of trials (first steps of clinical trials or about to enter):

- Some recombinant proteins using the RBD protein-based S protein trimer-Tag platform, including the AS02 adjuvant from GSK/Dynavax, are in Phase 2 clinical trials.
- Replicating viral vector vaccines using Measles virus vector-based (TMV-083) from the Pasteur Institute/Merck also in the early phases of the clinical trials.[24]
- Non-replicating viral vector using the modified Ankara vaccinia virus (MVA) coding the S protein with very good results in preclinical trials in mice that shows high protection against viral challenge and that in short, it will enter in Phase 1 clinical trial that will be produced by Biofabri/Zendal group in Spain.[46]
- DNA based vaccines using a new technology that produces a synthetic vaccine (Alonso et al., 2018) that codes for the S protein and can integrate; in this way, it mimics the mechanism of the virus to enter the cells and produce the S protein.[47]
- The attenuated SARS-CoV-2 virus is genetically modified to significantly reduce its virulence following a previously reported coronavirus technique.[48] This vaccine will enter soon in Phase 1 and has the advantage of being able to block SARS-CoV-2 infection[48]

It is expected that the virus turns into a seasonal virus and that vaccines will still be needed for several years or annually. In this regard, these ongoing vaccines not yet in clinical trials will be required, and higher production of the current vaccines. The variants of SARS-CoV-2 may affect the efficiency of the vaccines, and some of the vaccines will need to be reformulated.

The Delta Variant Mutation

The SARS-CoV-2 delta variant was first detected in India at the end of 2020. After a few months, it was responsible of a large surge of COVID-19 cases in India. The high transmission rate of this new variant along with low vaccination rates in the general population and limited health resources in a country with a high population density, all accounted for unprecedented mortality figures. During the summer of 2021, the delta variant became predominant almost worldwide causing a new wave in most countries and has become a significant cause of morbidity and mortality particularly among the unvaccinated.[49] Although most current approved vaccines largely remain active against the delta variant, their efficacy may be lower. A recent study demonstrated an improvement in efficacy of the BNT162b2 (Pfizer) and ChAdOx1 nCoV-19 (Astra Zeneca against the Delta variant when two injections are administered.[50,51]

SARS-CoV-2 (COVID-19) Prevention using Anti-Virals

The unprecedented success of antiretroviral therapy in the HIV/AIDS field has revolutionized the use of anti-virals for managing distinct viral illnesses. We are convinced that lessons learned from the HIV paradigm may well apply to COVID-19.[52,53]

Since it first appeared in 1981, AIDS has expanded globally with cumulative estimates of nearly 80 million people infected with HIV up to date, of whom only half remain alive. However, since the advent of antiretroviral therapy (ART) in the mid-nineties, the prognosis of HIV infection has changed dramatically. Indeed, under good adherence to medications, immunological damage no longer occurs, and the life expectancy of treated HIV-seropositive individuals approaches that seen in the general population. As a result, AIDS is rarely seen nowadays, mostly restricted to persons unaware of their infection presenting late to clinics.

During the past 25 years, improvements in ART have resulted in significant reductions in disease morbidities and mortality in HIV persons. Current HIV medications depict unique, appealing profiles, often in one single multi-drug pill given once daily.[54] Furthermore, ART is highly efficacious, well tolerated, and safe, with few and manageable drug interactions and a high barrier to resistance. As a result, ART is nowadays recommended for all HIV-positives, including those asymptomatic and with preserved immune status. Indeed, *'rapid initiation of ART'* is desirable and should be considered right after being diagnosed with HIV.

Following the widespread use of ART was the recognition of its power to halt HIV transmission. Infected persons treated with ART with undetectable viremia do not transmit the virus. This effect is known as *'treatment-as-prevention'* and globally has fostered the use of ART.[55]

Another further step for expanding the use of ART came from the recognition that HIV-seronegative persons at risk for viral acquisition could prevent infection by taking antiretrovirals. HIV *'pre-exposure prophylaxis'* (PrEP) is currently recommended for uninfected individuals engaged in risky behaviors, such as men having sex with men with multiple partners, sex workers, or injection drug users who share needles. PrEP is prescribed as single pills taken daily, two to three times per week, or at demand. These pills combine tenofovir and emtricitabine. They prevent HIV acquisition in more than 95% of users with good drug adherence.[56–58]

Efforts to make more effortless daily oral ART have resulted in the recent development of **long-acting (LA) antiretrovirals**, such as cabotegravir and rilpivirine, administered monthly intramuscularly.[59,60] In the clinic, these formulations are considered for both maintenance therapy in patients already suppressed under conventional daily ART and PrEP in HIV-negative persons at risk. However, these medications may produce local injection site reactions, may be associated with drug interactions, and require monthly visits to clinics.[61]

A Path Forward: XLA-Antivirals

There has been growing interest in the development of XLA-antiviral formulations and devices to manage chronic viral infections. Following intramuscular or subcutaneous administration, the placement site for therapies serves as a primary depot. The drug is slowly absorbed into the blood and redistributed into peripheral tissues serving as secondary drug storage sites. Therefore, unlike orally administered medicines for which clearance rates determine the drug half-life, the extended duration of activity for XLA-antivirals depends on the amount of drug absorbed/day from such depots to enable lower loading doses to last for months collectively. In one example, when a single dose intramuscular injection of a cabotegravir prodrug formulation is administered, drug concentrations above the protein-adjusted 90% inhibitory concentration can be sustained for 1 year in preclinical animal studies.[62] The agent exhibits unique properties for prolonged drug release, reflecting a selective depot formation at the injection site and within the reticuloendothelial system. Macrophages are the primary cell depot for drug uptake and wide biodistribution across lymphoid, mucosal, gut, and brain tissues.[63] Given the nanocrystal formulation, volumes of less than 1 mL would be needed for yearly administration in humans, reducing the likelihood of local injection site reactions.

There are several advantages of having XLA-antivirals. At first sight, they will solve the challenges of injection site reactions and needs to attend monthly clinic visits. Special populations that would primarily benefit from once a year injectables are persons in jail, children and adolescents, homeless, mentally ill, and refugees for whom regular attendance of visits at health care sites might be difficult. For similar reasons, infected people in some of the poorest regions would benefit the most yearly instead of monthly medications. Additional advantages would be lower risk for selecting drug resistance and increased efficacy.[64]

A second look at XLA-antivirals might be even more appealing. In the absence of a vaccine, these medications might act as chemical prophylaxis for uninfected people at risk. To some extent, XLA-antivirals might work as vaccine mimetics (**Fig. 4.2**) (Soriano et al., 2020).[64]

Prospects for XLA-Antivirals for Preventing Viral Infections other than HIV

Most viruses causing human diseases in the community are either respiratory or sexually transmitted. The most frequent pathogenic respiratory viruses include influenza, parainfluenza, respiratory syncytial virus, rhinoviruses, adenoviruses, and coronaviruses.

At least two clinical scenarios may be considered for prioritizing the use of XLA-antivirals. First, individuals engaged in high-risk behaviors for acquiring sexually or parenterally transmitted viruses, such as men having sex with men, sex workers, and injection drug users. Second, persons at high risk for developing severe respiratory viral infections, including the elderly and patients with chronic lung disease.

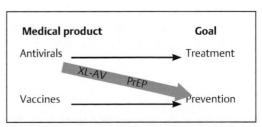

Fig. 4.2 The changing paradigm of anti-viral use: switching from treatment to prevention.

The new paradigm of XLA-antivirals originally being developed against HIV might well apply to other viral conditions, for which antivirals exist but no vaccines. Moreover, even when vaccines have been developed, XLA-antivirals may provide a significant benefit in at least three circumstances. First, when sustained and universal coverage is insufficient, as it occurs with hepatitis B, polio, and papillomavirus. Second, when immunity wanes over time, as described with influenza, mumps, or SARS-CoV-2. Third, when new viral escape mutant variants emerge, as reported for influenza and coronaviruses.[65]

XLA-antivirals are appealing viable approaches for mitigating the acquisition of SARS-CoV-2 infection, where prevention of contagions is challenged by the fact that the virus is transmissible from carriers during the incubation period before symptoms develop.[4] Scenarios where long-acting forms of remdesivir or molnupiravir could be prescribed once a year to prevent the acquisition of SARS-CoV-2 in persons at risk for disease severity and mortality could ease the burden of infection spread.[4,66,67] Furthermore, providing such medication with nebulizers to potential contacts of newly diagnosed individuals could help control COVID-19 outbreaks.

A further benefit of having extended-release formulations used once or just a few times is that anti-viral stocks can be ensured for larger population groups. This may be important when new viral pandemics emerge, and initial efforts with drug repurposing are looking for anti-virals that may depict some activity against the new agent. However, in contrast with antibiotics, the current anti-viral armamentarium is still relatively limited. The chances of future viral spillovers causing outbreaks and pandemics must be expected from the vast animal reservoirs.

Conclusion

We envision the use of **XLA-antivirals** for the prevention of SARS-CoV-2 infection. Implementing such "chemical vaccines" would fill an immediate need to provide sustained protection against viral infections when classical ('immune-protective') vaccines do not exist. This can be achieved by the blockade of essential steps in the viral replication cycle. The delivery of such extended-release formulations should be explored through injectables and nebulizers. They will complement the protection given by classical vaccines when viral escape mutants emerge or immunity wanes.

References

1. Morawska L, Tang JW, Bahnfleth W, et al. How can airborne transmission of COVID-19 indoors be minimised? Environ Int 2020;142:105832–105832

2. Chin AWH, Chu JTS, Perera MRA, et al. Stability of SARS-CoV-2 in different environmental conditions. Lancet Microbe 2020;1(1):e10

3. Guallar MP, Meiriño R, Donat-Vargas C, Corral O, Jouvé N, Soriano V. Inoculum at the time of SARS-CoV-2 exposure and risk of disease severity. Int J Infect Dis 2020;97:290–292

4. Gandhi M, Yokoe DS, Havlir DV. Asymptomatic transmission, the Achilles' heel of current strategies to control COVID-19. In: Cockerham WC, Cockerham GB, eds. The COVID-19 Reader: The Science and What It Says about the Social. Routledge; 2020:36–39

5. Hajj Hussein I, Chams N, Chams S, et al. Vaccines through centuries: major cornerstones of global health. Front Public Health 2015;3:269

6. Gerberding JL, Haynes BF. Vaccine innovations—past and future. N Engl J Med 2021; 384(5):393–396

7. Blok BA, Arts RJW, van Crevel R, Benn CS, Netea MG. Trained innate immunity as underlying mechanism for the long-term, nonspecific effects of vaccines. J Leukoc Biol 2015;98(3):347–356

8. Malone RW, Felgner PL, Verma IM. Cationic liposome-mediated RNA transfection. Proc Natl Acad Sci U S A 1989;86(16):6077–6081

9. Malone R, Kumar R, Felgner P. High levels of messenger RNA expression following cationic liposome mediated transfection tissue culture cells. Washington, DC: NIH Conference; June 1989

10. Coffman RL, Sher A, Seder RA. Vaccine adjuvants: putting innate immunity to work. Immunity 2010;33(4):492–503

11. Awate S, Babiuk LA, Mutwiri G. Mechanisms of action of adjuvants. Front Immunol 2013; 4:114

12. Di Pasquale A, Preiss S, Tavares Da Silva F, Garçon N. Vaccine adjuvants: from 1920 to 2015 and beyond. Vaccines (Basel) 2015; 3(2):320–343

13. Sharma O, Sultan AA, Ding H, Triggle CR. A review of the progress and challenges of developing a vaccine for COVID-19. Front Immunol 2020;11:585354

14. Khalil RH, Al-Humadi N. Types of acute phase reactants and their importance in vaccination. Biomed Rep 2020;12(4):143–152

15. Guimarães LE, Baker B, Perricone C, Shoenfeld Y. Vaccines, adjuvants and autoimmunity. Pharmacol Res 2015;100:190–209

16. Stone CA Jr, Rukasin CRF, Beachkofsky TM, Phillips EJ. Immune-mediated adverse reactions to vaccines. Br J Clin Pharmacol 2019;85(12):2694–2706

17. Dotan A, Muller S, Kanduc D, David P, Halpert G, Shoenfeld Y. The SARS-CoV-2 as an instrumental trigger of autoimmunity. Autoimmun Rev 2021;20(4):102792

18. Green MD, Al-Humadi NH. Preclinical toxicology of vaccines. In: Faqi AS, ed. A Comprehensive Guide to Toxicology in Preclinical Drug Development. Elsevier; 2012:619–645

19. Sanchez-Trincado JL, Gomez-Perosanz M, Reche PA. Fundamentals and methods for T- and B-cell epitope prediction. J Immunol Res 2017;2017:2680160

20. Hodgson SH, Mansatta K, Mallett G, Harris V, Emary KRW, Pollard AJ. What defines an efficacious COVID-19 vaccine? A review of the challenges assessing the clinical efficacy of vaccines against SARS-CoV-2. Lancet Infect Dis 2021;21(2):e26–e35

21. Li F. Structure, function, and evolution of coronavirus spike proteins. Annu Rev Virol 2016;3(1):237–261

22. Padron-Regalado E. Vaccines for SARS-CoV-2: lessons from other coronavirus strains. Infect Dis Ther 2020;9(2):1–20

23. Chiuppesi F, Salazar MD, Contreras H, et al. Development of a multi-antigenic SARS-CoV-2 vaccine candidate using a synthetic poxvirus platform. Nat Commun 2020;11(1):6121

24. Flanagan KL, Best E, Crawford NW, et al. Progress and pitfalls in the quest for effective SARS-CoV-2 (COVID-19) vaccines. Front Immunol 2020;11:579250

25. Huang Y, Yang C, Xu XF, Xu W, Liu SW. Structural and functional properties of SARS-CoV-2 spike protein: potential antivirus drug development for COVID-19. Acta Pharmacol Sin 2020;41(9):1141–1149

26. Wrapp D, Wang N, Corbett KS, et al. Cryo-EM structure of the 2019-nCoV spike in the prefusion conformation. Science 2020;367(6483):1260–1263

27. Yi C, Sun X, Ye J, et al. Key residues of the receptor binding motif in the spike protein of SARS-CoV-2 that interact with ACE2 and neutralizing antibodies. Cell Mol Immunol 2020;17(6):621–630

28. Schultze JL, Aschenbrenner AC. COVID-19 and the human innate immune system. Cell 2021;184(7):1671–1692

29. Shah VK, Firmal P, Alam A, Ganguly D, Chattopadhyay S. Overview of immune response during SARS-CoV-2 infection: lessons from the past. Front Immunol 2020; 11:1949

30. Costela-Ruiz VJ, Illescas-Montes R, Puerta-Puerta JM, Ruiz C, Melguizo-Rodríguez L. SARS-CoV-2 infection: the role of cytokines in COVID-19 disease. Cytokine Growth Factor Rev 2020;54:62–75

31. Tay MZ, Poh CM, Rénia L, MacAry PA, Ng LFP. The trinity of COVID-19: immunity, inflammation and intervention. Nat Rev Immunol 2020;20(6):363–374

32. Galipeau Y, Greig M, Liu G, Driedger M, Langlois M-A. Humoral responses and serological assays in SARS-CoV-2 infections. Front Immunol 2020;11:610688

33. Bal A, Pozzetto B, Trabaud M-A, et al; COVID SER Study Group. Evaluation of high-throughput SARS-CoV-2 serological assays in a longitudinal cohort of patients with mild COVID-19: clinical sensitivity, specificity, and association with virus neutralization test. Clin Chem 2021;67(5):742–752

34. Sette A, Crotty S. Adaptive immunity to SARS-CoV-2 and COVID-19. Cell 2021;184(4): 861–880

35. Diao B, Wang C, Tan Y, et al. Reduction and functional exhaustion of T cells in patients

with coronavirus disease 2019 (COVID-19). Front Immunol 2020;11:827–827

36. Dong Y, Dai T, Wei Y, Zhang L, Zheng M, Zhou F. A systematic review of SARS-CoV-2 vaccine candidates. Signal Transduct Target Ther 2020;5(1):237

37. Chung YH, Beiss V, Fiering SN, Steinmetz NF. COVID-19 vaccine frontrunners and their nanotechnology design. ACS Nano 2020; 14(10):12522–12537

38. Wu Z, Hu Y, Xu M, et al. Safety, tolerability, and immunogenicity of an inactivated SARS-CoV-2 vaccine (CoronaVac) in healthy adults aged 60 years and older: a randomised, double-blind, placebo-controlled, phase 1/2 clinical trial. Lancet Infect Dis 2021;21(6): 803–812

39. Logunov DY, Dolzhikova IV, Shcheblyakov DV, et al; Gam-COVID-Vac Vaccine Trial Group. Safety and efficacy of an rAd26 and rAd5 vector-based heterologous prime-boost COVID-19 vaccine: an interim analysis of a randomised controlled phase 3 trial in Russia. Lancet 2021;397(10275):671–681

40. American Society of Hematology. Thrombosis with thrombocytopenia syndrome (also termed vaccine-induced thrombotic thrombocytopenia). Available at: https://www.hematology.org/covid-19/vaccine-induced-immune-thrombotic-thrombocytopenia

41. Yang J, Wang W, Chen Z, et al. A vaccine targeting the RBD of the S protein of SARS-CoV-2 induces protective immunity. Nature 2020;586(7830):572–577

42. An Y, Li S, Jin X, et al. A tandem-repeat dimeric RBD protein-based COVID-19 vaccine ZF2001 protects mice and nonhuman primates. bioRxiv 2021 (e-pub ahead of print). doi:10.1101/2021.03.11.434928

43. McPherson C, Chubet R, Holtz K, et al. Development of a SARS coronavirus vaccine from recombinant spike protein plus delta inulin adjuvant. Methods Mol Biol 2016; 1403:269–284

44. Shinde V, Bhikha S, Hoosain Z, et al; 2019nCoV-501 Study Group. Efficacy of NVX-CoV2373 Covid-19 vaccine against the B.1.351 variant. N Engl J Med 2021;384(20):1899–1909

45. European Medicines Agency. Assessment report COVID-19 vaccine Moderna. Available at: https://www.ema.europa.eu/en/documents/assessment-report/ covid-19-vaccine-moderna-epar-public-assessment-report_en.pdf

46. García-Arriaza J, Garaigorta U, Pérez P, et al. COVID-19 vaccine candidates based on modified vaccinia virus Ankara expressing the SARS-CoV-2 spike induce robust T- and B-cell immune responses and full efficacy in mice. J Virol 2021;95(7):e02260–20

47. Alonso A, Larraga V, Alcolea PJ. The contribution of DNA microarray technology to gene expression profiling in Leishmania spp.: a retrospective view. Acta Trop 2018;187: 129–139

48. Enjuanes L, Zuñiga S, Castaño-Rodriguez C, Gutierrez-Alvarez J, Canton J, Sola I. Molecular basis of coronavirus virulence and vaccine development. Adv Virus Res 2016; 96:245–286

49. Thangaraj JWV, Yadav P, Kumar CG, et al. Predominance of delta variant among the COVID-19 vaccinated and unvaccinated individuals, India, May 2021. J Infect. Published online August 6, 2021. doi:10.1016/j.jinf. 2021.08.006

50. Barros-Martins J, Hammerschmidt SI, Cossmann A, et al. Immune responses against SARS-CoV-2 variants after heterologous and homologous ChAdOx1 nCoV-19/BNT162b2 vaccination. Nat Med 2021;27(9):1525–1529

51. Lopez Bernal J, Andrews N, Gower C, et al. Effectiveness of Covid-19 vaccines against the B.1.617.2 (delta) variant. N Engl J Med 2021;385(7):585–594

52. Elias C, Nkengasong JN, Qadri F. Emerging infectious diseases - learning from the past and looking to the future. N Engl J Med 2021; 384(13):1181–1184

53. De Cock KM, Jaffe HW, Curran JW. Reflections on 40 years of AIDS. Emerg Infect Dis 2021; 27(6):1553–1560

54. Saag MS, Gandhi RT, Hoy JF, et al. Antiretroviral drugs for treatment and prevention of HIV infection in adults: 2020 recommendations of the International Antiviral Society-USA Panel. JAMA 2020;324(16):1651–1669

55. Rodger AJ, Cambiano V, Bruun T, et al; PARTNER Study Group. Sexual activity without condoms and risk of HIV transmission in serodifferent couples when the HIV-positive partner is using suppressive antiretroviral therapy. JAMA 2016;316(2):171–181

56. Grant RM, Lama JR, Anderson PL, et al; iPrEx Study Team. Preexposure chemoprophylaxis

for HIV prevention in men who have sex with men. N Engl J Med 2010;363(27):2587–2599

57. Baeten JM, Donnell D, Ndase P, et al; Partners PrEP Study Team. Antiretroviral prophylaxis for HIV prevention in heterosexual men and women. N Engl J Med 2012;367(5):399–410

58. Mayer KH, Molina J-M, Thompson MA, et al. Emtricitabine and tenofovir alafenamide vs emtricitabine and tenofovir disoproxil fumarate for HIV pre-exposure prophylaxis (DISCOVER): primary results from a randomised, double-blind, multicentre, active-controlled, phase 3, non-inferiority trial. Lancet 2020;396(10246):239–254

59. Swindells S, Andrade-Villanueva J-F, Richmond GJ, et al. Long-acting cabotegravir and rilpivirine for maintenance of HIV-1 suppression. N Engl J Med 2020;382(12):1112–1123

60. Orkin C, Arasteh K, Górgolas Hernández-Mora M, et al. Long-acting cabotegravir and rilpivirine after oral induction for HIV-1 infection. N Engl J Med 2020;382(12):1124–1135

61. Benítez-Gutiérrez L, Soriano V, Requena S, Arias A, Barreiro P, de Mendoza C. Treatment and prevention of HIV infection with long-acting antiretrovirals. Expert Rev Clin Pharmacol 2018;11(5):507–517

62. Kulkarni TA, Bade AN, Sillman B, et al. A year-long extended release nanoformulated cabotegravir prodrug. Nat Mater 2020;19(8):910–920

63. Gautam N, McMillan JM, Kumar D, et al. Lipophilic nanocrystal prodrug-release defines the extended pharmacokinetic profiles of a year-long cabotegravir. Nature Communications. 2021;12(1):3453. doi:10.1038/s41467-021-23668-x

64. Soriano V, Barreiro P, de Mendoza C. Long-acting antiretroviral therapy. Nat Mater 2020;19(8):826–827

65. Hacisuleyman E, Hale C, Saito Y, et al. Vaccine breakthrough infections with SARS-CoV-2 variants. N Engl J Med 2021;384(23):2212–2218

66. Beigel JH, Tomashek KM, Dodd LE, et al; ACTT-1 Study Group Members. Remdesivir for the treatment of Covid-19—final report. N Engl J Med 2020;383(19):1813–1826

67. Rosenke K, Hansen F, Schwarz B, et al. Orally delivered MK-4482 inhibits SARS-CoV-2 replication in the Syrian hamster model. Nat Commun 2021;12(1):2295

05 — Cardinal Manifestations of COVID-19

Jose Iglesias and Paul Marik

The Patient: Initial Considerations and Brief Review of Clinical Findings

Although reports vary, the incubation period of COVID-19 averages about 5 days, and nearly all infected patients will exhibit symptoms by day 12.[1] In contrast to previous coronaviruses causing severe diseases such as SARS-CoV-1 (severe acute respiratory syndrome coronavirus 1) and MERS (Middle East respiratory syndrome), the asymptomatic and presymptomatic phases of COVID-19 are associated with the highest viral load.[2,3] Patients are more likely to be contagious in the asymptomatic and presymptomatic phases of COVID-19.[2,3] We propose that COVID-19 progresses from an asymptomatic phase to a symptomatic phase and then to an early pulmonary phase and, finally, to a late pulmonary phase in which symptomatology, laboratory parameters, and severity of the disease can be better understood employing this paradigm (**Fig. 5.1**). The following section is a brief overview of the clinical presentations of patients with COVID-19. Many of the clinical presentations that involve the cardiac, dermatologic, pulmonary, and gastrointestinal systems will be covered in detail in the ensuing chapters.

Presenting Symptoms

Although proportions of symptoms may differ depending on the geographic location, e.g., gastrointestinal symptoms seem to be more prominent in Western countries, the most common symptoms include fever, fatigue, dry cough, myalgias, chill, anosmia, and ageusia (**Table 5.1**).[4,5-9] In a small percentage of patients, anosmia and ageusia may be the only presenting symptoms.[10-12] Dyspnea develops in some patients within 5 to 8 days after the onset of symptoms.[4,6] Fever may be absent in 20% of patients; however, if patients require hospitalization, fever occurs in up to 89%.[4,6] In the majority of patients (80%), these symptoms are self-limiting and resolve by 7 to 10 days. Approximately 20% of patients progress to a pulmonary phase characterized by progressive dyspnea and progressive respiratory distress severe enough to require hospitalization; 5% of these patients develop advanced pulmonary phase associated with progressive hypoxemia, thereby increasing supplemental oxygen requirements, severe lung injury/pneumonia/respiratory failure, cytokine storm, and shock requiring intensive care admission.[4,13-15]

Physical Examination

Physical findings on examination vary with the severity of disease and systemic involvement. Patients in the early symptomatic disease may present with a relatively benign physical exam such as mild temperature elevation, sore throat, upper respiratory tract symptoms, and normal vital signs.[6,16,17] It is important to note that although major findings are consistent with an upper and lower respiratory tract illness, distal organ system involvement, including cardiac, neurologic, gastrointestinal, and integumentary, is not uncommon.[6,13,17,18] As the disease progresses in severity, patients may present with high-grade fever, tachypnea, tachycardia,

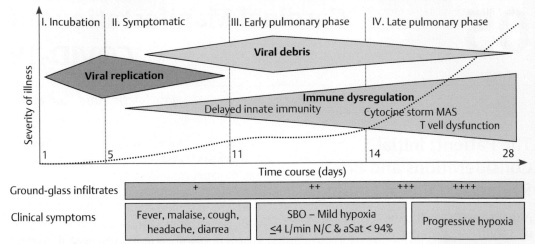

Fig. 5.1 The time frame of the clinical course of SARS-CoV-2 infection emphasizing the phases of COVID-19 disease.

Table 5.1   Common presenting signs and symptoms of patients with COVID-19*

Major presenting symptoms	Proportion
Fever	77%
Cough	68%
Anosmia	41%
Dyspnea	37%
Ageusia	34%
Fatigue/Myalgia	30%
Sputum production	18%
GI symptoms	18%
Odynophia/sore throat	16%
Headache	15%

Other symptoms: Chills, rhinorrhea, hemoptysis, rash
*Represented as proportion of patients will not add up to 100% as many patients have more than one symptom

hemodynamic instability (hypertension or hypotension), clinical evidence of volume depletion, and evidence of respiratory distress such as wheezing, rales, or decreased breath sounds.[18–20] Patients with myocarditis may present with clinical evidence of congestive heart failure.[21] The abdominal examination is usually benign despite abdominal pain, a common complaint in patients presenting with COVID-19.[9] Once hypercapnia and hypoxemia have been excluded, a change in mental status or lethargy may be indicative of COVID-19-associated encephalitis.[22] Patients with COVID-19-associated hypercoagulable state can present with deep vein thrombosis, arterial thrombosis, and stroke.[22-25] There are a multitude of skin lesions that may be present such as chilblain lesions on extremities, acral cyanosis, and maculopapular and vesicular rash.[26-28]

Laboratory Findings

Several laboratory parameters are correlated with severity and clinical outcome. In contrast to their less severely ill counterparts, typical laboratory parameters of patients hospitalized with COVID-19 demonstrate marked dysfunction in innate immunity and adaptive immunity.[29-31] Understanding this imbalance has therapeutic implications, which will be covered in the ensuing chapters. Elevations in interleukin 6, serum ferritin, and C-reactive protein indicate an unabated innate immune response and hyperinflammation.[29,31,32] The presence of lymphopenia or an elevated neutrophil-to-lymphocyte ratio is indicative of a dysfunctional adaptive immunity mediated by cytokine-induced apoptosis of lymphocytes and possible direct cytopathic effects of viral infection.[30,32-36] Endothelial damage and dysfunction, elevations in fibrinogen and D-dimer, and abnormalities in coagulation parameters are common.[37,38] Approximately 57% of patients with COVID-19 have elevated activated partial thromboplastin time and accompanying thrombocytopenia.[39,40] Despite anticoagulation, up to 20% of patients develop thrombotic and thromboembolic events.[41,42] Recently, there have been COVID-19 case series reporting the presence of antiphospholipid antibodies.[39,42,43] Progressive hypoxemia elevations in alanine aminotransferase, lactate dehydrogenase, and troponin I are early markers of progressive organ dysfunction possibly mediated by unabated inflammation and microvascular thrombosis.[25,39,44]

Radiographic Findings

Weinstock et al evaluated chest X-rays (CXR) of 636 ambulatory patients in an outpatient setting and described normal CXR in 58% of patients.[45] Abnormal CXR was found in 42% of patients, with the common finding being ground-glass opacities and interstitial markings mainly with a lower lobe predominance. Of those patients with abnormal findings, 73% were described as mild, 24% as moderate, and 3% as severe. Approximately 89% of the patients in their series had normal or only mild changes on CXR images.[45] Studies suggest that imaging abnormalities peak at around day 12, consistent with the pulmonary phase of the disease.[46-48] Computed tomography (CT) scans demonstrate that the severity of CT findings follows a time frame of progression from normal or ground-glass subpleural unilateral or bilateral lower lobe opacities to a progressive organization and consolidation with total lung involvement that generally peaks at day 12 to 14 from the onset of symptoms (**Fig. 5.2a–c** and **Fig. 5.3**).[48,49]

Conclusion

COVID-19 disease in symptomatic patients may range from mild symptoms involving the aerodigestive tract to markedly severe multisystem involvement and respiratory failure. In its most severe form, it is a highly inflammatory and coagulopathic disease. Understanding the manifold clinical manifestations of COVID-19 will assist the clinician in addressing potential complications that arise during the clinical course of the disease.

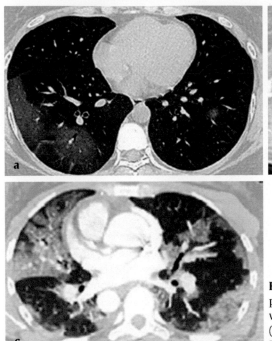
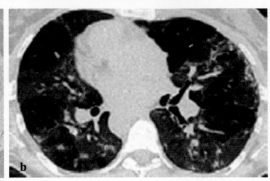

Fig. 5.2 **(a–c)** Serial CT scans of a patient with progressive severe COVID-19 pulmonary disease, who presented several days after symptom onset. (The images are provided courtesy of Paul Marik, MD, Eastern Virginia School of Medicine.)

Days from onset of symptoms	0–4	5–8	9->14
CT scan findings			
Normal	56%	9%	4%
Consolidation	9%	55%	60%
Bilateral disease	28%	76%	88%
Peripheral	64%	64%	72%
Linear	0%	9%	20%
will not add up to 100% as many patients have more than one symptom			

Fig. 5.3 CT scan findings demonstrate that the severity of CT findings follows a time frame of progression from normal or ground-glass subpleural unilateral or bilateral lower lobe opacities to a progressive organization and consolidation with total lung involvement that generally peaks at day 12 to 14 from the onset of symptoms.[48,49]

References

1. Lauer SA, Grantz KH, Bi Q, et al. The incubation period of coronavirus disease 2019 (COVID-19) from publicly reported confirmed cases: estimation and application. Ann Intern Med 2020;172(9):577–582

2. To KK-W, Tsang OT-Y, Leung W-S, et al. Temporal profiles of viral load in posterior oropharyngeal saliva samples and serum antibody responses during infection by SARS-CoV-2: an observational cohort study. Lancet Infect Dis 2020;20(5):565–574

3. He X, Lau EHY, Wu P, et al. Temporal dynamics in viral shedding and transmissibility of COVID-19. Nat Med 2020;26(5):672–675

4. Guan W-J, Ni Z-Y, Hu Y, et al; China Medical Treatment Expert Group for Covid-19. Clinical characteristics of coronavirus disease 2019 in China. N Engl J Med 2020; 382(18):1708–1720

5. Sun P, Qie S, Liu Z, Ren J, Li K, Xi J. Clinical characteristics of hospitalized patients with

SARS-CoV-2 infection: a single arm meta-analysis. J Med Virol 2020;92(6):612–617

6. Xie Y, Wang Z, Liao H, Marley G, Wu D, Tang W. Epidemiologic, clinical, and laboratory findings of the COVID-19 in the current pandemic: systematic review and meta-analysis. BMC Infect Dis 2020;20(1):640

7. Sun Y, Dong Y, Wang L, et al. Characteristics and prognostic factors of disease severity in patients with COVID-19: the Beijing experience. J Autoimmun 2020;112: 102473–102473

8. Huang C, Wang Y, Li X, et al. Clinical features of patients infected with 2019 novel coronavirus in Wuhan, China. Lancet 2020; 395(10223):497–506

9. Patel KP, Patel PA, Vunnam RR, et al. Gastrointestinal, hepatobiliary, and pancreatic manifestations of COVID-19. J Clin Virol 2020;128:104386–104386

10. Meng X, Deng Y, Dai Z, Meng Z. COVID-19 and anosmia: a review based on up-to-date knowledge. Am J Otolaryngol 2020;41(5): 102581

11. Gane SB, Kelly C, Hopkins C. Isolated sudden onset anosmia in COVID-19 infection. A novel syndrome? Rhinology 2020;58(3): 299–301

12. Hjelmesæth J, Skaare D. Loss of smell or taste as the only symptom of COVID-19. Tidsskr Nor Laegeforen 2020;140(7). doi:10.4045/ tidsskr.20.0287

13. Wu Z, McGoogan JM. Characteristics of and important lessons from the coronavirus disease 2019 (COVID-19) outbreak in China: summary of a report of 72 314 cases from the Chinese Center for Disease Control and Prevention. JAMA 2020;323(13):1239–1242

14. Cummings MJ, Baldwin MR, Abrams D, et al. Epidemiology, clinical course, and outcomes of critically ill adults with COVID-19 in New York City: a prospective cohort study. Lancet 2020;395(10239):1763–1770

15. CDC COVID-19 Response Team. Severe outcomes among patients with coronavirus disease 2019 (COVID-19)—United States, February 12-March 16, 2020. MMWR Morb Mortal Wkly Rep 2020;69(12):343–346

16. Struyf T, Deeks JJ, Dinnes J, et al; Cochrane COVID-19 Diagnostic Test Accuracy Group. Signs and symptoms to determine if a patient presenting in primary care or hospital outpatient settings has COVID-19

disease. Cochrane Database Syst Rev 2020; 7(7):CD013665–CD013665

17. Grant MC, Geoghegan L, Arbyn M, et al. The prevalence of symptoms in 24,410 adults infected by the novel coronavirus (SARS-CoV-2; COVID-19): a systematic review and meta-analysis of 148 studies from 9 countries. PLoS One 2020;15(6):e0234765

18. Zhu J, Ji P, Pang J, et al. Clinical characteristics of 3062 COVID-19 patients: a meta-analysis. J Med Virol 2020;92(10):1902–1914

19. Wang X, Fang J, Zhu Y, et al. Clinical characteristics of non-critically ill patients with novel coronavirus infection (COVID-19) in a Fangcang Hospital. Clin Microbiol Infect 2020;26(8):1063–1068

20. Baj J, Karakuła-Juchnowicz H, Teresiński G, et al. COVID-19: specific and non-specific clinical manifestations and symptoms: the current state of knowledge. J Clin Med 2020; 9(6):1753

21. Pirzada A, Mokhtar AT, Moeller AD. COVID-19 and myocarditis: what do we know so far? CJC Open 2020;2(4):278–285

22. Varatharaj A, Thomas N, Ellul MA, et al; CoroNerve Study Group. Neurological and neuropsychiatric complications of COVID-19 in 153 patients: a UK-wide surveillance study. Lancet Psychiatry 2020;7(10):875–882

23. Avula A, Nalleballe K, Toom S, et al. Incidence of thrombotic events and outcomes in COVID-19 patients admitted to intensive care units. Cureus 2020;12(10):e11079

24. Lodigiani C, Iapichino G, Carenzo L, et al; Humanitas COVID-19 Task Force. Venous and arterial thromboembolic complications in COVID-19 patients admitted to an academic hospital in Milan, Italy. Thromb Res 2020;191:9–14

25. Lu Y-F, Pan L-Y, Zhang W-W, et al. A meta-analysis of the incidence of venous thromboembolic events and impact of anticoagulation on mortality in patients with COVID-19. Int J Infect Dis 2020;100:34–41

26. Freeman EE, McMahon DE, Lipoff JB, et al. The spectrum of COVID-19-associated dermatologic manifestations: an international registry of 716 patients from 31 countries. J Am Acad Dermatol 2020;83(4):1118–1129

27. Gottlieb M, Long B. Dermatologic manifestations and complications of COVID-19. Am J Emerg Med 2020;38(9):1715–1721

28. Bandhala Rajan M, Kumar-M P, Bhardwaj A. The trend of cutaneous lesions during COVID-19 pandemic: lessons from a meta-analysis and systematic review. Int J Dermatol 2020; 59(11):1358–1370

29. Acharya D, Liu G, Gack MU. Dysregulation of type I interferon responses in COVID-19. Nat Rev Immunol 2020;20(7):397–398

30. Qin C, Zhou L, Hu Z, et al. Dysregulation of immune response in patients with coronavirus 2019 (COVID-19) in Wuhan, China. Clin Infect Dis 2020;71(15):762–768

31. Moutchia J, Pokharel P, Kerri A, et al. Clinical laboratory parameters associated with severe or critical novel coronavirus disease 2019 (COVID-19): a systematic review and meta-analysis. PLoS One 2020; 15(10):e0239802

32. Blanco-Melo D, Nilsson-Payant BE, Liu W-C, et al. Imbalanced host response to SARS-CoV-2 drives development of COVID-19. Cell 2020;181(5):1036–1045.e9

33. Liu J, Li S, Liu J, et al. Longitudinal characteristics of lymphocyte responses and cytokine profiles in the peripheral blood of SARS-CoV-2 infected patients. EBioMedicine 2020;55:102763

34. Azkur AK, Akdis M, Azkur D, et al. Immune response to SARS-CoV-2 and mechanisms of immunopathological changes in COVID-19. Allergy 2020;75(7):1564–1581

35. Cizmecioglu A, Akay Cizmecioglu H, Goktepe MH, et al. Apoptosis-induced T-cell lymphopenia is related to COVID-19 severity. J Med Virol 2021;93(5):2867–2874

36. Zheng M, Gao Y, Wang G, et al. Functional exhaustion of antiviral lymphocytes in COVID-19 patients. Cell Mol Immunol 2020; 17(5):533–535

37. Iba T, Connors JM, Levy JH. The coagulopathy, endotheliopathy, and vasculitis of COVID-19. Inflamm Res 2020;69(12):1181–1189

38. Levi M, Thachil J, Iba T, Levy JH. Coagulation abnormalities and thrombosis in patients with COVID-19. Lancet Haematol 2020; 7(6):e438–e440

39. Borghi MO, Beltagy A, Garrafa E, et al. Antiphospholipid antibodies in COVID-19 are different from those detectable in the antiphospholipid syndrome. Front Immunol 2020;11:584241

40. Tang N, Bai H, Chen X, Gong J, Li D, Sun Z. Anticoagulant treatment is associated with decreased mortality in severe coronavirus disease 2019 patients with coagulopathy. J Thromb Haemost 2020;18(5):1094–1099

41. Middeldorp S, Coppens M, van Haaps TF, et al. Incidence of venous thromboembolism in hospitalized patients with COVID-19. J Thromb Haemost 2020;18(8):1995–2002

42. El Hasbani G, Taher AT, Jawad A, Uthman I. COVID-19, antiphospholipid antibodies, and catastrophic antiphospholipid syndrome: a possible association? Clin Med Insights Arthritis Musculoskelet Disord 2020;13: 1179544120978667

43. Harzallah I, Debliquis A, Drénou B. Lupus anticoagulant is frequent in patients with Covid-19. J Thromb Haemost 2020;18(8): 2064–2065

44. Hu J, Wang Y. The clinical characteristics and risk factors of severe COVID-19. Gerontology 2021;67(3):255–266

45. Weinstock WB, Echenique A, Russell JW, et al. Chest X-ray findings in 636 ambulatory patients with COVID-19 presenting to an urgent care center: a normal chest X-ray is no guarantee. J Urgent Care Med 2020; 14(7):13–18

46. Rousan LA, Elobeid E, Karrar M, Khader Y. Chest x-ray findings and temporal lung changes in patients with COVID-19 pneumonia. BMC Pulm Med 2020;20(1):245

47. Cheng Z, Lu Y, Cao Q, et al. Clinical features and chest CT manifestations of coronavirus disease 2019 (COVID-19) in a single-center study in Shanghai, China. AJR Am J Roentgenol 2020;215(1):121–126

48. Bernheim A, Mei X, Huang M, et al. Chest CT findings in coronavirus disease-19 (COVID-19): relationship to duration of infection. Radiology 2020;295(3):200463

49. Ding X, Xu J, Zhou J, Long Q. Chest CT findings of COVID-19 pneumonia by duration of symptoms. Eur J Radiol 2020;127:109009

06 Cardiovascular Manifestations of COVID-19

Rajesh Mohan

Introduction

Severe acute respiratory syndrome coronavirus 2 (SARS-CoV-2) has been responsible for the worst pandemic in the past 100 years. Initially thought to be primarily a respiratory system disease, Coronavirus Disease 2019 (Covid-19) has generally been accepted as a disease with systemic manifestations. Understanding the pathophysiology of this disease makes us realize that SARS-CoV-2 targets and utilizes angiotensin-converting enzyme 2 (ACE-2) receptors as the initial point of invasion into the human body, which eventually results in the devastating cascade that has become the hallmark of this disease. ACE-2 receptors are expressed not only in type 1 and type 2 pneumocytes but also in endothelial cells, vascular smooth muscle cells, and migratory angiogenic cells in the vascular system and cardiac fibroblasts, cardiomyocytes, and endothelial cells, pericytes, and epicardial adipose cells in the heart. Therefore, it becomes very evident that SARS-CoV-2 targets the entire cardiovascular system characterized by a cytokine storm that is distinct in patients with COVID-19, which results in endothelial dysfunction, endothelial inflammation, microvascular thrombosis, and multiorgan failure,[1] in addition to the lungs, thereby not limited to being a respiratory disease causing pneumonia and respiratory failure.[2–5] Myocardial injury, defined as elevated cardiac troponin levels, is present in almost one in four hospitalized COVID-19 patients.[6–9] The mortality rate of COVID-19 among all patients was deemed to be about 3.4 and 1.4% among patients without underlying disease.[2] However, in patients with pre-existing cardiovascular disease (CVD), the mortality rate was 13.2%.[2] The cardiovascular complications covered in this chapter are summarized in **Fig. 6.1**.

Pathophysiology

Cardiovascular manifestations of COVID-19 are due to both direct infection and invasion of myocardial cells and endothelial dysfunction and inflammation, and microvascular thrombosis resulting in indirect injury to the cardiovascular system.

Direct Myocardial Injury

SARS-Cov-2 is a single-stranded ribonucleic acid (RNA) virus. The Spike protein (S) of SARS-CoV-2 binds to the ACE-2 receptors, allowing the virus to enter the cells. Cell entry of the virus requires priming the spike protein by cellular serine protease transmembrane protease series 2 (TMPRSS2) or other proteases such as cathepsin L, cathepsin B, factor X, trypsin, elastase, and furin.[10,11] Patients with pre-existing CVD are associated with more severe COVID-19 disease because they have higher plasma levels of ACE-2.[12] After gaining entry into the host cell, the virus uses the cell's machinery to translate RNA to polypeptides, including an RNA-dependent RNA polymerase that the virus uses to replicate its own RNA.[13] Thereafter, a new virus is released from the cell by exocytosis. Host cells subsequently are disabled or destroyed, potentially triggering an innate immune response.[14] However, only a few reports confirm the presence of viral inclusion bodies or SARS-CoV-2 genomic RNA from myocardial tissue in biopsy-proven COVID-19 myocarditis cases that are associated with typical features of myocarditis, including intramyocardial inflammation, microvascular thrombosis, and

Risks
Older age, obesity, hypertension, diabetes, cardiovascular disease, cerebrovascular disease, immobility, critical illness, chronic respiratory disease

Systemic Inflammation · Direct viral injury · COVID drug side effects

Thrombo-embolism	Acute Coronary Syndromes	Myocardial injury, myocarditis	Heart Failure, Cardiomyopathy	Arrhythmias
Prevalence 25% Mortality 23%	Prevalence 1% Mortality 27%	Prevalence 36% Mortality 60%	Prevalence 29% Mortality 47%	Prevalence 17% Mortality 20%

Fig. 6.1 Cardiovascular complications of Covid-19 and associated risk of mortality. Licensed under creative commons license *Creative Commons–Attribution 4.0 International–CC BY 4.0.* Lee CCE, Ali K, Connell D, Mordi IR, George J, Lang EM, Lang CC. COVID-19-associated cardiovascular complications. Diseases 2021;9:47. https://doi.org/10.3390/diseases9030047[144]

myocardial necrosis.[15–20] An autopsy series of consecutive patients showed SARS-CoV-2 in cardiac tissues in 61.5% of those patients.[21]

Indirect Injury by SARS-CoV-2

ACE-2 converts angiotensin II (Ang II) to angiotensin (Ang)-(1-7), which in turn acts by activating its receptor MAS—a G-protein-coupled receptor (GPCR).[22] This ACE-2/Ang-(1-7)/Mas axis counteracts and is an inverse regulator of the renin-angiotensin-aldosterone system (RAAS) counterbalancing the vasoconstrictive and proinflammatory actions of classical RAAS, which includes renin, ACE, Ang II, and its receptors AT1 and AT2 while acting as the protective arm of the RAAS.[22] The interaction between the Spike protein of SARS-CoV-2 and ACE-2 extracellular domains leads to downregulation of surface ACE-2 expression while allowing SARS CoV-2 into cells.[23] Downregulation of ACE-2 activity leads to an increase in the accumulation of Ang II since it is responsible for the conversion of Ang II to Ang-(1-7).[13]

ACE-2 and Inflammation

A disintegrin and metalloproteinase domain 17 (ADAM-17), a transmembrane protease, which is also responsible for the proteolysis and ectodomain shedding of ACE-2, spurs the activation of macrophages which are integral to the immune system and are a source of inflammatory cytokine tumor necrosis factor alpha (TNF-α).[24,25] Downregulation of ACE-2 results in an increase in Ang-II/angiotensin 1 receptor (AT1R) at the expense of ACE-2/Ang-1-7/Mas axis, which is the protective arm of the RAAS, and is essential in maintaining the physiological and pathophysiological equilibrium of the body.[23] Accumulation of Ang II leads to increased binding of Ang II to Ang II type I receptor, triggering a signaling cascade that leads to ADAM-17 phosphorylation and enhanced catalytic activity.[5,24] Activated ADAM-17 increases ACE-2 shedding, resulting in further reductions of Ang II clearance, increased Ang II-mediated inflammatory responses, and a vicious positive feedback cycle.[13] This deleterious imbalance leads to comprehensive negative consequences, including aldosterone secretin, fibrosis, proinflammation, hypertrophy, vasoconstriction, enhanced reactive oxygen species and vascular permeability, cardiac remolding, gut dysbiosis, and multiple organ dysfunction syndrome (MODS).[5,23,26] Downregulation of ACE-2 expression has been seen in myocardial cells in both SARS-CoV-2-infected mice and humans.[27] A positive correlation between elevated circulating Ang II levels in COVID-19 patients and lung injury and increased viral load has also been seen.[23] Therefore, it has been surmised that a direct link between tissue ACE-2 downregulation and upregulation of Ang II is at least partially responsible for the development of cardiovascular complications or multiorgan failure following SARS-Cov-2 infection.[28,29]

Endothelial Inflammation, Endothelial Dysfunction, and Thrombosis

It is known that the endothelium of both venous and arterial vasculature express ACE-2.[30] Microscopic evidence of SARS-CoV-2 viral particles in endothelial cells of the kidney and endotheliitis characterized by activated neutrophils and macrophages in numerous organs, including the lung, intestine, and heart, has been obtained from histopathological studies.[31,32] The release of interleukin-1β (IL-1β) and IL-6 causes endothelial activation and the expression of cell adhesion molecules.

Endothelial inflammation and subsequent endothelial dysfunction make it proadhesive and prothrombotic with an increased expression of tissue factor and plasminogen activator inhibitor-1.[32] It has also been shown that von Willebrand factor (vWF), a circulating blood coagulation glycoprotein associated with endothelial dysfunction, is significantly elevated in COVID-19 patients compared with normal individuals, indicating ongoing endothelial activation and dysfunction.[33-35] vWF, being a carrier of coagulation factor VIII, can trigger platelet aggregation and blood coagulation[36] (**Fig. 6.2**). Evidence of endotheliitis caused by SARS-CoV-2 infection has been shown by histological studies.[31] Interaction of platelets and neutrophils and macrophage activation thereafter can then lead to proinflammatory responses, including cytokine storm and the formation of neutrophil extracellular traps (NETs).[37] NETs then damage the endothelium and stimulate both extrinsic and intrinsic coagulation pathways, which result in microthrombus formation and microvascular dysfunction. High levels of NETs were reportedly seen in hospitalized

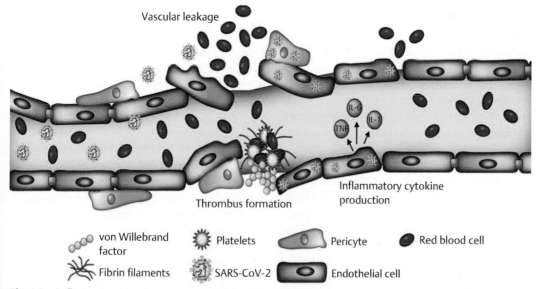

Fig. 6.2 Inflammatory response at the endothelial level direct viral injury and cytokine-mediated factors activate endothelial cell resulting in local release of cytokines, netosis (NET), and endotheliitis associated microthrombosis. Modified from Farshidfar F, Koleini N, Ardehali H. Cardiovascular complications of COVID-19. https://doi.org/10.1172/jci.insight.148980 http://creativecommons.org/licenses/by/4.0/

patients with COVID-19, which correlated positively with disease severity.[38]

Both indirect generation of inflammation and prothrombotic conditions resulting in vasculopathy and the direct invasion of endothelial cells by SARS-CoV-2 infection contribute to the pathophysiological mechanisms of COVID-19.[30,31,39] Hyperinflammation and the cytokine storm are hallmarks of severe COVID-19. Rapid viral replication, interference with interferon signaling, and recruitment of inflammatory cells (neutrophils and monocytes/macrophages) are mediators of hyperinflammation as per previous studies with human coronaviruses.[40] White blood cells, neutrophils, lymphocyte subtypes, and inflammation parameters (CRP and procalcitonin), which are measurements of immunity, were independently related to acute cardiac injury in patients with COVID-19.[41]

A sharp rise in levels of multiple proinflammatory cytokines triggered by infection has been observed following infection with H1N1 (44), SARS,[40,42] and MERS, and is characteristic of a cytokine storm.[40,42–44] The SARS-CoV-2 infection causes an increase in chemokines, high levels of interleukin-6 (IL-6), and decreased levels of type I and III interferons, resulting in an atypical inflammatory reaction. A reduction in innate antiviral defenses and raised proinflammatory responses contribute to COVID-19 pathology. SARS-CoV-2 infection results in pathogenic T-helper 1 cells, and inflammatory CD14, CD16 monocytes induce high granulocyte macrophage colony-stimulating factor (GM-CSF) and IL-6 expression. IL-6 is known to activate coagulation, induce thrombosis, inhibit heart function, cause endothelial dysfunction leading to vascular leakage, tissue ischemia, and hypoxia, resulting in a drop in blood pressure, disseminated intravascular coagulation (DIC), and MODS.[45–49] Higher serum levels of IL-6 have been linked to worse prognosis and have been found to correlate with fibrinogen levels in patients with COVID-19.[50–54]

Since hypoxemia is the preeminent clinical manifestation of COVID-19, an oxygen supply–demand mismatch resulting in myocardial injury is frequently seen.[55] The pathophysiology of cardiac injury among many COVID-19 patients does not involve the acute disruption of atheromatous plaque. It is similar to type 2 myocardial infarction resulting from an imbalance of oxygen supply and demand caused by cytokine storm and endothelial dysfunction.[56,57] The cytokine storm causes the release of IL-6 and catecholamines that increase core body temperature, heart rate, and cardiac oxygen consumption.[23] In addition, endothelial dysfunction and cytokine storm cause pathological changes such as coronary artery spasm and thrombosis, which lead to decreased coronary artery blood flow.[23] Reflex tachycardia, severe hypoxemia, hypotension, and anemia in critically ill COVID-19 patients with increased cardiometabolic demand further compromise oxygen supply. Therefore, an oxygen supply and demand mismatch due to the confluence of factors in COVID-19 patients leads to acute cardiac injury.[23]

Clinical Cardiovascular Manifestations of COVID-19

Understanding the wide-ranging manifestations of the pathophysiology of COVID-19 affecting the cardiovascular system brings the realization that clinical cardiovascular manifestations of COVID-19 would involve a broad spectrum of disease. Pre-existing CVD could worsen, or COVID-19 could precipitate new cardiovascular complications. This would include ischemic and nonischemic myocardial injury (based upon elevation of cardiac biomarkers), arrhythmias, venous thromboembolism, acute heart failure and cardiomyopathy, and shock. A clear and established association of severity of COVID-19 with cardiovascular manifestations of the disease makes it incumbent to recognize and understand the spectrum of clinical cardiovascular expressions of the disease process.

According to the definition of myocardial injury in the Fourth Universal Definition of Myocardial Infarction, myocardial injury has been clinically identified by the presence of at least one cardiac troponin value above the 99th percentile upper reference limit (URL).[58] Myocardial injury is generally identified by elevation of cardiac troponin, including all conditions that cause cardiomyocyte death with or without accompanying electrocardiographic or echocardiographic evidence of acute ischemia.[6,7,58–61] Even after controlling for other comorbidities, increased levels of hs-cTn correlate with disease severity and mortality rate in COVID-19.[27,62]

With abnormal serum troponins, it could be challenging. However, it is essential to differentiate type I myocardial infarction (MI), which is due to plaque rupture or thrombosis, type II myocardial infarction, which is due to supply–demand mismatch, myocardial injury in disseminated intravascular coagulation (DIC), acute myocarditis, and Takotsubo (stress) cardiomyopathy.

Ischemic Myocardial Injury

Ischemic myocardial injury can be caused by epicardial coronary artery disease (CAD) due to plaque rupture or demand ischemia, cardiac microvascular dysfunction, small vessel cardiac vasculitis, and endotheliitis.[31,63]

The Fourth Universal Definition of MI also provides clinical classification based upon the cause of myocardial ischemia.[58]

1. Type 1 MI is due to acute atherothrombotic CAD, usually precipitated by atherosclerotic plaque rupture or erosion.
2. Type 2 MI is due to oxygen supply and demand mismatch.
3. Type 3 MI is sudden or unexplained death suspicious of MI in which biomarker confirmation could not be obtained.

Acute Coronary Syndrome (Type 1 MI)

The acute coronary syndrome includes patients with either ST-elevation myocardial infarction (STEMI) or non-ST-elevation myocardial infarction (NSTEMI), or unstable angina. The Fourth Universal Definition of MI states that the term "acute MI" should be used when there is an acute myocardial injury with clinical evidence of acute myocardial ischemia and with detection of a rise or fall of cardiac troponin values with at least one value above the 99th percentile URL and at least one of the following[58]:

1. Symptoms of myocardial ischemia.
2. New ischemic electrocardiographic (ECG) changes.
3. Development of pathological Q waves.
4. Imaging evidence of new loss of viable myocardium or new regional wall motion abnormality in a pattern consistent with an ischemic etiology.
5. Identification of a coronary thrombus by angiography or autopsy (not for type II or III MI).

Type I acute myocardial infarction (AMI) due to plaque rupture or erosion can result from the systemic inflammation and catecholamine surge inherent to COVID-19 disease.[64,65] Coronary thrombosis has been identified as a possible cause of acute coronary syndrome in COVID-19 patients.[66] Severe viral infections can cause a systemic inflammatory response syndrome that increases the risk of plaque rupture and thrombus formation, resulting in AMI.[65,67,68] Viral products known as pathogen-associated molecular patterns entering the systemic circulation activate immune receptors on cells in existing atherosclerotic plaques and predispose them to plaque rupture.[65,69] They are also believed to activate the inflammasome and convert nascent pro-cytokines into biologically active cytokines.[70] In addition, viral infection and inflammation may also lead to dysregulation of coronary vascular endothelial function and cause vasoconstriction and thrombosis.[71] Extensive inflammation, endothelial dysfunction, and hypercoagulability in patients with COVID-19 may increase the risk of AMI.[42,72] Some studies have shown an increased risk of AMI in patients with COVID-19.[73–75] However, the actual incidence of AMI in COVID-19 patients is unknown so far. Newly diagnosed AMI was reported in 5.3% of cases in an electrocardiographic study of COVID-19.[76] AMI was seen in 2.9% in an echocardiography study.[77] However, in 33.3 to 39.3% of patients with COVID-19 who had STEMI were found to have nonobstructive coronary artery disease.[74,78]

The American College of Cardiology (ACC) recommendations for AMI in COVID-19 patients gives the option of fibrinolysis for patients with low-risk STEMI defined as inferior wall STEMI with no right ventricular involvement or lateral AMI without hemodynamic compromise while recognizing that the treatment of choice remains percutaneous coronary intervention (PCI).[42] The ACC recommends that hemodynamically unstable COVID-19 patients with NSTEMI be managed similarly to those with STEMI.[42] Real-time reverse transcriptase polymerase chain reaction (RT-PCR) assays for testing for COVID-19 should be readily and easily available, as waiting for test results in patients with uncertain COVID-19 status would exceed the time frame within which primary revascularization is beneficial for myocardial salvage. As the airborne transmission of SARS-CoV-2 is no longer a mystery, it goes without saying that staff should don appropriate personal protective equipment (PPE), and full decontamination of the catheterization laboratory should be performed following each procedure. According to the ACC for COVID-19 patients with NSTEMI, diagnostic testing before catheterization is recommended, and conservative therapy may be sufficient.[42]

Supply–Demand Mismatch (Type 2 MI)

As stated, type 2 MI is due to myocardial oxygen supply–demand mismatch, also known as demand ischemia. With the understanding of the pathophysiology of COVID-19, four specific mechanisms in the context of COVID-19 have been proposed.[13] They are:

1. Fixed coronary atherosclerosis limiting myocardial perfusion.

2. Endothelial dysfunction within the coronary microcirculation.
3. Severe systemic hypertension resulting from elevated circulating Ang-II levels and intense arteriolar vasoconstriction.
4. Hypoxemia resulting from acute respiratory distress syndrome (ARDS) or from in situ pulmonary vascular thromboses.

It has been seen that patients with underlying atherosclerosis are susceptible to myocardial infarction or injury in conditions such as systemic inflammatory response syndrome (SIRS), coronavirus pneumonia, and HINI influenza.[79,80] It has been seen in conditions involving severe physiological stress such as respiratory failure, sepsis, and lung injury that biomarkers of myocardial injury are elevated even in the absence of atherosclerotic plaques.[81-83] Inflammatory profile in patients with cardiomyopathy associated with sepsis exhibits high serum levels of cytokines that include IL-6 and TNF-α.[79,80,84]

The Suspicion of Death due to MI in CVD (Type 3 MI)

This unfortunate clinical scenario explains unexplained sudden cardiac death among patients with known coronary artery disease suspected of having COVID-19.[85-89] In these patients, there is a suspicion of MI as the cause of death without obtaining cardiac biomarker confirmation. During the multiple surges of COVID-19, many patients avoided hospital care, some of whom died without confirmation of either COVID-19 or myocardial infarction.[85-89]

Stress-Induced (Takotsubo) Cardiomyopathy

Patients with stress-induced cardiomyopathy have elevated cardiac troponin with echocardiographic findings. It has been observed that the incidence of Takotsubo cardiomyopathy significantly increased from 1.5 to 1.8% during prepandemic periods to 7.8% during the COVID-19 pandemic.[90] It appears that in addition to the pathophysiology of COVID-19 resulting in a hypersympathetic state, cytokine storm, endotheliitis, and microvascular dysfunction, a rise in social, mental, and financial stress may have contributed to an association between Takotsubo cardiomyopathy and COVID-19.

A single-center study in New York City with 118 consecutive laboratory-confirmed COVID-19 patients who underwent transthoracic echocardiographic evaluation showed imaging features compatible with the diagnosis of Takotsubo cardiomyopathy (e.g., circumferential hypokinesis or akinesis of the apical and midwall segments without a discrete epicardial coronary artery distribution) in 4.2% of these patients.[91] These patients with Takotsubo cardiomyopathy had higher degrees of cardiac troponin elevation than patients with myocardial injury who did not have features of Takotsubo cardiomyopathy on transthoracic echocardiography. Patients with myocardial injury and features of Takotsubo cardiomyopathy had higher rates of in-hospital mortality and major complications from COVID-19 compared with patients without myocardial injury.[13]

Acute Myocarditis

Patients with acute myocarditis can present as a diagnostic challenge in the COVID-19 era. These patients can present with chest pain, shortness of breath, along with abnormal serum troponins levels. The ECG findings can be nonspecific ST-segment changes, ST-segment depression or elevation, and PR segment deviation. COVID-19 patients with acute myocarditis may also present with a third-degree atrioventricular block.[76] In COVID-19 patients, pericardial involvement with cardiac tamponade and acute myopericarditis with elevated levels of cardiac biomarkers have been reported.[2,64,92–94] In one study, myocarditis was thought to be the cause of 7% of COVID-19-related deaths.[51] Echocardiographic evaluation could help differentiate acute myocarditis from an acute coronary syndrome, with focal wall motion abnormalities being present more in acute coronary syndrome. Acute myocarditis would either have no wall motion abnormality or will have global wall motion dysfunction.[42,72] Both direct injury to the cardiomyocytes by SARS-CoV-2 and immune-mediated hyperinflammation are considered the causes of acute myocarditis (**Fig. 6.3**). COVID-19-related myocarditis cases have been confirmed by cardiac magnetic resonance (CMR) imaging.[15,95] SARS-CoV-2 particles were found in interstitial cells of the myocardium.[18] Endomyocardial biopsy found evidence of lymphocytic inflammatory infiltrates in the myocardium.[96] In a prospective cohort study conducted in Germany of 100 patients who recovered from COVID-19 and underwent CMR imaging at a median time interval of 71 days since infection, CMR revealed cardiac involvement in nearly 80% of patients and ongoing myocardial inflammation in 60%. CMR abnormalities included low left ventricular ejection fraction, greater left ventricular volumes, raised native T1 and T2, late gadolinium enhancement, and pericardial enhancement.[97] These findings correlated with higher levels of high-sensitivity troponin and active lymphocytic inflammation on endomyocardial biopsy specimens.[13] It appears that myocardial injury in acute myocarditis is more because of systemic effects of COVID-19 and less due to direct viral injury to cardiomyocytes.[38]

Incidence and Outcomes of Myocardial Injury in COVID-19

Elevated cardiac troponin levels were seen in about 10 to 30% of hospitalized COVID-19 patients and are associated with higher mortality.[7,50,59,98] The prevalence of acute myocardial injury is higher in patients admitted to the intensive care unit (ICU) at 22.2 versus 2% in patients who are not.[6] Also, acute cardiac injury is seen in 59% of nonsurvivors versus 1% among survivors.[50] One early

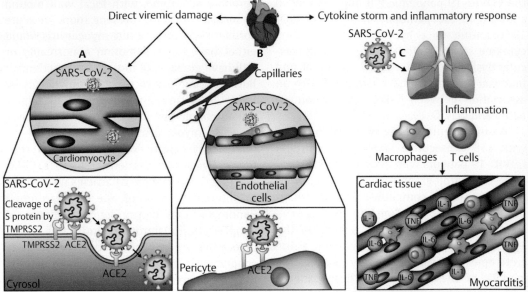

Fig. 6.3   Summary of mechanisms involved in Covid-19-associated myocarditis. **(a)** Direct viral injury to cardiac myocytes and **(b)** endotheliitis. **(c)** Cytokine-mediated injury and inflammation may also predominate. Modified from Farshidfar F, Koleini N, Ardehali H. Cardiovascular complications of COVID-19. https://doi.org/10.1172/jci.insight.148980 http://creativecommons.org/licenses/by/4.0

observational study showed that acute myocardial injury as determined by elevated troponin levels exhibited a strong association of CVD (CAD, hypertension, or cardiomyopathy) and mortality.[59] In this study, a history of CVD was present in 35% of patients, and troponin was elevated in 28% of all patients. Troponin elevation was seen in 55% of patients with CVD. The mortality rate was 69% in patients with CVD who had elevated troponin. Among patients without CVD and normal troponin, the mortality rate was 7.6%. The mortality rate was 13.3% among patients with CVD and normal troponin. Patients without CVD and elevated troponin had a mortality rate of 37.5%. The mortality rate of 69.4% was the highest among patients who had both CVD and elevated troponin. A higher troponin level was associated with increase in mortality. It has been shown that the pattern in the rise of cTn levels is significant from a prognostic standpoint. Higher levels of cTn elevation with continued rise until death (mean time from symptom answer to death was 18.5 days) were seen in nonsurvivors, while in survivors, cTn levels remained unchanged.[50] Therefore, trending off cTn levels in hospitalized COVID-19 patients would be significant.

Many patients with COVID-19 who have elevated cardiac troponin, or ECG cardiac abnormalities, or cardiac imaging abnormalities do not have classic anginal symptoms of heart disease, especially in the initial stages, including among hospitalized patients. Most patients with myocardial injury do not have previously diagnosed CVD and frequently present without chest pain.[59,60] It is also seen that myocardial injury and other manifestations of end-organ damage appeared to occur later (greater than 14 days) after the onset of initial symptoms.[13] There are only small-sized studies that have echocardiographic findings in patients with COVID-19. The most common echocardiographic abnormality found was right ventricular dilatation and right ventricular dysfunction, with only a small percentage of patients having left lenticular systolic dysfunction.[13,99–101] The true incidence of type 1 MI is still unknown in COVID-19 patients. Troponin and D-dimer levels were higher in COVID-19 patients with type 1 MI, but these type 1 MI patients had lower in-hospital mortality than COVID-19 patients who had a nonischemic myocardial injury.[13] Nonobstructive CAD in patients with COVID-19 presenting with STEMI had a high prevalence, as seen in an extensive series of 28 patients who underwent invasive coronary angiography in northern Italy.[78]

A multicenter retrospective analysis in New York City is the largest available outcome study of myocardial injury.[7] In this study, a total of 2,736 patients were included, of whom 36% had evidence of myocardial injury at the time of presentation based on the elevation of cardiac troponin. Only 30% of patients who had myocardial injury had a history of coronary artery disease. Patients who had troponin elevations (signifying myocardial injury) were associated with increased risk of in-hospital mortality (adjusted odds ratio [OR]: 1.75; 95% confidence interval [CI]: 1.37–2.24 and adjusted OR: 3.03; 95% CI: 2.42–3.80, respectively). Cardiac troponin elevation has shown a correlation with higher levels of inflammatory biomarkers (e.g., ferritin, IL-6, C-reactive protein), coagulation biomarkers (e.g., D-dimer), and severity of hypoxemia and respiratory illness (e.g., need for mechanical ventilation).[13]

Arrhythmias in COVID-19 Patients

Acute myocardial injury is seen in about 10 to 27.8% of admitted COVID-19 patients.[6–8,59,60,102] With a myocardial injury, the incidents of arrhythmias increase substantially. Arrhythmias were reported in 17.3% of hospitalized COVID-19 patients with myocardial injury and 1.5% of patients with no myocardial injury.[59,60] In another study, arrhythmias were present in 16.7% of hospitalized COVID-19 patients, with an increased prevalence of 44.4% among patients admitted to the ICU versus 6.9% in non-ICU hospitalized COVID-19 patients.[6] Ventricular arrhythmias were seen in 17.3% of COVID-19 patients with acute myocardial injury compared to 1.5%

COVID-19 patients without acute myocardial injury.[59] Atrial arrhythmias were seen in 17.7% of COVID-19 patients who required mechanical ventilation compared to 1.9% of hospitalized COVID-19 patients who did not require mechanical ventilation.[103] In a New York cohort of hospitalized COVID-19 patients, prolonged corrected QT (500 ms) was found in 6% of 4,250 patients.[95] Asystole was the most common initial rhythm reported in 89.7% of hospitalized COVID-19 patients who suffered cardiac arrest compared to shockable rhythms in 5.9% of such patients.[104] Third-degree atrioventricular block has also been reported in a COVID-19 patient with acute myocarditis.[76]

In addition to the increased risk of incidence of arrhythmias associated with myocardial injury, other mechanisms for arrhythmias in COVID-19 patients should be considered, especially seen in patients with worsening renal function.[105,106] These include arrhythmias that may develop due to electrolyte abnormalities, including hypokalemia, hypomagnesemia, hypoxemia, and QT-prolonging medications. COVID-19 patients with previously present myocardial scar could experience monomorphic ventricular tachycardia due to the prevalence of hyperadrenergic state in such patients.[13] Arrhythmias in hospitalized COVID-19 patients have also been found to be due to the direct electrophysiological effects of cytokines on the myocardium due to the hyperinflammatory state that is characteristic of COVID-19.[13] The ventricular action potential duration is prolonged due to the modulation of the expression/activity of cardiomyocyte K+ and Ca++ ion channels by the inflammatory cytokines upregulated in patients with COVID-19. In such patients with increased expression of inflammatory cytokines, IL-6 inhibits the human ether-a-go-go-related gene (hERG)-K+ channel resulting in the prolongation of the ventricular action potential.[107] IL-6 also inhibits cytochrome 450 (CYP) 3A4, increasing the bioavailability of several QT-prolonging medications. In addition to the direct cardiac effects of inflammatory cytokines, cardiac sympathetic system hyperactivation is also provoked centrally (an inflammatory reflex mediated by the hypothalamus) and peripherally (by activating the left stellate ganglia), which can then trigger life-threatening arrhythmias in the setting of long QT.[108]

Heart Failure and Shock in COVID-19 Patients

An increase in biomarkers for heart failure, BNP/NT-proBNP in hospitalized COVID-19 patients is associated with a poor prognosis.[51] Nonsurvivors had a higher (52%) incidence of heart failure than survivors (12%), heart failure being present in 23% of hospitalized COVID-19 patients.[50,109] Biventricular failure was reported in 7 to 33% of hospitalized COVID-19 patients.[51,110] Isolated right ventricular failure was also observed in patients with and without pulmonary embolism (PE).[111,112] It becomes apparent that heart failure in COVID-19 patients may be the culmination of the pathogenic cascade of COVID-19 as well as its insults on the myocardium along the way. This not only may have immediate and short-term consequences for COVID-19 patients but long-term sequelae in patients infected by SARS-CoV-2.

Shock, including cardiogenic, septic, or mixed shock, was found in 8.7% of 138 COVID-19 patients in a study wherein 30.6% of such patients were ICU patients, and 1.0% were non-ICU patients.[61] In such patients with shock, a recognition of cardiogenic constituent would be critical to assist in clinical decision making, especially as it would impact device selection (venoarterial vs. venovenous) when mechanical respiratory and circulatory assistance with extracorporeal membranous oxygenation (ECMO) is considered.[113]

Thromboembolic Disease in COVID-19 Patients

Proinflammatory and prothrombotic conditions resulting in thromboembolic disease are associated with COVID-19.[72,114-116] Among ICU patients with COVID-19, according to studies done in the Netherlands and China, there was a similar result with about 25% incidence of venous thromboembolism (VTE).[117,118] In addition, 71.4% of COVID-19 patients who died were diagnosed with DIC.[89] It was reported that despite prophylactic anticoagulation, 31% of patients with COVID-19 still developed VTE, of which 16.7% of patients were diagnosed with PE.[46] It was also reported that the incidents of PE were higher (11.7%) in COVID-19 patients with ARDS than in patients with ARDS who did not have COVID-19 (2.1%).[54]

Small case series and retrospective single-center data have shown trends of association and an increase in the incidence of arterial thromboembolic events among hospitalized COVID-19 patients, acute cerebrovascular events, ischemic stroke, and acute limb ischemia.[119-121] In a single-center retrospective study, the incidence of acute cerebrovascular events among hospitalized COVID-19 patients and severe infection was about 5%. The incidence of acute ischemic stroke in COVID-19 patients is about 1 to 3%.[6] In addition to arterial strokes, cerebral venous sinus thrombosis has been reported.[33]

Hyperinflammation, endothelial dysfunction, prothrombotic, or a hypercoagulable state observed in COVID-19 patients may result in both arterial and venous thrombosis. In addition, hypoxemia that is ubiquitous in moderate and severe COVID-19 patients decreases S protein production, which increases the risk of thrombosis.[122] A higher incidence of supraventricular tachyarrhythmias, as reviewed, may also contribute to increased incidence of arterial thromboembolism despite adequate thromboembolic prophylaxis.[123,124] In a multicenter retrospective cohort study, elevated D-dimer levels (>1 µg/mL) were associated with thromboembolic disease and were independent predictors of in-hospital deaths among COVID-19 patients[50] (**Fig. 6.4**). D-dimer was identified as one of the risk factors for death in COVID-19 patients and is associated with 18 times increased risk for mortality.[50] Both

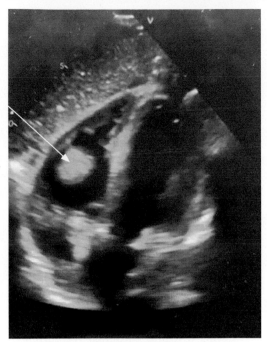

Fig. 6.4 Echocardiogram demonstrating a large right ventricular thrombus (*white arrow*) in a 52-year-old man who presented with cardiogenic shock and Covid-19.

inflammatory biomarkers—D-dimer and fibrinogen—are associated with thromboembolic disease and increased mortality.

Anticoagulation with heparin and low-molecular-weight heparin is used to prevent and manage thromboembolic disease in COVID-19 patients. They both have theoretical benefits over vitamin K antagonists and direct oral anticoagulants.[125–128] Heparin has specific anti-inflammatory properties and can downregulate IL-6. This may be particularly helpful in COVID-19 patients because heparin binds the S protein of SARS-CoV-2, although the superiority of heparin cannot be confirmed due to the absence of a direct comparison with oral anticoagulants.[127,128] Treatment dose anticoagulation was associated with reduced mortality in a study from New York. In this study, in-hospital mortality was 23%, with a median survival of 21 days in COVID-19 patients who received anticoagulation versus a mortality rate of 23% with a median survival of 14 days in patients who did not receive treatment dose anticoagulation. In COVID-19 patients on mechanical ventilation, in-hospital mortality was 29% in patients who received treatment dose anticoagulation with a median survival of 21 days compared to in-hospital mortality of 63% with a median survival of 9 days in patients who did not receive treatment dose anticoagulation.[129] Fibrin deposition in the pulmonary vasculature seen in animal models of ARDS may suggest the possibility of pulmonary microvascular and macrovascular thrombi influencing the pathophysiology of ARDS in some COVID-19 patients, leading to the possible benefit of tissue plasminogen activator in severe COVID-19 patients with ARDS.[130–134]

Multisystem Inflammatory Syndrome in Children and Adults

Multisystem inflammatory syndrome in adults (MIS-A) is a rare but severe postacute COVID-19 complication of SARS-CoV-2 infection.[135] A similar condition was first described in children as multisystem inflammatory syndrome in children (MIS-C).[68,136,137]

MIS-C is seen in children whom SARS-CoV-2 has infected with very high inflammatory markers (CRP, procalcitonin, neutrophilia, lymphopenia), proinflammatory cytokine levels, IL-6, IL-10, soluble IL-2 receptor, ferritin levels and D-dimers, and multisystem organ involvement, persistent fever, with no other plausible diagnosis.[68,136,137] It is also termed Kawasaki-like disease as it appears to share clinical, pathogenetic, and laboratory features with Kawasaki disease (KD), toxic shock syndrome, and macrophage activation syndrome.[138] KD is an acute inflammatory disease, causing medium vessel systemic vasculitis with a predilection for coronary arteries mostly in early childhood (<5 y). Diagnosis of KD is clinical and is based upon AHA clinical criteria and is confirmed by the presence of coronary artery aneurysms. MIS-C, on the other hand, affects children from early childhood to late adolescence.

MIS-C has more frequent gastrointestinal involvement, myocarditis, cardiogenic shock, heart failure requiring inotropic support and circulatory assistance. MIS-C is a cytokine storm with predominant inflammatory mediators being IL-6 and IL-8, unlike in patients with KD, wherein IL-1 appears to be the main mediator of coronary artery inflammation.[138] MIS-C has no known treatment, whereas timely infusion of intravenous immunoglobulin (IVIg) in the acute phase of the disease in KD reduces the risk of development of coronary artery abnormalities from 25% to about 4%.[139–143]

MIS-A is seen in adults whom SARS-CoV-2 has infected and present with fever and primary or secondary clinical criteria that may include: severe cardiac illness (includes myocarditis, pericarditis, coronary artery aneurysm/dilatation, or new-onset right or left ventricular dysfunction, second or third-degree atrioventricular block, or ventricular tachycardia), rash and nonpurulent conjunctivitis, new-onset neurologic signs and symptoms (encephalopathy, seizures, meningeal signs, or peripheral neuropathy), shock or hypotension, abdominal pain/vomiting/diarrhea, thrombocytopenia. In addition, there should be elevated levels of at least two of the following inflammatory markers: C-reactive protein, ferritin, IL-6, erythrocyte sedimentation rate, procalcitonin.[135]

Perspective

SARS-Cov-2, initially thought to primarily cause lung infection, is now accepted to have systemic manifestations and consequences that may include multiorgan dysfunction, including the cardiovascular system. Although the virus may cause direct injury and invasion of cells upon entry, it is the cascade of indirect injury that it sets in motion, which eventually may lead to catastrophic and tragic consequences to the human body, both in the acute and long post-COVID phases. Endothelial activation with subsequent endothelial dysfunction leading to a hyperinflammatory state, hypercoagulability, microvascular and macrovascular thrombosis, myocardial injury and its sequelae, and multiorgan dysfunction or failure, at various stages, present challenges and opportunities for mitigating the mayhem that has become the hallmark of this 100-year pandemic. MIS-C and MIS-A have shown that the apparent randomness of this disease is still confounding the best of minds. Moreover, it may only worsen with the emergence of more contagious and lethal variants of a virus mutating at its own time and place of choosing. Vaccines are beneficial but must not be the only option. If we can develop effective vaccines as marvelously as we have, then there is no reason we should not be able to develop or repurpose drugs for prophylaxis and treatments for COVID-19. Despite the vaccines, if we do not have effective drugs against the virus for prophylaxis and treatment, we will be fighting a losing battle—as we currently are. A multifaceted approach is not only the best approach to defeat the virus and end the pandemic; it is the only approach.

References

1. McElvaney OJ, McEvoy NL, McElvaney OF, et al. Characterization of the inflammatory response to severe COVID-19 illness. Am J Respir Crit Care Med 2020;202(6):812–821

2. World Health Organization. Report of the WHO: China Joint Mission on Coronavirus Disease 2019 (COVID-19). 2020

3. Peiris JS, Chu CM, Cheng VC, et al; HKU/UCH SARS Study Group. Clinical progression and viral load in a community outbreak of coronavirus-associated SARS pneumonia: a prospective study. Lancet 2003;361(9371):1767–1772

4. Pizzini A, Burkert F, Theurl I, Weiss G, Bellmann-Weiler R. Prognostic impact of high sensitive Troponin T in patients with influenza virus infection: a retrospective analysis. Heart Lung 2020;49(1):105–109

5. Gheblawi M, Wang K, Viveiros A, et al. Angiotensin-converting enzyme 2: SARS-CoV-2 receptor and regulator of the renin-angiotensin system: celebrating the 20th anniversary of the discovery of ACE2. Circ Res 2020;126(10):1456–1474

6. Wang D, Hu B, Hu C, et al. Clinical characteristics of 138 hospitalized patients with 2019 novel coronavirus-infected pneumonia in Wuhan, China. JAMA 2020;323(11): 1061–1069

7. Lala A, Johnson KW, Januzzi JL, et al; Mount Sinai COVID Informatics Center. Prevalence and impact of myocardial injury in patients hospitalized with COVID-19 infection. J Am Coll Cardiol 2020;76(5):533–546

8. Richardson S, Hirsch JS, Narasimhan M, et al; The Northwell COVID-19 Research Consortium. Presenting characteristics, comorbidities, and outcomes among 5700 patients hospitalized with COVID-19 in the New York City area. JAMA 2020;323(20):2052–2059

9. Bavishi C, Bonow RO, Trivedi V, Abbott JD, Messerli FH, Bhatt DL. Special article—acute myocardial injury in patients hospitalized with COVID-19 infection: a review. Prog Cardiovasc Dis 2020;63(5):682–689

10. Hoffmann M, Kleine-Weber H, Schroeder S, et al. SARS-CoV-2 cell entry depends on ACE2 and TMPRSS2 and is blocked by a clinically proven protease inhibitor. Cell 2020;181(2):271–280.e8

11. Lei C, Qian K, Li T, et al. Neutralization of SARS-CoV-2 spike pseudotyped virus by recombinant ACE2-Ig. Nat Commun 2020; 11(1):2070

12. Walters TE, Kalman JM, Patel SK, Mearns M, Velkoska E, Burrell LM. Angiotensin converting enzyme 2 activity and human atrial fibrillation: increased plasma angiotensin converting enzyme 2 activity is associated with atrial fibrillation and more advanced left atrial structural remodelling. Europace 2017;19(8):1280–1287

13. Giustino G, Pinney SP, Lala A, et al. Coronavirus and cardiovascular disease, myocardial injury, and arrhythmia: JACC Focus Seminar. J Am Coll Cardiol 2020;76(17):2011–2023

14. Liu PP, Blet A, Smyth D, Li H. The science underlying COVID-19: implications for the cardiovascular system. Circulation 2020; 142(1):68–78

15. Kim IC, Kim JY, Kim HA, Han S. COVID-19-related myocarditis in a 21-year-old female patient. Eur Heart J 2020;41(19):1859

16. Meyer P, Degrauwe S, Van Delden C, Ghadri JR, Templin C. Typical takotsubo syndrome triggered by SARS-CoV-2 infection. Eur Heart J 2020;41(19):1860

17. Inciardi RM, Lupi L, Zaccone G, et al. Cardiac involvement in a patient with coronavirus disease 2019 (COVID-19). JAMA Cardiol 2020;5(7):819–824

18. Tavazzi G, Pellegrini C, Maurelli M, et al. Myocardial localization of coronavirus in COVID-19 cardiogenic shock. Eur J Heart Fail 2020;22(5):911–915

19. Escher F, Pietsch H, Aleshcheva G, et al. Detection of viral SARS-CoV-2 genomes and histopathological changes in endomyocardial biopsies. ESC Heart Fail 2020;7(5):2440–2447

20. Wenzel P, Kopp S, Göbel S, et al. Evidence of SARS-CoV-2 mRNA in endomyocardial biopsies of patients with clinically suspected myocarditis tested negative for COVID-19 in nasopharyngeal swab. Cardiovasc Res 2020;116(10):1661–1663

21. Lindner D, Fitzek A, Bräuninger H, et al. Association of cardiac infection with SARS-CoV-2 in confirmed COVID-19 autopsy cases. JAMA Cardiol 2020;5(11):1281–1285

22. Alenina N, dos Santos RAS. Angiotensin-(1–7) and Mas: a brief history. The Protective Arm of the Renin-Angiotensin System 2015;155–159: 10.1016/B978-0-12-801364-9.00021-3 (RAS)

23. Dou Q, Wei X, Zhou K, Yang S, Jia P. Cardiovascular manifestations and mechanisms in patients with COVID-19. Trends Endocrinol Metab 2020;31(12):893–904

24. Scott AJ, O'Dea KP, O'Callaghan D, et al. Reactive oxygen species and p38 mitogen-activated protein kinase mediate tumor necrosis factor α-converting enzyme (TACE/ADAM-17) activation in primary human monocytes. J Biol Chem 2011;286(41):35466–35476

25. Patel VB, Clarke N, Wang Z, et al. Angiotensin II induced proteolytic cleavage of myocardial ACE2 is mediated by TACE/ADAM-17: a positive feedback mechanism in the RAS. J Mol Cell Cardiol 2014;66:167–176

26. Tan WSD, Liao W, Zhou S, Mei D, Wong WF. Targeting the renin-angiotensin system as novel therapeutic strategy for pulmonary diseases. Curr Opin Pharmacol 2018;40:9–17

27. Oudit GY, Kassiri Z, Jiang C, et al. SARS-coronavirus modulation of myocardial ACE2 expression and inflammation in patients with SARS. Eur J Clin Invest 2009;39(7):618–625

28. Wang K, Gheblawi M, Oudit GY. Angiotensin converting enzyme 2: a double-edged sword. Circulation 2020;142(5):426–428

29. Liu Y, Yang Y, Zhang C, et al. Clinical and biochemical indexes from 2019-nCoV infected patients linked to viral loads and lung injury. Sci China Life Sci 2020;63(3):364–374

30. Ackermann M, Verleden SE, Kuehnel M, et al. Pulmonary vascular endothelialitis, thrombosis, and angiogenesis in COVID-19. N Engl J Med 2020;383(2):120–128

31. Varga Z, Flammer AJ, Steiger P, et al. Endothelial cell infection and endotheliitis in COVID-19. Lancet 2020;395(10234):1417–1418

32. Boisramé-Helms J, Kremer H, Schini-Kerth V, Meziani F. Endothelial dysfunction in sepsis. Curr Vasc Pharmacol 2013;11(2):150–160

33. Panigada M, Bottino N, Tagliabue P, et al. Hypercoagulability of COVID-19 patients in intensive care unit: a report of thromboelastography findings and other parameters of hemostasis. J Thromb Haemost 2020;18(7): 1738–1742

34. Escher R, Breakey N, Lämmle B. Severe COVID-19 infection associated with endothelial activation. Thromb Res 2020;190:62

35. Zachariah U, Nair SC, Goel A, et al. Targeting raised von Willebrand factor levels and macrophage activation in severe COVID-19: consider low volume plasma exchange and low dose steroid. Thromb Res 2020;192:2

36. Löf A, Müller JP, Brehm MA. A biophysical view on von Willebrand factor activation. J Cell Physiol 2018;233(2):799–810

37. Tomar B, Anders HJ, Desai J, Mulay SR. Neutrophils and neutrophil extracellular traps drive necroinflammation in COVID-19. Cells 2020;9(6):1383

38. Zuo Y, Yalavarthi S, Shi H, et al. Neutrophil extracellular traps in COVID-19. JCI Insight 2020;5(11):5

39. Teuwen LA, Geldhof V, Pasut A, Carmeliet P. COVID-19: the vasculature unleashed. Nat Rev Immunol 2020;20(7):389–391

40. Channappanavar R, Perlman S. Pathogenic human coronavirus infections: causes and consequences of cytokine storm and immunopathology. Semin Immunopathol 2017;39(5):529–539

41. Li D, Chen Y, Jia Y, et al. SARS-CoV-2-induced immune dysregulation and myocardial injury risk in China: insights from the ERS-COVID-19 study. Circ Res 2020;127(3):397–399

42. Welt FGP, Shah PB, Aronow HD, et al; American College of Cardiology's Interventional Council and the Society for Cardiovascular Angiography and Interventions. Catheterization laboratory considerations during the coronavirus (COVID-19) pandemic: from the ACC's Interventional Council and SCAI. J Am Coll Cardiol 2020; 75(18):2372–2375

43. Bermejo-Martin JF, Ortiz de Lejarazu R, Pumarola T, et al. Th1 and Th17 hypercytokinemia as early host response signature in severe pandemic influenza. Crit Care 2009; 13(6):R201

44. Kindler E, Thiel V, Weber F. Interaction of SARS and MERS coronaviruses with the antiviral interferon response. Adv Virus Res 2016;96:219–243

45. Zhou YG. Pathogenic T cells and inflammatory monocytes incite inflammatory storms in severe COVID-19 patients. Natl Sci Rev 2020;7:998–1002

46. Pathan N, Hemingway CA, Alizadeh AA, et al. Role of interleukin 6 in myocardial dysfunction of meningococcal septic shock. Lancet 2004;363(9404):203–209

47. Tanaka T, Narazaki M, Kishimoto T. Immunotherapeutic implications of IL-6 blockade for cytokine storm. Immunotherapy 2016;8(8): 959–970

48. Blanco-Melo D, Nilsson-Payant BE, Liu WC, et al. Imbalanced host response to SARS-CoV-2 drives development of COVID-19. Cell 2020;181(5):1036–1045.e9

49. Stone RL, Nick AM, McNeish IA, et al. Paraneoplastic thrombocytosis in ovarian cancer. N Engl J Med 2012;366(7):610–618

50. Zhou F, Yu T, Du R, et al. Clinical course and risk factors for mortality of adult inpatients with COVID-19 in Wuhan, China: a retrospective cohort study. Lancet 2020;395(10229): 1054–1062

51. Ruan Q, Yang K, Wang W, Jiang L, Song J. Clinical predictors of mortality due to COVID-19 based on an analysis of data of 150 patients from Wuhan, China. Intensive Care Med 2020;46(5):846–848

52. Wu C. Heart injury signs are associated with higher and earlier mortality in coronavirus disease 2019 (COVID-19) MedRxiv. 2020 doi: 10.1101/2020.02.26.20028589. Published online Feb 29, 2020

53. Cummings MJ, Baldwin MR, Abrams D, et al. Epidemiology, clinical course, and outcomes of critically ill adults with COVID-19 in New

York City: a prospective cohort study. Lancet 2020;395(10239):1763–1770

54. Ranucci M, Ballotta A, Di Dedda U, et al. The procoagulant pattern of patients with COVID-19 acute respiratory distress syndrome. J Thromb Haemost 2020;18(7): 1747–1751

55. Zhou K, Yang S, Jia P. Towards precision management of cardiovascular patients with COVID-19 to reduce mortality. Prog Cardiovasc Dis 2020;63(4):529–530

56. Musher DM, Abers MS, Corrales-Medina VF. Acute infection and myocardial infarction. N Engl J Med 2019;380(2):171–176

57. Sandoval Y, Jaffe AS. Type 2 myocardial infarction: JACC review topic of the week. J Am Coll Cardiol 2019;73(14):1846–1860

58. Thygesen K, Alpert JS, Jaffe AS, et al; Executive Group on behalf of the Joint European Society of Cardiology (ESC)/American College of Cardiology (ACC)/American Heart Association (AHA)/World Heart Federation (WHF) Task Force for the Universal Definition of Myocardial Infarction. Fourth Universal Definition of Myocardial Infarction (2018). J Am Coll Cardiol 2018;72(18):2231–2264

59. Guo T, Fan Y, Chen M, et al. Cardiovascular implications of fatal outcomes of patients with coronavirus disease 2019 (COVID-19). JAMA Cardiol 2020;5(7):811–818

60. Shi S, Qin M, Shen B, et al. Association of cardiac injury with mortality in hospitalized patients with COVID-19 in Wuhan, China. JAMA Cardiol 2020;5(7):802–810

61. Huang C, Wang Y, Li X, et al. Clinical features of patients infected with 2019 novel coronavirus in Wuhan, China. Lancet 2020; 395(10223):497–506

62. Zheng Y-Y, Ma YT, Zhang JY, Xie X. COVID-19 and the cardiovascular system. Nat Rev Cardiol 2020;17(5):259–260

63. Fox SE, Lameira FS, Rinker EB, Vander Heide RS. Cardiac endotheliitis and multisystem inflammatory syndrome after COVID-19. Ann Intern Med 2020;173(12):1025–1027

64. Xiong TY, Redwood S, Prendergast B, Chen M. Coronaviruses and the cardiovascular system: acute and long-term implications. Eur Heart J 2020;41(19):1798–1800

65. Schoenhagen P, Tuzcu EM, Ellis SG. Plaque vulnerability, plaque rupture, and acute coronary syndromes: (multi)-focal

manifestation of a systemic disease process. Circulation 2002;106(7):760–762

66. Dominguez-Erquicia P, Dobarro D, Raposeiras-Roubín S, Bastos-Fernandez G, Iñiguez-Romo A. Multivessel coronary thrombosis in a patient with COVID-19 pneumonia. Eur Heart J 2020;41(22):2132

67. Warren-Gash C, Hayward AC, Hemingway H, et al. Influenza infection and risk of acute myocardial infarction in England and Wales: a CALIBER self-controlled case series study. J Infect Dis 2012;206(11):1652–1659

68. https://www.cdc.gov/mis/hcp/index.html

69. Mogensen TH. Pathogen recognition and inflammatory signaling in innate immune defenses. Clin Microbiol Rev 2009;22(2): 240–273

70. van de Veerdonk FL, Netea MG, Dinarello CA, Joosten LA. Inflammasome activation and IL-1β and IL-18 processing during infection. Trends Immunol 2011;32(3):110–116

71. Vallance P, Collier J, Bhagat K. Infection, inflammation, and infarction: does acute endothelial dysfunction provide a link? Lancet 1997;349(9062):1391–1392

72. Driggin E, Madhavan MV, Bikdeli B, et al. Cardiovascular considerations for patients, health care workers, and health systems during the COVID-19 pandemic. J Am Coll Cardiol 2020;75(18):2352–2371

73. Modin D, Claggett B, Sindet-Pedersen C, et al. Acute COVID-19 and the incidence of ischemic stroke and acute myocardial infarction. Circulation 2020;142(21):2080–2082

74. Bangalore S, Sharma A, Slotwiner A, et al. ST-segment elevation in patients with Covid-19: a case series. N Engl J Med 2020; 382(25):2478–2480

75. Bilaloglu S, Aphinyanaphongs Y, Jones S, Iturrate E, Hochman J, Berger JS. Thrombosis in hospitalized patients with COVID-19 in a New York City Health System. JAMA 2020;324(8):799–801

76. Li Y, Liu T, Tse G, et al. Electrocardiograhic characteristics in patients with coronavirus infection: a single-center observational study. Ann Noninvasive Electrocardiol 2020; 25(6):e12805

77. Dweck MR, Bularga A, Hahn RT, et al. Global evaluation of echocardiography in patients with COVID-19. Eur Heart J Cardiovasc Imaging 2020;21(9):949–958

78. Stefanini GG, Montorfano M, Trabattoni D, et al. ST-elevation myocardial infarction in patients with COVID-19: clinical and angiographic outcomes. Circulation 2020; 141(25):2113–2116

79. Harrington RA. Targeting inflammation in coronary artery disease. N Engl J Med 2017;377(12):1197–1198

80. Kwong JC, Schwartz KL, Campitelli MA, et al. Acute myocardial infarction after laboratory-confirmed influenza infection. N Engl J Med 2018;378(4):345–353

81. Lim W, Qushmaq I, Devereaux PJ, et al. Elevated cardiac troponin measurements in critically ill patients. Arch Intern Med 2006;166(22):2446–2454

82. Sarkisian L, Saaby L, Poulsen TS, et al. Prognostic impact of myocardial injury related to various cardiac and noncardiac conditions. Am J Med 2016;129(5):506–514.e1

83. Sarkisian L, Saaby L, Poulsen TS, et al. Clinical characteristics and outcomes of patients with myocardial infarction, myocardial injury, and nonelevated troponins. Am J Med 2016;129(4):446.e5–446.e21

84. Kumar A, Thota V, Dee L, Olson J, Uretz E, Parrillo JE. Tumor necrosis factor alpha and interleukin 1 beta are responsible for in vitro myocardial cell depression induced by human septic shock serum. J Exp Med 1996;183(3):949–958

85. Ebinger JE, Shah PK. Declining admissions for acute cardiovascular illness: the Covid-19 paradox. J Am Coll Cardiol 2020;76(3): 289–291

86. Metzler B, Siostrzonek P, Binder RK, Bauer A, Reinstadler SJ. Decline of acute coronary syndrome admissions in Austria since the outbreak of COVID-19: the pandemic response causes cardiac collateral damage. Eur Heart J 2020;41(19):1852–1853

87. De Rosa S, Spaccarotella C, Basso C, et al; Società Italiana di Cardiologia and the CCU Academy investigators group. Reduction of hospitalizations for myocardial infarction in Italy in the COVID-19 era. Eur Heart J 2020;41(22):2083–2088

88. Pessoa-Amorim G, Camm CF, Gajendragadkar P, et al. Admission of patients with STEMI since the outbreak of the COVID-19 pandemic: a survey by the European Society of Cardiology. Eur Heart J Qual Care Clin Outcomes 2020; 6(3):210–216

89. Bhatt AS, Moscone A, McElrath EE, et al. Fewer hospitalizations for acute cardiovascular conditions during the COVID-19 pandemic. J Am Coll Cardiol 2020;76(3):280–288

90. Jabri A, Kalra A, Kumar A, et al. Incidence of stress cardiomyopathy during the coronavirus disease 2019 pandemic. JAMA Netw Open 2020;3(7):e2014780

91. Giustino G, Croft LB, Oates CP, et al. Takotsubo cardiomyopathy in COVID-19. J Am Coll Cardiol 2020;76(5):628–629

92. Hua A, O'Gallagher K, Sado D, Byrne J. Life-threatening cardiac tamponade complicating myo-pericarditis in COVID-19. Eur Heart J 2020;41(22):2130

93. Dabbagh MF, Aurora L, D'Souza P, Weinmann AJ, Bhargava P, Basir MB. Cardiac tamponade secondary to COVID-19. JACC Case Rep 2020;2(9):1326–1330

94. Atkins JL, Masoli JAH, Delgado J, et al. Pre-existing comorbidities predicting COVID-19 and mortality in the UK Biobank Community cohort. J Gerontol A Biol Sci Med Sci 2020; 75(11):2224–2230

95. Doyen D, Moceri P, Ducreux D, Dellamonica J. Myocarditis in a patient with COVID-19: a cause of raised troponin and ECG changes. Lancet 2020;395(10235):1516

96. Sala S, Peretto G, Gramegna M, et al. Acute myocarditis presenting as a reverse Tako-Tsubo syndrome in a patient with SARS-CoV-2 respiratory infection. Eur Heart J 2020;41(19):1861–1862

97. Puntmann VO, Carerj ML, Wieters I, et al. Outcomes of cardiovascular magnetic resonance imaging in patients recently recovered from coronavirus disease 2019 (COVID-19). JAMA Cardiol 2020;5(11): 1265–1273

98. Clerkin KJ, Fried JA, Raikhelkar J, et al. COVID-19 and cardiovascular disease. Circulation 2020;141(20):1648–1655

99. Sud K, Vogel B, Bohra C, et al. Echocardiographic findings in patients with COVID-19 with significant myocardial injury. J Am Soc Echocardiogr 2020;33(8): 1054–1055

100. Mahmoud-Elsayed HM, Moody WE, Bradlow WM, et al. Echocardiographic findings in patients with COVID-19 pneumonia. Can J Cardiol 2020;36(8):1203–1207

101. Szekely Y, Lichter Y, Taieb P, et al. Spectrum of cardiac manifestations in COVID-19:

a systematic echocardiographic study. Circulation 2020;142(4):342–353

102. Smeeth L, Thomas SL, Hall AJ, Hubbard R, Farrington P, Vallance P. Risk of myocardial infarction and stroke after acute infection or vaccination. N Engl J Med 2004;351(25):2611–2618

103. Goyal P, Choi JJ, Pinheiro LC, et al. Clinical characteristics of COVID-19 in New York City. N Engl J Med 2020;382(24):2372–2374

104. Shao F, Xu S, Ma X, et al. In-hospital cardiac arrest outcomes among patients with COVID-19 pneumonia in Wuhan, China. Resuscitation 2020;151:18–23

105. Hirsch JS, Ng JH, Ross DW, et al; Northwell COVID-19 Research Consortium; Northwell Nephrology COVID-19 Research Consortium. Acute kidney injury in patients hospitalized with COVID-19. Kidney Int 2020;98(1):209–218

106. Batlle D, Soler MJ, Sparks MA, et al; COVID-19 and ACE2 in Cardiovascular, Lung, and Kidney Working Group. Acute kidney injury in COVID-19: emerging evidence of a distinct pathophysiology. J Am Soc Nephrol 2020;31(7):1380–1383

107. Lazzerini PE, Laghi-Pasini F, Boutjdir M, Capecchi PL. Cardioimmunology of arrhythmias: the role of autoimmune and inflammatory cardiac channelopathies. Nat Rev Immunol 2019;19(1):63–64

108. Lazzerini PE, Boutjdir M, Capecchi PL. COVID-19, arrhythmic risk and inflammation: mind the gap! Circulation 2020; 142(1):7–9

109. Chen T, Wu D, Chen H, et al. Clinical characteristics of 113 deceased patients with coronavirus disease 2019: retrospective study. BMJ 2020;368:m1091

110. Arentz M, Yim E, Klaff L, et al. Characteristics and outcomes of 21 critically Ill patients with COVID-19 in Washington state. JAMA 2020;323(16):1612–1614

111. Ullah W, Saeed R, Sarwar U, Patel R, Fischman DL. COVID-19 complicated by acute pulmonary embolism and right-sided heart failure. JACC Case Rep 2020;2(9): 1379–1382

112. Creel-Bulos C, Hockstein M, Amin N, Melhem S, Truong A, Sharifpour M. Acute cor pulmonale in critically ill patients with COVID-19. N Engl J Med 2020;382(21):e70

113. MacLaren G, Fisher D, Brodie D. Preparing for the most critically ill patients with COVID-19: the potential role of extracorporeal membrane oxygenation. JAMA 2020;323(13):1245–1246

114. Kollias A, Kyriakoulis KG, Dimakakos E, Poulakou G, Stergiou GS, Syrigos K. Thromboembolic risk and anticoagulant therapy in COVID-19 patients: emerging evidence and call for action. Br J Haematol 2020;189(5):846–847

115. Han H, Yang L, Liu R, et al. Prominent changes in blood coagulation of patients with SARS-CoV-2 infection. Clin Chem Lab Med 2020;58(7):1116–1120

116. Bikdeli B, Madhavan MV, Jimenez D, et al; Global COVID-19 Thrombosis Collaborative Group, Endorsed by the ISTH, NATF, ESVM, and the IUA, Supported by the ESC Working Group on Pulmonary Circulation and Right Ventricular Function. COVID-19 and thrombotic or thromboembolic disease: implications for prevention, antithrombotic therapy, and follow-up: JACC State-of-the-Art Review. J Am Coll Cardiol 2020;75(23): 2950–2973

117. Klok FA, Kruip MJHA, van der Meer NJM, et al. Incidence of thrombotic complications in critically ill ICU patients with COVID-19. Thromb Res 2020;191:145–147

118. Cui S, Chen S, Li X, Liu S, Wang F. Prevalence of venous thromboembolism in patients with severe novel coronavirus pneumonia. J Thromb Haemost 2020;18(6):1421–1424

119. Mao L, Jin H, Wang M, et al. Neurologic manifestations of hospitalized patients with coronavirus disease 2019 in Wuhan, China. JAMA Neurol 2020;77(6):683–690

120. Oxley TJ, Mocco J, Majidi S, et al. Large-vessel stroke as a presenting feature of covid-19 in the young. N Engl J Med 2020; 382(20):e60

121. Bellosta R, Luzzani L, Natalini G, et al. Acute limb ischemia in patients with COVID-19 pneumonia. J Vasc Surg 2020; 72(6):1864–1872

122. Pilli VS, Datta A, Afreen S, Catalano D, Szabo G, Majumder R. Hypoxia downregulates protein S expression. Blood 2018; 132(4):452–455

123. Kashi M, Jacquin A, Dakhil B, et al. Severe arterial thrombosis associated with Covid-19 infection. Thromb Res 2020;192:75–77

124. Lodigiani C, Iapichino G, Carenzo L, et al; Humanitas COVID-19 Task Force. Venous and arterial thromboembolic complications in COVID-19 patients admitted to an academic hospital in Milan, Italy. Thromb Res 2020;191:9–14

125. Young E. The anti-inflammatory effects of heparin and related compounds. Thromb Res 2008;122(6):743–752

126. Mummery RS, Rider CC. Characterization of the heparin-binding properties of IL-6. J Immunol 2000;165(10):5671–5679

127. de Haan CA, Li Z, te Lintelo E, Bosch BJ, Haijema BJ, Rottier PJ. Murine coronavirus with an extended host range uses heparan sulfate as an entry receptor. J Virol 2005; 79(22):14451–14456

128. Belouzard S, Chu VC, Whittaker GR. Activation of the SARS coronavirus spike protein via sequential proteolytic cleavage at two distinct sites. Proc Natl Acad Sci U S A 2009;106(14):5871–5876

129. Paranjpe I, Fuster V, Lala A, et al. Association of treatment dose anticoagulation with in-hospital survival among hospitalized patients with COVID-19. J Am Coll Cardiol 2020;76(1):122–124

130. Hardaway RM, Williams CH, Marvasti M, et al. Prevention of adult respiratory distress syndrome with plasminogen activator in pigs. Crit Care Med 1990;18(12):1413–1418

131. Stringer KA, Hybertson BM, Cho OJ, Cohen Z, Repine JE. Tissue plasminogen activator (tPA) inhibits interleukin-1 induced acute lung leak. Free Radic Biol Med 1998;25(2): 184–188

132. Wang J, Hajizadeh N, Moore EE, et al. Tissue plasminogen activator (tPA) treatment for COVID-19 associated acute respiratory distress syndrome (ARDS): A case series. J Thromb Haemost 2020;18(7):1752–1755

133. Poor HD, Ventetuolo CE, Tolbert T, et al. COVID-19 critical illness pathophysiology driven by diffuse pulmonary thrombi and pulmonary endothelial dysfunction responsive to thrombolysis. Clin Transl Med 2020;10(2):e44

134. Ackermann M, Verleden SE, Kuehnel M, et al. Pulmonary vascular endothelialitis, thrombosis, and angiogenesis in Covid-19. N Engl J Med 2020;383(2):120–128

135. https://www.cdc.gov/mis/mis-a/hcp.html

136. Alunno A, Carubbi F, Rodríguez-Carrio J. Storm, typhoon, cyclone or hurricane in patients with COVID-19? Beware of the same storm that has a different origin. RMD Open 2020;6(1):e001295

137. Lee PY, Day-Lewis M, Henderson LA, et al. Distinct clinical and immunological features of SARS-CoV-2-induced multisystem inflammatory syndrome in children. J Clin Invest 2020;130(11):5942–5950

138. Gkoutzourelas A, Bogdanos DP, Sakkas LI. Kawasaki Disease and COVID-19. Mediterr J Rheumatol 2020; 31(2, Suppl 2):268–274

139. McCrindle BW, Rowley AH, Newburger JW, et al; American Heart Association Rheumatic Fever, Endocarditis, and Kawasaki Disease Committee of the Council on Cardiovascular Disease in the Young; Council on Cardiovascular and Stroke Nursing; Council on Cardiovascular Surgery and Anesthesia; and Council on Epidemiology and Prevention. Diagnosis, treatment, and long-term management of Kawasaki Disease: a scientific statement for health professionals from the American Heart Association. Circulation 2017;135(17):e927–e999 Erratum in: Circulation. 2019 Jul 30;140(5):e181-e184. PMID: 28356445

140. Newburger JW, Takahashi M, Beiser AS, et al. A single intravenous infusion of gamma globulin as compared with four infusions in the treatment of acute Kawasaki syndrome. N Engl J Med 1991;324(23):1633–1639

141. Newburger JW, Takahashi M, Burns JC, et al. The treatment of Kawasaki syndrome with intravenous gamma globulin. N Engl J Med 1986;315(6):341–347

142. Terai M, Shulman ST. Prevalence of coronary artery abnormalities in Kawasaki disease is highly dependent on gamma globulin dose but independent of salicylate dose. J Pediatr 1997;131(6):888–893

143. Furusho K, Kamiya T, Nakano H, et al. High-dose intravenous gammaglobulin for Kawasaki disease. Lancet 1984;2(8411): 1055–1058

144. Lee CCE, Ali K, Connell D, et al. COVID-19-Associated Cardiovascular Complications. Diseases. 2021;9(3). doi:10.3390/diseases 9030047

07 Pulmonary Manifestations of COVID-19

Jose Iglesias, Pierre Kory, and Paul Marik

Introduction

Respiratory failure progressing to multiorgan failure is the primary cause of death in patients with COVID-19 infection. In most cases of COVID-19 disease, infection occurs when severe acute respiratory syndrome coronavirus 2 (SARS-CoV-2) enters the aerodigestive tract via aerosols or droplets.[1] The major cell receptor necessary for the cellular entry of SARS-CoV-2 is the angiotensin-converting enzyme 2 (ACE2) in conjunction with cellular transmembrane protease serine 2 (TMPRSS2) found on the surface of epithelial cells lining the aerodigestive tract and the alveoli of the lungs.[1,2] Initially, infection occurs in the nasopharynx and sinus epithelial cells and then in the bronchial tree and, in severe cases, in the distal airways and alveoli, resulting in bronchopneumonia.[1,3–5] Although nasopharyngeal infection may result in anosmia, from a pathophysiologic standpoint, viral replication in the nasopharyngeal tract may be considered the asymptomatic phase, as the innate and adaptive immune system of the nasopharyngeal tract serves as the mainline of defense against progressive disease.[1,5–7]

Disease Progression

As the disease progresses into the distal lung, patients become symptomatic as a robust innate immune response occurs via the activation of interferon response genes and inflammasomes, followed by the release of interferons and proinflammatory cytokines.[4,8,9] This host innate immune response results in viral clearance and resolution of the infection.[4,10–12] However, SARS-CoV-2 encodes several proteins that allow the virus to evade host responses and blunt host interferon signaling.[4,8,13,14] In approximately 20% of patients, perhaps due to impaired host viral recognition pathways, a blunted interferon response due to the possible formation of autoantibodies results in the virus not being cleared, followed by a pulmonary phase with the development of increasing pulmonary opacities and hypoxemia.[15–19] During the pulmonary phase, viral infection of the gas exchange units of the lung consisting of type I and type II epithelial cells and endothelial cells is thought to occur. SARS-CoV-2 demonstrates a greater affinity to type II epithelial cells.[20-23] Infection and inflammation results in a dysregulated immune response increasing type II epithelial cell apoptosis, pyroptosis, severe endothelial damage, and endothelial dysfunction.[20-23] Increased activation and dysregulation of the innate immune response occurs due to type II epithelial apoptosis and pyroptosis with the increasing release of viable and nonviable viral particles and viral RNAemia into the alveolar unit.[20–22,24]

Approximately 5% of severely ill patients develop increasing pulmonary infiltrates, progressive hypoxemia, hyperinflammation, and coagulopathy, and are commonly described as developing COVID-19-associated acute respiratory distress syndrome (CARDS).[20,25–27] Although labeled as ARDS, this is a misnomer due to the fact that in COVID this diagnosis of ARDS is based solely on the acute presence of bilateral opacities and hypoxemia, yet the traditional pathognomonic feature of alveolar edema is absent, as evidenced by the widely described high compliance of the lung in the early phase.[28–31]

Epidemiology

Several epidemiological studies reveal that among those COVID-19 patients who progress to the pulmonary phase and develop increasing severity of respiratory failure, approximately 29 to 89% require invasive mechanical ventilation (MV).[32-36] In patients who require MV, variable and high mortality rates are observed.[32-34,36] The variability observed in these studies is multifactorial and includes the timing of MV, the determination of the need for MV, availability of intensive care unit (ICU) resources, and burden of patient comorbidities.[32-34,36,37] In ICU patients in general and in patients requiring MV in particular, predictors of mortality include age, lymphopenia, the burden of comorbidities, obesity, male gender, the persistent presence of viral RNAemia, and the severity of inflammation.[20,24,38-41] The association between the presence of SARS-CoV-2 RNAemia and clinical outcome is controversial, with some studies demonstrating the association of RNAemia with respiratory failure and progressive organ dysfunction, and others demonstrating no association.[24,42] Bermejo-Martin et al and others have demonstrated that higher levels of RNAemia are associated with the development of respiratory failure, multiorgan dysfunction, and coagulopathy.[24] Schlesinger et al demonstrated that RNAemia was found in tracheal aspirates of critically ill patients with respiratory failure but there was no association with patient mortality.[42] Although RNAemia may be accounted by increased viral load, it is most likely that the effects seen are most likely related to host response, immune dysregulation, and cytokine storm–associated inflammation.[8,16,43,44]

CARDS—Atypical ARDS or ARDS? Understanding Possible Variability

From the beginning of the pandemic, the observation was made that in many patients with severe COVID-19 pneumonia and associated respiratory failure (CARDS), there was a significant disconnect between the severity of hypoxemia, laboratory values, and the clinical presentation of the patient.[45,46] Many patients were profoundly hypoxemic while having very little dyspnea (happy hypoxemics).[45,47-49] However, the exact mechanism of asymptomatic hypoxemia has yet to be defined. A major potential cause is thought to involve pulmonary platelet activation and release of excess serotonin, which then causes abnormal hyperperfusion to the involved lung due to the lack of hypoxic vasoconstriction (serotonin causes vasodilation).[47,50-53] Other factors include the development of distal fibroblast plugs consistent with organizing pneumonia (OP), possible viral effects on carotid body chemoreceptors and microvascular thrombosis.[47,50-53] Many of these patients demonstrate preserved lung mechanics, including normal lung compliance. Rapid deterioration of clinical status has been observed in these patients.[47,50-53]

The major pulmonary pathologic findings in postmortem studies are, unsurprisingly, diffuse alveolar damage, given that this is the end result of all forms of lung injury, and a surprisingly high incidence of OP or acute fibrinous organizing pneumonia (AFOP) (**Fig. 7.1a–d**).[52,54,55] A critical limitation of the pathologic literature is the near-complete lack of tissue biopsy in the early pulmonary phase. This is important because the radiology literature strongly suggests that, in virtually all cases, OP is the initial form of lung injury observed, likely explaining the profound response to corticosteroids.[52,56] Furthermore, in most autopsy studies, COVID-19 patients who died of respiratory failure in contrast to historical controls of patients expiring from other forms of ARDS had a predominance of endotheliitis, microvascular injury, microthrombi, and thromboembolic disease.[3,50,57] One study showed microvascular thrombosis affecting greater than 25% of the lung parenchyma in 87% of cases.[3,50,57] Borczuk et al reported that although 71% of patients in their study received some form of anticoagulation,

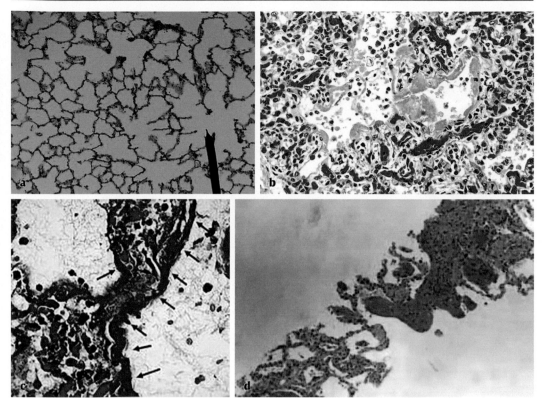

Fig. 7.1 (a) Normal alveoli. (https://www.newworldencyclopedia.org/entry/New_World_ Encyclopedia:Creative_Commons_CC-by-sa_3.0; https://www.newworldencyclopedia.org/p/index. php?title=Pulmonary_alveolus&oldid=988660) **(b)** Diffuse alveolar damage (DAD). (https://www. newworldencyclopedia.org/p/index.php?title=Pulmonary_alveolus&oldid=988660; https://commons. wikimedia.org/wiki/User:Nephron / https://fhs.mcmaster.ca/pathology/contact_us/faculty/faculty_ bios/Bonert.html) **(c)** Diffuse alveolar damage with hyaline membranes (arrows). (Maiese, A., Manetti, A. C., La Russa, R., Di Paolo, M., Turillazzi, E., Frati, P., & Fineschi, V. (2021). Autopsy findings in COVID-19-related deaths: a literature review. Forensic science, medicine, and pathology, 17(2), 279–296. https:// doi.org/10.1007/s12024-020-00310-8 http://creativecommons.org/licenses/by/4.0) **(d)** DAD with acute fibrinous and organizing pneumonia. (Gomes, R., Padrão, E., Dabó, H., Soares Pires, F., Mota, P., Melo, N., Jesus, J. M., Cunha, R., Guimarães, S., Souto Moura, C., & Morais, A. (2016). Acute fibrinous and organizing pneumonia: A report of 13 cases in a tertiary university hospital. Medicine, 95(27), e4073. http:// creativecommons.org/licenses/by/4.0)

46% demonstrated large vessel thrombosis, and 88% demonstrated microthrombosis in the pulmonary microcirculation.[3]

It is essential to note that during the SARS-CoV-1 epidemic OP and AFOP were reported in 30 to 60% of ICU cases, and in many respects, the clinical presentation, chest computed tomography (CT) radiographic findings, and postmortem studies suggest that CARDS represents a viral triggered OP.[52,58] COVID-19 chest CT findings reveal the archetypal form of OP as evidenced by a temporal progression of disease from peripheral ground-glass opacities (GGO) to progressive bilateral GGO, organizing consolidations, and dense consolidations (**Fig. 7.2**).[56,59–61]

The initial clinical presentation of CARDS can be quite heterogeneous. Patients can be profoundly hypoxemic with no evidence of distress, or severely hypoxemic with normocapnia, hypocapnia, or hypercapnia. The response to nitrous oxide, ventilator recruitment procedures, and prone ventilation can be variable.[28,29,62–65]

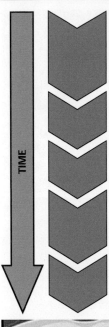

- Peripheral, patchy, predominantly basal ground glass opacification (GGO). GGO is defined an increase in density of lung with visualization of bronchial and vascular structures through it.
- Progressive widespread bilateral GGO.

- Crazy paving (CGO with interlobular and intralobular septal thickening).
- Air space consolidation (air bronchograms).

- Dense airspace consolidation.
- Coalescent consolidation.

- Segmental/subsegmental pulmonary vessel dilatation
- Bronchial wall thickening.
- Linear opacities.

- Traction bronchiectasis.
- Cavitation.
- Fibrotic changes with bullae and reticulation.

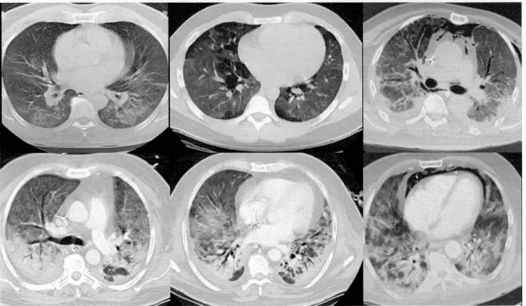

Fig. 7.2 Progression of severity of pulmonary disease during the clinical course of COVID-19 pulmonary disease. (Images provided courtesy of Paul Marik and Pierre Kory)

Given that CARDS is distinct from "traditional" ARDS in that it initially presents with a lack of alveolar edema in early phases, a central focus of debate has been on the relative importance of the need to adhere to strict ARDS net protocols.[28,29,64] Some observations and studies support little or no difference in CARDS versus ARDS patients, emphasizing there should be no deviation from lung-protective strategies and alveolar recruitment techniques.[30,34,64,66] In contrast to ARDS from other causes, Gattinoni and colleagues reporting on 150 CARDS patients from northern Italy identified two different phenotypes of patients with CARDS, termed L and H phenotypes. Differing from ARDS, CARDS L phenotype representing 50% of their series demonstrated normal compliance for the degree of PaO_2/FiO_2 (low elastance), normal or near-normal lung water (low lung water), normal or near-normal expired gas volumes, low V/Q (low V/Q ratio), and poor recruitability of alveoli to maneuvers such as PEEP (low recruitability).[28,29,31] CARDS H phenotype representing approximately 20 to 30% of cases are not dissimilar to ARDS from other causes manifesting low compliance (high elastance), high lung water, high right to left shunt, and high recruitability. It has been proposed that type L phenotype will progress to type H phenotype due to the severity of infection, host factors, immune phenomena, and self-induced lung injury (SILI) due to rising negative intrathoracic pressures as patients become increasingly dyspneic.[28,29,67,68]

The implementation of positive pressure of noninvasive positive-pressure ventilation or MV may also precipitate ventilator-induced lung injury.[67,68] Chiumello et al compared chest CT scans and physiologic variables in CARDS patients and two different ARDS populations, and found that CARDS patients demonstrated higher compliance and nearly double the end-expiratory gas volume, CARDS patients had lower PaO_2/FiO_2 ratios when matched with ARDS patients with the same compliance, and, in contrast to ARS patients in whom PaO_2/FiO_2 decreases linearly with decreases in compliance, there was no such relationship in patients with CARDS.[31] The investigators noted that increasing PEEP from 5 to 15 mm Hg in PaO_2/FiO_2 matched ARDS patients' improved dead space, improved $PACO_2$ and respiratory mechanics, and remained unchanged or worsened in patients with CARDS, suggesting that CARDS patients are at risk for alveolar overdistension and barotrauma.[31] Grasselli et al, in a study comparing CARDS patients to a previously collected dataset of patients with ARDS, discovered that compliance was 28% higher, and up to 6% of patients with CARDS had compliance greater than 95%.[30] Similar

to the Chiumello cohort of patients, as PaO_2/FiO_2 decreased, static compliance decreased in the ARDS group, while in the CARDS group, this relationship with PaO_2/FiO_2 was not observed.[30,31]

Thus, the major cause of hypoxemic respiratory failure in CARDS is V/Q mismatch, with the major driving force of hypoxemia likely being the dysregulated microcirculatory function as opposed to the alveolar compartment in typical ARDS.[28,29,31,69,70] In addition to the theory that excess serotonin from platelet activation underlies the pulmonary vasodilation in affected areas, other causes may be due to disruption of the normal homeostatic mechanism mediated by the local renin–angiotensin system of the microvascular endothelium.[53,71] Although this occurs when the SARS-CoV-2 virus invades cells of the alveolar-capillary units, a common misconception of the pulmonary phase is that the opacities result from viral invasion and are then described as "viral pneumonia." This is yet another misnomer, given that in only 20% of autopsies can viral cytopathic changes be found.[72]

Thus, although viral invasion is not common, it should be noted that it disrupts the healthy state when it occurs. Homeostasis is maintained by a balance of vasodilatory and vasoconstrictor molecules. Membrane bound ACE2 catalyzes angiotensin 2 (A2), a vasoconstrictive, inflammatory prothrombotic peptide, into Ang 1-7, which has anti-inflammatory, antithrombotic, vasodilatory properties.[71,73,74] ACE2 also catalyzes A1 into Ang 1-9, a powerful activator of the vasodilatory bradykinin system. The binding of SARS-CoV-2 to membrane bound (ACE2) on susceptible cells of alveolar-capillary unit results in downregulation of ACE2; ADAM17 proteolytically cleaves soluble ACE2, resulting in further downregulation of ACE2. The result is a vasoplegic, proinflammatory, and prothrombotic state inducing microvascular thrombosis and loss of appropriate hypoxia-induced vasoconstriction.[71,73,74]

From the beginning of the pandemic, there has been a paradigm shift from early intubation in CARDS patients to a more step-wise approach favoring late intubation when necessary. Initially, due to fears of a rapid and sometimes unpredictable deterioration of CARDS patients, experts recommended early MV in patients who demonstrated severe hypoxemia that did not improve within 2 hours of increasing oxygen or other forms of noninvasive ventilation (NIV).[75,76] Another concern was the development of SILI as a result of rapid swings in intrathoracic pressures due to increasing dyspnea and respiratory drive of spontaneously breathing hypoxemic CARDS patients receiving oxygenation with high-flow nasal cannula (HFNC) and other forms of NIV.[28,67,68] Gattinoni et al, in a small series of patients, observed that patients transitioned from an L phenotype to an H phenotype after 1 week on NIV, suggesting that SILI was a potential initiating event.[28] Furthermore, data from the LUNG SAFE study demonstrated increased mortality in patients with ARDS on NIV, which generated spontaneous tidal volumes greater than 9 mL/kg.[77] Thus, there is no clear-cut threshold as to when a patient with CARDS should be initiated on MV. A recent meta-analysis and systematic review involving 12 studies and over 8,000 patients found no difference between the timing of MV and patient morbidity or mortality.[78] Given the known higher mortality of MV, it appears reasonable to delay initiation as long as tolerable. Thus, current evidence is mounting supporting a stepwise conservative approach alongside close clinical monitoring of patients' respiratory status in the decision to initiate MV.[68,76,79-83]

Management

Details on treatment and management of hospitalized patients will be extensively covered in other chapters and will briefly be mentioned in this section. Hypoxemia should not be the major criterion for MV. Therefore, we recommend a stepwise approach to respiratory support and try to delay intubation if at all possible, accepting permissive hypoxemia keeping O_2 saturations greater than 80% unless there is evidence of oxygen debt demonstrated by lactic acidosis or desaturations of central venous blood (**Table 7.1**).[84-90] Other causes of worsening or refractory hypoxemia should be sought as secondary bacterial infections, and large vessel thromboembolic events are not uncommon.[91-94] Initial employment of oxygen support should begin with the administration of O_2 via nasal cannula 1 to 6 L/min and escalation to HFNC up to 60 to 80 L/min if oxygenation goals are not met.[86,87,95] One should consider MV in patients on NIV who generate tidal volumes of greater than 9 mL/kg despite measures to attenuate large swings in intrathoracic pressures.[77] If tolerated, awake prone positioning should be attempted. Should patients require MV, volume-protective strategies should be employed with the lowest driving pressure (<15 cm H_2O) and lowest possible PEEP. If the decision to employ prone MV is made, it should be maintained for 16 to 18 hours.[86,87,95] Neuromuscular blockade and sedation may be needed (**Table 7.1**).

COVID-19 respiratory disease, best described as secondary OP in its early stages and CARDS later, is a severe inflammatory disease highly responsive to glucocorticoid therapy.[96-100] The benefits of therapy appear to be time-dependent.[97-99,101] Early aggressive treatment is critical to prevent disease progression, as delays in therapy may limit disease reversibility. Thus, the first task of the clinician is to determine the reversibility of the pulmonary disease by assessing the time of onset of symptoms and employing chest CT to determine the extent and stage of pulmonary involvement as GGO pattern is significantly more prevalent in early-phase disease compared with the late-phase disease. In contrast, consolidation patterns are significantly more common in the late phase.[61,102-105] Monitoring D-dimer and C-reactive protein (CRP) may assist in predicting outcome.[20,106] Intubated patients who have low pulmonary compliance and elevated D-dimers or progressive elevations in D-dimer are associated with poor prognosis.[30] Elevated CRP levels with declines in levels upon initiation

Table 7.1 Strategies for respiratory support with a focus on preventing intubation

General schema for respiratory support in patients with COVID-19
Try to avoid intubation if posible

DETERIORATION → ← **RECOVERY**

Low flow nasal cannula
- Typically set at 1–6 L/minute

High flow nasal cannula
- Accept permissive hypoxemia (O_2 Saturation > 86%)
- Titrate FiO_2 based on patient's saturation
- Accept flow rates of 60 to 80 L/min
- Trial of inhaled Flolan (epoprostenol)
- Attempt proning (cooperative proning)

Invasive mechanical ventilation
- Target tidal volumes of –6 cc/kg
- Lowest driving pressure and PEEP
- Sedation to avoid self-extubation
- Trial of inhaled Flolan

Prone positioning
- Exact indication for prone ventilation is unclear.
Consider in patients with PaO_2/FiO_2 ratio <150.

Salvage Therapies
- High dose corticosteroids; 120–250 mg methylprednisolone q6-8
- Plasma exchange
- "Half-dose" rTPA

of anti-inflammatory/immunomodulatory therapy suggest reversibility of pulmonary disease.[97,105,107,108]

In patients requiring respiratory support, glucocorticoid therapy has been shown to reduce mortality.[100] The RECOVERY trial randomized 2,104 patients to receive dexamethasone 6 mg (equivalent to 32-mg methylprednisolone) once daily (by mouth or intravenous injection) for 10 days, versus 4,321 patients who received standard treatment.[100] In ventilated patients, dexamethasone reduced mortality by roughly 30% (rate ratio, 0.65 [95% confidence interval, 0.48– 0.88]; p = 0.01).[100] A recent study from the COVID-19 SPANISH ICU Network demonstrated that pre-ICU corticosteroids and corticosteroids administered within 48 hours of admission to the ICU reduced mortality.[101] However, patients who received late corticosteroids had an increase in mortality and a high risk for secondary infection.[101] Their study underscores the importance of early anti-inflammatory therapy in the pulmonary phase of COVID-19. Furthermore (and most importantly), early high-dose corticosteroids, far higher than those employed in the RECOVERY trial of dexamethasone (>1 mg/kg methylprednisolone eq/day), were associated with far more reduced mortality compared to early low-dose corticosteroids.[101]

Studies employing methylprednisolone and hydrocortisone in CARDS are described in **Table 7.2**.[97,98,109–114]

Table 7.2 Published studies on corticosteroid in the treatment of CARDS

Published RCT's/Cohort Studies of Corticosteroid Therapy in COVID-19		Absolute Difference in Mortality Rate (Rx Group vs. Control Group)	Estimated Number Needed to Treat to Save One Life
Methylprednisone—Hospital patients (Edalatifard et al, Iran)		5.9% vs. 42.9%	2.7
Methylprednisone—ICU patients (Salton et al, Italy)		7.2% vs. 23.3%	6.2
Methlprednisone—Hospital patients, (Fadel et al, USA)		13.6% vs 26.3%	7.8
Methylprednisone—Ards patients (Wu C et al, China)		46.0% vs 61.8%	6.3
Methylpredinsone—Pts on oxygen – (Fernandez-Cruz, Spain)		13.9% vs 23.9%	10.0
CoDEX—dexamethasone—mechanical ventilation		56.3% vs 61.5%	**19.2**
Recovery trial (dexamathasone)	PTS ON oxygen	23.3% vs 26.2%	**28.6**
	PTS ON MV	29.3% vs 41.4%	**8.4**
Hydrocortisone-cape-COVID—ICU patients (DEQUIN et al France)		14.7% vs 27.4%	7.9
Hydrocortisone—remap-CAP—ICU patients		28% vs 33%	20.0

Source: Courtesy of Pierre Kory.

Combatting the thrombotic manifestations of COVID-19 in general and CARDS in particular is essential. Observational studies have demonstrated that therapeutic anticoagulation was associated with survival, and a longer duration of anticoagulation was associated with a survival benefit in CARDS patients on MV. Interim analysis of the ATTACC, ACTIVE IV-1, and REMAP-CAP trial revealed that in critically ill COVID-19 patients with CARDS on organ support, therapeutic anticoagulation did not improve survival compared to thromboprophylaxis doses of heparin.[115] In contrast, regardless of D-dimer levels, in patients with moderate disease not in the ICU, full-dose anticoagulation resulted in a significant survival benefit.[115]

In ICU patients with severe COVID-19, if full-dose anticoagulation has not already been started before ICU admission, initiation of full dose should be avoided, and these patients should instead receive thromboprophylactic doses of heparin.[115] Patients who have been transitioned from medical floors to the ICU should remain on full-dose anticoagulation unless a contraindication has occurred.[115] Given the role of activated platelets in the pathogenesis of immunothrombosis observed with COVID-19, aspirin administration should be considered. In a recent observational trial, it was reported that the use of aspirin within 24 hours of hospital admission or in the 7 days before hospital admission was associated with a decreased need for MV, ICU admission, and in-hospital mortality.[116]

Conclusion

Respiratory failure progressing to multiorgan failure is the primary cause of death in patients with COVID-19 infection. Although increasing viral load may play a factor, the development of CARDS is mainly due to the host immune response rather than virulence of SARS-CoV-2. CARDS displays many pathologic features of an OP and is very responsive to corticosteroids and anti-inflammatory, immune modulating therapy. CARDS, in the early phases, may present with some atypical features and phenotypes of not commonly seen in classic ARDS. When compared to classic ARDS, CARDS patients' pulmonary pathology is much more vasculocentric manifesting with endotheliitis, microvascular, and macrovascular thrombosis and injury. Despite these differences, lung-protective strategies should be employed and recruitment strategies (PEEP) should be modified according to the patient's response. Delaying endotracheal intubation and tolerating moderate hypoxemia has not resulted in worsening outcome. CARDS is a highly inflammatory and coagulopathic disease, and corticosteroids, anti-inflammatory, and antithrombotic strategies should be initiated during the pulmonary phase of this disease.

References

1. Gengler I, Wang JC, Speth MM, Sedaghat AR. Sinonasal pathophysiology of SARS-CoV-2 and COVID-19: a systematic review of the current evidence. Laryngoscope Investig Otolaryngol 2020;5(3):354–359

2. Singh H, Choudhari R, Nema V, Khan AA. ACE2 and TMPRSS2 polymorphisms in various diseases with special reference to its impact on COVID-19 disease. Microb Pathog 2021;150:104621

3. Borczuk AC, Salvatore SP, Seshan SV, et al. COVID-19 pulmonary pathology: a multi-institutional autopsy cohort from Italy and New York City. Mod Pathol 2020;33(11): 2156–2168

4. Shah VK, Firmal P, Alam A, Ganguly D, Chattopadhyay S. Overview of immune response during SARS-CoV-2 infection: lessons from the past. Front Immunol 2020; 11:1949

5. Sungnak W, Huang N, Bécavin C, et al; HCA Lung Biological Network. SARS-CoV-2 entry factors are highly expressed in nasal epithelial cells together with innate immune genes. Nat Med 2020;26(5):681–687

6. Gallo O, Locatello LG, Mazzoni A, Novelli L, Annunziato F. The central role of the nasal microenvironment in the transmission, modulation, and clinical progression of SARS-CoV-2 infection. Mucosal Immunol 2021;14(2):305–316

7. Chua RL, Lukassen S, Trump S, et al. COVID-19 severity correlates with airway epithelium-immune cell interactions identified by single-cell analysis. Nat Biotechnol 2020;38(8):970–979

8. Azkur AK, Akdis M, Azkur D, et al. Immune response to SARS-CoV-2 and mechanisms of immunopathological changes in COVID-19. Allergy 2020;75(7):1564–1581

9. Chowdhury MA, Hossain N, Kashem MA, Shahid MA, Alam A. Immune response in COVID-19: a review. J Infect Public Health 2020;13(11):1619–1629

10. García LF. Immune response, inflammation, and the clinical spectrum of COVID-19. Front Immunol 2020;11:1441

11. Schreiber G. The role of type I interferons in the pathogenesis and treatment of COVID-19. Front Immunol 2020;11:595739

12. Schultze JL, Aschenbrenner AC. COVID-19 and the human innate immune system. Cell 2021;184(7):1671–1692

13. Mu J, Fang Y, Yang Q, et al. SARS-CoV-2 N protein antagonizes type I interferon signaling by suppressing phosphorylation and nuclear translocation of STAT1 and STAT2. Cell Discov 2020;6(1):65

14. Catanzaro M, Fagiani F, Racchi M, Corsini E, Govoni S, Lanni C. Immune response in COVID-19: addressing a pharmacological challenge by targeting pathways triggered by SARS-CoV-2. Signal Transduct Target Ther 2020;5(1):84

15. Acharya D, Liu G, Gack MU. Dysregulation of type I interferon responses in COVID-19. Nat Rev Immunol 2020;20(7):397–398

16. Blanco-Melo D, Nilsson-Payant BE, Liu W-C, et al. Imbalanced host response to SARS-CoV-2 drives development of COVID-19. Cell 2020;181(5):1036–1045.e9

17. Calabrese LH, Winthrop K, Strand V, Yazdany J, Walter JE. Type I interferon, anti-interferon antibodies, and COVID-19. Lancet Rheumatol 2021;3(4):e246–e247

18. Bastard P, Rosen LB, Zhang Q, et al; HGID Lab; NIAID-USUHS Immune Response to COVID Group; COVID Clinicians; COVID-STORM

Clinicians; Imagine COVID Group; French COVID Cohort Study Group; Milieu Intérieur Consortium; CoV-Contact Cohort; Amsterdam UMC Covid-19 Biobank; COVID Human Genetic Effort. Autoantibodies against type I IFNs in patients with life-threatening COVID-19. Science 2020;370 (6515):eabd4585

19. Zhang Q, Bastard P, Liu Z, et al; COVID-STORM Clinicians; COVID Clinicians; Imagine COVID Group; French COVID Cohort Study Group; CoV-Contact Cohort; Amsterdam UMC Covid-19 Biobank; COVID Human Genetic Effort; NIAID-USUHS/TAGC COVID Immunity Group. Inborn errors of type I IFN immunity in patients with life-threatening COVID-19. Science 2020;370(6515):eabd4570

20. Huang C, Wang Y, Li X, et al. Clinical features of patients infected with 2019 novel coronavirus in Wuhan, China. Lancet 2020; 395(10223):497–506

21. Yang M. Cell pyroptosis, a potential pathogenic mechanism of 2019-nCoV infection. January 29, 2020. Available at: http://dx.doi.org/10.2139/ssrn.3527420

22. Chen I-Y, Moriyama M, Chang M-F, Ichinohe T. Severe acute respiratory syndrome coronavirus viroporin 3a activates the NLRP3 inflammasome. Front Microbiol 2019;10:50

23. Carcaterra M, Caruso C. Alveolar epithelial cell type II as main target of SARS-CoV-2 virus and COVID-19 development via NF-Kb pathway deregulation: a physio-pathological theory. Med Hypotheses 2021;146:110412

24. Bermejo-Martin JF, González-Rivera M, Almansa R, et al. Viral RNA load in plasma is associated with critical illness and a dysregulated host response in COVID-19. Crit Care 2020;24(1):691

25. Cummings MJ, Baldwin MR, Abrams D, et al. Epidemiology, clinical course, and outcomes of critically ill adults with COVID-19 in New York City: a prospective cohort study. Lancet 2020;395(10239):1763–1770

26. Du R-H, Liu L-M, Yin W, et al. Hospitalization and critical care of 109 decedents with COVID-19 pneumonia in Wuhan, China. Ann Am Thorac Soc 2020;17(7):839–846

27. Wu Z, McGoogan JM. Characteristics of and important lessons from the coronavirus disease 2019 (COVID-19) outbreak in China: summary of a report of 72 314 cases from the Chinese Center for Disease Control and Prevention. JAMA 2020;323(13):1239–1242

28. Gattinoni L, Chiumello D, Caironi P, et al. COVID-19 pneumonia: different respiratory treatments for different phenotypes? Intensive Care Med 2020;46(6):1099–1102

29. Gattinoni L, Coppola S, Cressoni M, Busana M, Rossi S, Chiumello D. COVID-19 does not lead to a "typical" acute respiratory distress syndrome. Am J Respir Crit Care Med 2020;201(10):1299–1300

30. Grasselli G, Tonetti T, Protti A, et al; collaborators. Pathophysiology of COVID-19-associated acute respiratory distress syndrome: a multicentre prospective observational study. Lancet Respir Med 2020; 8(12):1201–1208

31. Chiumello D, Busana M, Coppola S, et al. Physiological and quantitative CT-scan characterization of COVID-19 and typical ARDS: a matched cohort study. Intensive Care Med 2020;46(12):2187–2196

32. Wunsch H. Mechanical ventilation in COVID-19: interpreting the current epidemiology. Am J Respir Crit Care Med 2020;202(1):1–4

33. Richardson S, Hirsch JS, Narasimhan M, et al; the Northwell COVID-19 Research Consortium. Presenting characteristics, comorbidities, and outcomes among 5700 patients hospitalized with COVID-19 in the New York City Area. JAMA 2020;323(20): 2052–2059

34. Grasselli G, Zangrillo A, Zanella A, et al; COVID-19 Lombardy ICU Network. Baseline characteristics and outcomes of 1591 patients infected with SARS-CoV-2 admitted to ICUs of the Lombardy region, Italy. JAMA 2020;323(16):1574–1581

35. Petrilli CM, Jones SA, Yang J, et al. Factors associated with hospital admission and critical illness among 5279 people with coronavirus disease 2019 in New York City: prospective cohort study. BMJ 2020; 369:m1966

36. Wang Y, Lu X, Li Y, et al. Clinical course and outcomes of 344 intensive care patients with COVID-19. Am J Respir Crit Care Med 2020;201(11):1430–1434

37. Zhou F, Yu T, Du R, et al. Clinical course and risk factors for mortality of adult inpatients with COVID-19 in Wuhan, China: a retrospective cohort study. Lancet 2020; 395(10229):1054–1062

38. Jutzeler CR, Bourguignon L, Weis CV, et al. Comorbidities, clinical signs and symptoms, laboratory findings, imaging features, treatment strategies, and outcomes in adult and pediatric patients with COVID-19: a systematic review and meta-analysis. Travel Med Infect Dis 2020;37:101825

39. Huang Y, Lu Y, Huang Y-M, et al. Obesity in patients with COVID-19: a systematic review and meta-analysis. Metabolism 2020;113:154378

40. Ortiz-Prado E, Simbaña-Rivera K, Gómez-Barreno L, et al. Clinical, molecular, and epidemiological characterization of the SARS-CoV-2 virus and the Coronavirus Disease 2019 (COVID-19), a comprehensive literature review. Diagn Microbiol Infect Dis 2020;98(1):115094

41. Ruan Q, Yang K, Wang W, Jiang L, Song J. Clinical predictors of mortality due to COVID-19 based on an analysis of data of 150 patients from Wuhan, China. Intensive Care Med 2020;46(5):846–848

42. Schlesinger T, Weißbrich B, Wedekink F, et al. Biodistribution and serologic response in SARS-CoV-2 induced ARDS: a cohort study. PLoS One 2020;15(11):e0242917

43. Dorward DA, Russell CD, Um IH, et al. Tissue-specific immunopathology in fatal COVID-19. Am J Respir Crit Care Med 2021; 203(2):192–201

44. Booz GW, Altara R, Eid AH, et al. Macrophage responses associated with COVID-19: a pharmacological perspective. Eur J Pharmacol 2020;887:173547

45. Xie J, Covassin N, Fan Z, et al. Association between hypoxemia and mortality in patients with COVID-19. Mayo Clin Proc 2020;95(6):1138–1147

46. Zubieta-Calleja G, Zubieta-DeUrioste N. Pneumolysis and "silent hypoxemia" in COVID-19. Indian J Clin Biochem 2020; 36(1):1–5

47. Tobin MJ, Laghi F, Jubran A. Why COVID-19 silent hypoxemia is baffling to physicians. Am J Respir Crit Care Med 2020;202(3): 356–360

48. Nouri-Vaskeh M, Sharifi A, Khalili N, Zand R, Sharifi A. Dyspneic and non-dyspneic (silent) hypoxemia in COVID-19: possible neurological mechanism. Clin Neurol Neurosurg 2020;198:106217

49. Simonson TS, Baker TL, Banzett RB, et al. Silent hypoxaemia in COVID-19 patients. J Physiol 2021;599(4):1057–1065

50. Nicolai L, Leunig A, Brambs S, et al. Immunothrombotic dysregulation in COVID-19 pneumonia is associated with respiratory failure and coagulopathy. Circulation 2020; 142(12):1176–1189

51. Iba T, Connors JM, Levy JH. The coagulopathy, endotheliopathy, and vasculitis of COVID-19. Inflamm Res 2020;69(12):1181–1189

52. Kory P, Kanne JP. SARS-CoV-2 organising pneumonia: 'Has there been a widespread failure to identify and treat this prevalent condition in COVID-19?'. BMJ Open Respir Res 2020;7(1):e000724

53. Jalali F, Rezaie S, Rola P, Kyle-Sidell C. COVID-19 pathophysiology: are platelets and serotonin hiding in plain sight? February 5, 2021. Available at: http://dx.doi.org/10.2139/ssrn.3800402

54. Hariri LP, North CM, Shih AR, et al. Lung histopathology in coronavirus disease 2019 as compared with severe acute respiratory sydrome and H1N1 influenza: a systematic review. Chest 2021;159(1):73–84

55. Copin M-C, Parmentier E, Duburcq T, Poissy J, Mathieu D; Lille COVID-19 ICU and Anatomopathology Group. Time to consider histologic pattern of lung injury to treat critically ill patients with COVID-19 infection. Intensive Care Med 2020;46(6):1124–1126

56. Kanne JP, Little BP, Chung JH, Elicker BM, Ketai LH. Essentials for radiologists on COVID-19: an update-*Radiology* Scientific Expert Panel. Radiology 2020;296(2):E113–E114

57. Ackermann M, Verleden SE, Kuehnel M, et al. Pulmonary vascular endothelialitis, thrombosis, and angiogenesis in Covid-19. N Engl J Med 2020;383(2):120–128

58. Hwang DM, Chamberlain DW, Poutanen SM, Low DE, Asa SL, Butany J. Pulmonary pathology of severe acute respiratory syndrome in Toronto. Mod Pathol 2005;18(1):1–10

59. Ooi GC, Khong PL, Müller NL, et al. Severe acute respiratory syndrome: temporal lung changes at thin-section CT in 30 patients. Radiology 2004;230(3):836–844

60. Ye Z, Zhang Y, Wang Y, Huang Z, Song B. Chest CT manifestations of new coronavirus disease 2019 (COVID-19): a pictorial review. Eur Radiol 2020;30(8):4381–4389

61. Pan F, Ye T, Sun P, et al. Time course of lung changes at chest CT during recovery from coronavirus disease 2019 (COVID-19). Radiology 2020;295(3):715–721

62. Tavazzi G, Pozzi M, Mongodi S, Dammassa V, Romito G, Mojoli F. Inhaled nitric oxide in patients admitted to intensive care unit with COVID-19 pneumonia. Crit Care 2020; 24(1):508

63. Abou-Arab O, Huette P, Debouvries F, Dupont H, Jounieaux V, Mahjoub Y. Inhaled nitric oxide for critically ill Covid-19 patients: a prospective study. Crit Care 2020;24(1):645

64. Fan E, Beitler JR, Brochard L, et al. COVID-19-associated acute respiratory distress syndrome: is a different approach to management warranted? Lancet Respir Med 2020;8(8):816–821

65. Maley JH, Winkler T, Hardin CC. Heterogeneity of acute respiratory distress syndrome in COVID-19: "typical" or not? Am J Respir Crit Care Med 2020;202(4):618–619

66. Ziehr DR, Alladina J, Petri CR, et al. Respiratory pathophysiology of mechanically ventilated patients with COVID-19: a cohort study. Am J Respir Crit Care Med 2020; 201(12):1560–1564

67. Cruces P, Retamal J, Hurtado DE, et al. A physiological approach to understand the role of respiratory effort in the progression of lung injury in SARS-CoV-2 infection. Crit Care 2020;24(1):494

68. Windisch W, Weber-Carstens S, Kluge S, Rossaint R, Welte T, Karagiannidis C. Invasive and non-invasive ventilation in patients with COVID-19. Dtsch Arztebl Int 2020;117(31–32):528–533

69. Gattinoni L, Chiumello D, Rossi S. COVID-19 pneumonia: ARDS or not? Crit Care 2020; 24(1):154

70. Ridge CA, Desai SR, Jeyin N, et al. Dual-energy CT pulmonary angiography (DECTPA) quantifies vasculopathy in severe COVID-19 pneumonia. Radiol Cardiothorac Imaging 2020;2(5):e200428

71. Amraei R, Rahimi N. COVID-19, renin-angiotensin system and endothelial dysfunction. Cells 2020;9(7):E1652

72. Polak SB, Van Gool IC, Cohen D, von der Thüsen JH, van Paassen J. A systematic review of pathological findings in COVID-19: a pathophysiological timeline and possible mechanisms of disease progression. Mod Pathol 2020;33(11):2128–2138

73. Cheng H, Wang Y, Wang G-Q. Organ-protective effect of angiotensin-converting enzyme 2 and its effect on the prognosis of COVID-19. J Med Virol 2020;92(7):726–730

74. Bourgonje AR, Abdulle AE, Timens W, et al. Angiotensin-converting enzyme 2 (ACE2), SARS-CoV-2 and the pathophysiology of coronavirus disease 2019 (COVID-19). J Pathol 2020;251(3):228–248

75. Zuo M-Z, Huang Y-G, Ma W-H, et al; Airway Management Chinese Society of Anesthesiology Task Force on; Chinese Society of Anesthesiology Task Force on Airway Management. Expert recommendations for tracheal intubation in critically ill patients with noval coronavirus disease 2019. Chin Med Sci J 2020;35(2):105–109

76. Rola P, Farkas J, Spiegel R, et al. Rethinking the early intubation paradigm of COVID-19: time to change gears? Clin Exp Emerg Med 2020;7(2):78–80

77. Bellani G, Laffey JG, Pham T, et al; LUNG SAFE Investigators; ESICM Trials Group. Noninvasive ventilation of patients with acute respiratory distress syndrome. Insights from the LUNG SAFE study. Am J Respir Crit Care Med 2017;195(1):67–77

78. Papoutsi E, Giannakoulis VG, Xourgia E, Routsi C, Kotanidou A, Siempos II. Effect of timing of intubation on clinical outcomes of critically ill patients with COVID-19: a systematic review and meta-analysis of non-randomized cohort studies. Crit Care 2021;25(1):121

79. Lee YH, Choi K-J, Choi SH, et al. Clinical significance of timing of intubation in critically ill patients with COVID-19: a multi-center retrospective study. J Clin Med 2020;9(9):E2847

80. Voshaar T, Stais P, Köhler D, Dellweg D. Conservative management of COVID-19 associated hypoxaemia. ERJ Open Res 2021; 7(1):00026-2021

81. Tobin MJ, Laghi F, Jubran A. Caution about early intubation and mechanical ventilation in COVID-19. Ann Intensive Care 2020; 10(1):78

82. Brusasco C, Corradi F, Di Domenico A, et al. Continuous positive airway pressure in COVID-19 patients with moderate-to-severe

respiratory failure. Eur Respir J 2021; 57(2):2002524

83. Oranger M, Gonzalez-Bermejo J, Dacosta-Noble P, et al. Continuous positive airway pressure to avoid intubation in SARS-CoV-2 pneumonia: a two-period retrospective case-control study. Eur Respir J 2020; 56(2):2001692

84. He HW, Liu DW, Long Y, Wang XT. High central venous-to-arterial CO_2 difference/arterial-central venous O_2 difference ratio is associated with poor lactate clearance in septic patients after resuscitation. J Crit Care 2016;31(1):76–81

85. He H-W, Liu D-W. Permissive hypoxemia/conservative oxygenation strategy: Dr. Jekyll or Mr. Hyde? J Thorac Dis 2016;8(5):748–750

86. Hajjar LA, Costa IBSDS, Rizk SI, et al. Intensive care management of patients with COVID-19: a practical approach. Ann Intensive Care 2021;11(1):36

87. Alhazzani W, Møller MH, Arabi YM, et al. Surviving sepsis campaign: guidelines on the management of critically ill adults with coronavirus disease 2019 (COVID-19). Intensive Care Med 2020;46(5):854–887

88. Abdelsalam M, Cheifetz IM. Goal-directed therapy for severely hypoxic patients with acute respiratory distress syndrome: permissive hypoxemia. Respir Care 2010; 55(11):1483–1490

89. Panwar R, Hardie M, Bellomo R, et al; CLOSE Study Investigators; ANZICS Clinical Trials Group. Conservative versus liberal oxygenation targets for mechanically ventilated patients. A pilot multicenter randomized controlled trial. Am J Respir Crit Care Med 2016;193(1):43–51

90. Raoof S, Nava S, Carpati C, Hill NS. High-flow, noninvasive ventilation and awake (nonintubation) proning in patients with coronavirus disease 2019 with respiratory failure. Chest 2020;158(5):1992–2002

91. Klok FA, Kruip MJHA, van der Meer NJM, et al. Incidence of thrombotic complications in critically ill ICU patients with COVID-19. Thromb Res 2020;191:145–147

92. Helms J, Tacquard C, Severac F, et al; CRICS TRIGGERSEP Group (Clinical Research in Intensive Care and Sepsis Trial Group for Global Evaluation and Research in Sepsis). High risk of thrombosis in patients with severe SARS-CoV-2 infection: a multicenter prospective cohort study. Intensive Care Med 2020;46(6):1089–1098

93. Maes M, Higginson E, Pereira-Dias J, et al. Ventilator-associated pneumonia in critically ill patients with COVID-19. Crit Care 2021;25(1):25

94. Suarez-de-la-Rica A, Serrano P, De-la-Oliva R, et al. Secondary infections in mechanically ventilated patients with COVID-19: an overlooked matter? Rev Esp Quimioter 2021; 34(4):330–336

95. Möhlenkamp S, Thiele H. Ventilation of COVID-19 patients in intensive care units. Herz 2020;45(4):329–331

96. Bani-Sadr F, Hentzien M, Pascard M, et al. Corticosteroid therapy for patients with COVID-19 pneumonia: a before-after study. Int J Antimicrob Agents 2020;56(2):106077

97. Salton F, Confalonieri P, Meduri GU, et al. Prolonged low-dose methylprednisolone in patients with severe COVID-19 pneumonia. Open Forum Infect Dis 2020;7(10):a421

98. Fadel R, Morrison AR, Vahia A, et al; Henry Ford COVID-19 Management Task Force. Early short-course corticosteroids in hospitalized patients with COVID-19. Clin Infect Dis 2020;71(16):2114–2120

99. Mongardon N, Piagnerelli M, Grimaldi D, Perrot B, Lascarrou JB; COVADIS study group investigators. Impact of late administration of corticosteroids in COVID-19 ARDS. Intensive Care Med 2021;47(1):110–112

100. Horby P, Lim WS, Emberson JR, et al; RECOVERY Collaborative Group. Dexamethasone in hospitalized patients with Covid-19. N Engl J Med 2021;384(8):693–704

101. Monedero P, Gea A, Castro P, et al; COVID-19 Spanish ICU Network. Early corticosteroids are associated with lower mortality in critically ill patients with COVID-19: a cohort study. Crit Care 2021;25(1):2

102. Ding X, Xu J, Zhou J, Long Q. Chest CT findings of COVID-19 pneumonia by duration of symptoms. Eur J Radiol 2020;127:109009

103. Yang R, Li X, Liu H, et al. Chest CT severity score: an imaging tool for assessing severe COVID-19. Radiol Cardiothorac Imaging 2020;2(2):e200047

104. Parry AH, Wani AH, Yaseen M, Shah NN, Dar KA. Clinicoradiological course in coronavirus disease-19 (COVID-19) patients who are

asymptomatic at admission. BJR Open 2020; 2(1):20200033

105. Francone M, Iafrate F, Masci GM, et al. Chest CT score in COVID-19 patients: correlation with disease severity and short-term prognosis. Eur Radiol 2020;30(12): 6808–6817

106. Kermali M, Khalsa RK, Pillai K, Ismail Z, Harky A. The role of biomarkers in diagnosis of COVID-19—a systematic review. Life Sci 2020;254:117788

107. Cui Z, Merritt Z, Assa A, et al. Early and significant reduction in C-reactive protein levels after corticosteroid therapy is associated with reduced mortality in patients with COVID-19. J Hosp Med 2021;16(3): 142–148

108. Letelier P, Encina N, Morales P, et al. Role of biochemical markers in the monitoring of COVID-19 patients. J Med Biochem 2021; 40(2):115–128

109. Edalatifard M, Akhtari M, Salehi M, et al. Intravenous methylprednisolone pulse as a treatment for hospitalised severe COVID-19 patients: results from a randomised controlled clinical trial. Eur Respir J 2020; 56(6):2002808

110. Fernández-Cruz A, Ruiz-Antorán B, Muñoz-Gómez A, et al. A retrospective controlled cohort study of the impact of glucocorticoid treatment in SARS-CoV-2 infection mortality. Antimicrob Agents Chemother 2020;64(9):e01168-20

111. Tomazini BM, Maia IS, Cavalcanti AB, et al; COALITION COVID-19 Brazil III Investigators. Effect of dexamethasone on days alive and ventilator-free in patients with moderate or severe acute respiratory distress syndrome and COVID-19: the CoDEX randomized clinical trial. JAMA 2020;324(13):1307–1316

112. Wu C, Hou D, Du C, et al. Corticosteroid therapy for coronavirus disease 2019–related acute respiratory distress syndrome: a cohort study with propensity score analysis. Crit Care 2020;24(1):643

113. Dequin P-F, Heming N, Meziani F, et al; CAPE COVID Trial Group and the CRICS-TriGGERSep Network. Effect of hydrocortisone on 21-day mortality or respiratory support among critically ill patients with COVID-19: a randomized clinical trial. JAMA 2020;324(13):1298–1306

114. Angus DC, Derde L, Al-Beidh F, et al; Writing Committee for the REMAP-CAP Investigators. Effect of hydrocortisone on mortality and organ support in patients with severe COVID-19: the REMAP-CAP COVID-19 corticosteroid domain randomized clinical trial. JAMA 2020;324(13):1317–1329

115. ATTACC, ACTIV-4a and REMAP-CAP Investigators. Results of interim analysis. March 26, 2021. Available at: https://static1.squarespace.com/static/5cde3c7d9a69340001d79ffe/t/6013892709de942b53f6e3da/1611893037749/mpRCT+interim+presentation_v21-slides+22+and+23+corrected.pdf

116. Chow JH, Khanna AK, Kethireddy S, et al. Aspirin use is associated with decreased mechanical ventilation, intensive care unit admission, and in-hospital mortality in hospitalized patients with coronavirus disease 2019. Anesth Analg 2021;132(4):930–941

COVID-19–Associated Renal Involvement and Acute Kidney Injury

Jose Iglesias and Jerrold S. Levine

Introduction

Acute kidney injury (AKI) is one of the most common extrapulmonary complications in patients hospitalized with COVID-19 infection and is associated with a significant increase in patient morbidity and mortality.[1] Early in the pandemic, reports from China demonstrated AKI rates ranging from 0.3 to 25%, contrasting with rates in the United States, Korea, and European nations, which ranged from 4.7% to as high as 72%.[2–7] The rate of AKI increases with increases in the severity of illness and with the need for escalation to critical care.[3–5,8] Differences in the incidence of AKI between China and other geographical locations are most likely due to differences in the age, race, severity of illness, genetic factors, and comorbidities of cohorts.[1,4,9] Cheng et al prospectively evaluated 701 hospitalized patients with COVID-19 and reported an incidence of AKI of 5.1%.[10] Proteinuria and hematuria were present in 44 and 23% of their patients, respectively.[10] In their study, the high prevalence of proteinuria and hematuria on admission may indicate glomerular involvement or chronic kidney disease (CKD) in those patients. Many patients were hospitalized after having symptoms for approximately 10 days, supporting the theory that direct virally induced tubular injury may have occurred prior to admission.[10] On biopsy, the most common pathologic finding is acute tubular necrosis (ATN), predominantly affecting the proximal tubule. In most series, a marked increase in mortality was observed in patients who developed ATN, with mortality increasing as the severity of AKI increased.[5–7,10] Patients requiring renal replacement therapy (RRT) have mortality rates as high as 70%.[1,11] Of those patients on RRT who survived hospitalization, many were discharged from the hospital still requiring dialysis, with no recovery of renal function.[5–7]

Overall, AKI in COVID-19 involves several mediators of injury. Risk factors for the development of AKI include elevated serum creatinine on admission, proteinuria, hematuria, elevated inflammatory markers, male sex, and black race.[1,3,6] Additional risk factors for AKI development are comorbidities such as hypertension and diabetes mellitus, hypoxemia, the need for vasopressor support, and mechanical ventilation (MV).[1,3,6] Initially, there had been considerable controversy regarding the continued use of angiotensin-converting enzyme 2 (ACE2) inhibitors and angiotensin 2 receptor antagonists, with some observations demonstrating an increased risk for AKI. Currently, however, there is overwhelming evidence that the use of these agents does not increase the risk of AKI.[12] Some evidence implicates the use of nonsteroidal anti-inflammatory drugs (NSAIDs) and vancomycin as independent risk factors for AKI development.[12,13] It seems likely that COVID-19-associated AKI is the result of multiple hits. These include the usual hemodynamic and nephrotoxic factors predisposing to ATN, pulmonary–renal crosstalk as observed in acute respiratory distress syndrome (ARDS), tubular and endothelial injury induced by the host response to severe acute respiratory syndrome coronavirus 2 (SARS-CoV-2), and direct virally induced damage. The role played by each of these potential hits may vary with the phase of the disease and is phase specific. By way of example, during the viremic phase, viral tropism for renal tubular epithelial cells and podocytes as well as prerenal factors may predominate, whereas during the early pulmonary phase and the later hyperinflammatory phase of the infection, pulmonary–renal crosstalk, cytokine storm–induced shock, endothelial injury with associated vascular dysregulation, and microvascular thrombosis may predominate (**Fig. 8.1**).

Viral Tropism and Potential Viral Cytopathic Effects

The relatively large amount of cellular ACE2 in renal tissue makes the kidney a potential nonpulmonary target of SARS-CoV-2.[14] Many

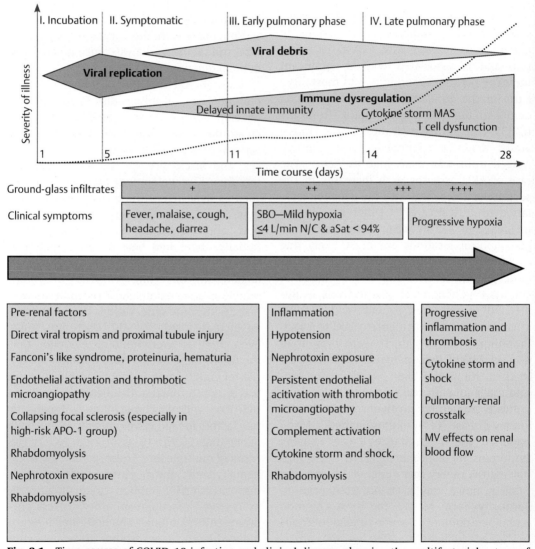

Fig. 8.1 Time course of COVID-19 infection and clinical disease, showing the multifactorial nature of AKI, with potential hits assuming greater or lesser importance at different stages of the disease. Renal insults do not strictly conform to the timeline, as significant overlap exists. However, during the viremic phase, viral tropic effects predominate. MAS, macrophage activation syndrome.

patients hospitalized with COVID-19 infection present with proteinuria and hematuria on admission.[10,15–17] Whether SARS-CoV-2 kidney infection occurs and results in viral cytopathic effect has been a matter of debate, with some studies demonstrating viral tropism and injury and others not.[18–22] Recent evidence supports viral renal tropism. The presence of SARS-CoV-2 in glomeruli and proximal tubules has been demonstrated in several ways, including immunostaining and hybridization of viral RNA.[21,22] Moreover, autopsy studies have retrieved replication-competent SARS-CoV-2.[23,24] Finally, electron microscopic imaging has revealed possible viral spike protein in renal tubular epithelial cells and glomerular visceral epithelial cells (podocytes). Recently, investigators demonstrated evidence of proximal tubular dysfunction, including low-molecular-weight proteinuria, abnormalities in urate and phosphate excretion, and aminoaciduria, in a subset of patients with COVID-19 infection.[25] Among patients infected with COVID-19, renal tissue obtained at autopsy or by biopsy has shown injury to glomerular podocytes.[21,26] Collapsing focal segmental glomerulosclerosis (CFSGS), not uncommonly observed with HIV and other viral infections, has been observed in some patients.[21,26] While the incidence of CFSGS is markedly increased in patients of African origin, especially in those with homozygosity in the high-risk ApoL1 allele, CFSGS is not restricted to this population (**Fig. 8.2a, b**).[26,27]

It remains controversial whether tubular and podocyte injury is related to direct viral cytopathic effects or to cytokine-driven toxicity.[23,24] Su et al, employing electron microscopic analysis of postmortem renal tissue, demonstrated cytoplasmic vesicular structures resembling coronavirus viral particles in both proximal tubular epithelial cells and podocytes.[21] The investigators concluded that these vesicular structures supply direct evidence of viral tropism.[21] However, direct viral tropism and viral cytopathic effects have been challenged by other investigators, who have shown that clathrin-coated pits in noninfected patients can resemble viral particles.[18,21,23,28,29]

Employing in situ hybridization and immunohistochemistry, Diao et al demonstrated the presence of viral RNA, nucleocapsid protein, and spike protein deposits in proximal tubular epithelial cells.[30] Furthermore, there was infiltration of the interstitium by CD68+ macrophages, along with deposition of the terminal complement complex C5–C9 localized to proximal

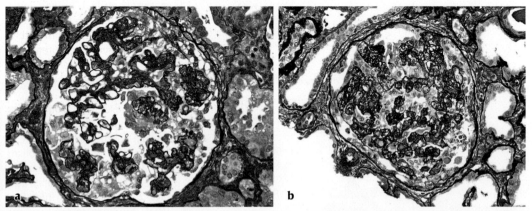

Fig. 8.2 **(a, b)** Collapsing variant of focal segmental sclerosis in a 55-year-old African American patient who presented with AKI and nephrotic range proteinuria. (The images are provided courtesy of Glen Markowitz, MD, Section of Renal Pathology, Department of Pathology, Columbia University College of Physicians and Surgeons.)

tubules.[30] Immunohistochemistry revealed colocalization of viral nucleocapsid and spike proteins, as well as the hypoxia-inducible proteins prostaglandin synthase and DP2 (prostaglandin D2 receptor-2).[30] Thus, SARS-CoV-2 potentially induces hypoxia-mediated tubular injury.[30] These findings support the concept of direct viral infection of proximal tubular epithelial cells with complement- and hypoxia-mediated initiation of inflammatory cascades.

In healthy individuals, macrovascular and microvascular homeostasis is maintained by a balance of opposing effects, including vasoconstrictive/vasodilatory, anti-inflammatory/proinflammatory, and antithrombotic/prothrombotic elements.[31,32] The major driver of vascular homeostasis at both a systemic and a local level is the renin–angiotensin system (RAS). Within this system, angiotensin II (AII) is the major effector.[31-34] An intact RAS system is essential for renal microcirculatory autoregulation, glomerular filtration, and overall homeostasis.[34-36] Among other properties, AII is a powerful vasoconstrictive and proinflammatory agent.[34,37,38] These effects[21,39] are mediated by binding of AII to its type 1 cell-surface receptor found on endothelial cells. Cell-surface ACE2 catalyzes the conversion of AII into angiotensin 1-7 (Ang 1-7). Ang 1-7 acting via its G-coupled receptor, MasR, mediates vasodilatory and anti-inflammatory effects, thereby counterbalancing the effects of AII[34,40] (**Fig. 8.3a, b**). The binding of SARS-CoV-2 to cell-surface ACE2 leads to the downregulation of ACE2. The resulting decreased conversion of AII to Ang 1-7 may produce an imbalance in the amounts of AII and Ang 1-17, with an increased ratio of AII to Ang 1-7 favoring the vasoconstrictive, proinflammatory, and prothrombotic effects of AII.[41-43] Such an imbalance is most likely to occur during the initial viremic phase of COVID-19, and the resulting homeostatic disruption of the renal microcirculation could predispose the kidney to the development of AKI.

In addition to ATN, AKI may also be the result of intrarenal thrombotic microangiopathy. Severe SARS-CoV-2 infection is associated with a dysregulated thromboinflammatory state characterized by thrombosis in microvascular and macrovascular systems.[44-49] Postmortem studies

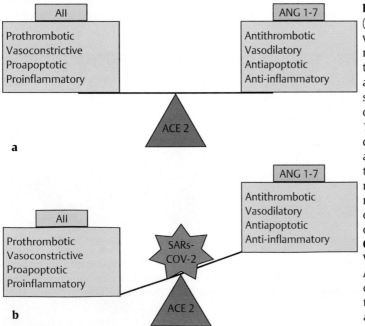

Fig. 8.3 (a) Angiotensin II (AII), a potent prothrombotic, vasoconstrictor, and proinflammatory peptide, is broken down to angiotensin 1-7 (Ang 1-7) and other peptides by cell-surface enzyme angiotensin II converting enzyme (ACE2). Ang 1-7 is itself antithrombotic, vasodilatory, and anti-inflammatory and therefore counteracts the effects of AII. Thus, under normal conditions, a balance is maintained by the metabolism of AII. **(b)** ACE2 on the surface of cells is a receptor for **SARS-CoV-2** during host infection. Viral binding to cell-surface ACE2 results in downregulation of surface ACE2 expression, thereby leading to a preponderance of the effects of AII.

have revealed endotheliitis and extensive thrombosis in the microcirculation of multiple organs.[39,50,51] Several lines of evidence suggest that the microvascular bed may be involved in COVID-19-associated AKI. Varga et al demonstrated endotheliitis and possible viral inclusion bodies in glomerular endothelial cells.[39] The postmortem study by Su et al described endothelial cell swelling and foamy degeneration in 5 out of 26 patients with AKI and glomerular fibrin thrombi in 3 out of 26 patients.[21] In addition, these same investigators described significant erythrocyte stagnation in glomerular capillary loops.[21] Together, these findings are consistent with virally mediated injury to the vascular endothelium. Similar findings of inflammatory injury, organ failure, and thrombosis have been observed in patients with disease states characterized by elevated levels of proinflammatory cytokines, such as macrophage activation syndrome and hemophagocytic lymphohistiocytic syndromes.[52-54]

Prerenal Insults, Other Causes of AKI, and Pulmonary Renal Crosstalk

During the symptomatic phase of COVID-19 infection, the patient may develop fever, loss of appetite, loss of taste and smell, and prominent gastrointestinal symptoms, resulting in a volume-depleted state. In this setting, the concurrent use of NSAIDs, diuretics, and agents that impact the renin–angiotensin–aldosterone system (RAAS), such as ACE2 inhibitors and angiotensin 2 receptor blockers, may lead to a prerenal state.[14,55-59] The risk and severity of prerenal states may be particularly pronounced in patients with preexisting endothelial dysfunction, as occurs with advanced age or in patient with comorbidities such as diabetes mellitus, CKD, or congestive heart failure.[1,3,60,61] Patients with COVID-19 are at increased risk for the development of a wide variety of nephrotoxic AKI.[1,14,58,62] In particular, AKI may occur because of rhabdomyolysis.[21,58]

The development of severe AKI usually coincides with the development of respiratory failure during the pulmonary phase of the illness.[55,63] Many patients with COVID-19-associated ARDS (CARDS) demonstrate the L phenotype of lung injury, characterized by low lung water (dry lungs) and low elastance.[64,65] These patients are either euvolemic or volume-depleted, and administration of diuretics in this setting may be detrimental.[59] In contrast, strategies employing prolonged aggressive volume expansion may lead to volume overload and the development of pulmonary edema, especially in association with cytokine-mediated inflammation and capillary leak. In this setting, volume overload can result in venous congestion, increases in intra-abdominal pressure, renal vein congestion, renal parenchymal interstitial edema, and further endothelial injury.[60,63,66,67] Persistent renal interstitial edema may result in loss of renal autoregulation, both of renal blood flow and of glomerular filtration rate (GFR).[68,69]

To prevent the deleterious effects of excessive volume expansion, we recommend clinical assessment of volume status, such as passive leg raising maneuvers, central venous pressure monitoring, assessment of capillary refill, and other available measures. Judicious fluid challenges of 500 to 1,000 mL of crystalloid solution should be administered to patients who are fluid responsive, particularly during the early phases of CARDS when many display the L phenotype. In fluid-responsive patients, volume expansion may be used to manage hypotension. During the later stages of illness, when patients demonstrate decreasing pulmonary compliance and recruiting ability, more restrictive fluid management should be employed, and active diuresis or ultrafiltration may need to be initiated.

Although patients with severe COVID-19 requiring hospitalization may present with renal dysfunction, severe AKI usually develops with the onset of respiratory failure progressing to CARDS and the need for MV. MV causes many physiologic changes, which impact renal hemodynamics and function.[63,66,68–71] MV increases intrathoracic pressure, leading to an increase in right ventricular afterload and a decrease in right ventricular preload. As a result, patients may develop fluid-responsive hypotension. Increasing intrathoracic pressures, particularly when positive end-expiratory pressure (PEEP) is employed, also results in increase release of antidiuretic hormone, aldosterone, and renin, leading to decreased urine output and GFR.[63,66,68,70–72] Theoretically, the release of renin induced by increasing intrathoracic pressure may worsen the imbalance between AII and Ang (1-7) in an already dysregulated renal micro-circulation.[71,73] As patients develop worsening CARDS with stiff lungs, MV and PEEP can increase intra-abdominal pressure, resulting in renal venous congestion and decreasing GFR.[63,66,68] Lung-protective ventilatory strategies result in permissive hypercapnia, often employed as a lung-protective strategy. It has the potential to impair autoregulation further.[66,74] Finally, worsening hypoxia can induce the release of hypoxia-inducible factors, resulting in proximal tubular injury.[72]

Crosstalk between the kidneys and lungs can result in worsening failure of both organs. The development of AKI increases proapoptotic pulmonary endothelial cell gene expression and apoptosis. The release of pro-inflammatory cytokines (interleukin 6 [IL-6], IL-1β, IL-12, IL-10, and granulocyte colony-stimulating factor) and vascular endothelial growth factor (VEGF) enhances pulmonary endothelial permeability, with worsening pulmonary edema.[75–80] Similarly, as in H1N1 influenza–associated ARDS, CARDS can increase the circulating levels of such pro-inflammatory chemokines and cytokines as VEGF, monocyte chemo-attractant protein-1 (MCP-1), IL-6, and IL-8, which have deleterious downstream renal effects.[77,79]

In summary, AKI is a multifactorial/multihit process that in some degree parallels the phases of SARS-CoV-2 infection. During the viremic and early symptomatic phase, viral tropism and cytopathic effects predominate and initiate injury. During the pulmonary phase, cytokine storm, ventilator-associated increases in intrathoracic pressure and hypotension, crosstalk between the lungs and kidneys, widespread inflammation, and thrombotic events exacerbate injury. Other "hits" include viral myositis and possibly rhabdomyolysis.[21,58,81,82] Superimposed nephrotoxic tubular injury has also been reported.[55,57,58,62] As organ failure progresses, patients with COVID-19-associated AKI develop oliguria and severe electrolyte abnormalities.

Electrolyte-Associated Abnormalities during the Clinical Course during Severe COVID-19

Electrolyte disturbances during COVID-19 illness are attributable to many causes and can have multiple downstream adverse effects, such as worsening respiratory failure, rhabdomyolysis, muscle weakness, and myocardial irritability. Hypokalemia, hyperkalemia, hyponatremia, and hypocalcemia are the most common electrolyte abnormalities in patients with COVID-19 illness. Evaluating the incidence of electrolyte abnormalities in COVID-19, hypokalemia and hyponatremia tend to predominate as the most common electrolyte abnormalities.[83–85] In a cohort of 594 patients admitted from the emergency room, the incidence of hypokalemia and hyponatremia was significantly increased compared to historical controls. Chen et al found that 37% of 175 patients had severe hypokalemia (less than 3 mEq/L), which correlated with increased C-reactive protein, elevated lactate dehydrogenase (LDH), increased creatinine kinase myocardial band (MB) fraction, and disease severity.[84] In a Spanish study involving 305 patients, hypokalemia within 72 hours of admission was associated with the need for MV.[85] While the development of hypokalemia may be related to diuretic use, gastrointestinal losses from diarrhea, vomiting, and insufficient dietary intake, renal potassium wasting was documented in many of the patients described by Chen et al.[84] It is possible that SARS-CoV-2 binding to the surface ACE2 leads to unopposed AII effects and activation of the RAAS.[84] Cellular shifts resulting in hypokalemia and hypophosphatemia may occur in alkalemic states, whereas hyperkalemia and hyperphosphatemia may develop with acidemia.[86–91] In particular, MV employing lung-protective strategies generally results in permissive hypercapnia and respiratory acidosis with hyperkalemia development. This experience with COVID-19-infected patients may differ from that in other patients, in whom respiratory acidosis is thought to result in only minor shifts of intracellular potassium.[92] If renal failure is present, a blunted renal compensatory response to respiratory acidosis occurs, and hyperkalemia may be refractory due to progressive acidemia.[93]

Hyponatremia is common and associated with the syndrome of inappropriate antidiuretic hormone release (SIADH), a decrease in solute intake, and sodium restriction.[94,95] In at least one study, hyponatremia correlated with the severity of renal injury.[96] Hyponatremia from SIADH may develop with worsening hypoxemia and is associated with worse clinical outcomes.[95] A Fanconi-like syndrome associated with hypophosphatemia, renal phosphate wasting, glycosuria, and metabolic acidosis has been described.[25]

Medical Management and Dialysis

The first approach to the patient with AKI in the setting of COVID-19 infection is optimization of the medical management of volume and electrolytes. One should recognize that proteinuria, hematuria, and electrolyte abnormalities represent a high-risk phenotype for AKI, which is itself a harbinger of a worse clinical outcome.[10,16,84,85,97] Attention should be focused on electrolyte replacement, avoidance of volume overload, and maintenance of hemodynamic stability.[98,99] In nonoliguric patients with CARDS, volume overload, and hypoproteinemia, administration of loop diuretics with 25% albumin may temporarily improve oxygenation.[100,101] Medical treatment of hyperkalemia should be no different than in non-COVID-19 patients and should be attempted in a time-limited manner. If acidemia is present, sodium bicarbonate may be given, either as a bolus or as an isotonic sodium bicarbonate solution. It is important to note that by the time significant hyperkalemia and AKI develop, many patients are already critically ill and volume overloaded.[1,102] If the patient has a functioning gastrointestinal tract, potassium-binding resins (patiromer and sodium zirconium cyclosilicate) can be administered.[103] Despite the absence of oliguria and response to medical therapy, many patients with COVID-19-associated AKI may still fail to achieve a net negative fluid balance or euvolemia. The decision to initiate RRT should therefore be made on an individual basis, although in the absence of an appropriate response to medical therapy, RRT should be initiated in a timely manner, within 24 to 48 hours of the onset of advanced AKI (**Fig. 8.4**).

To date, clinical experience demonstrates a wide variability in the percentage of patients with AKI who require dialytic support, ranging from 0.8 to 27%, with 6 to 73% of AKI patients requiring admission to intensive care unit. Conventional dialysis is a reasonable option for hemodynamically stable patients requiring little or no vasopressor support and without significant volume overload. For critically ill patients with volume overload, hemodynamic instability, and/or hypercatabolic states, continuous RRT should be employed. Because COVID-19 infection is a hypercoagulable state, anticoagulation should be instituted to prevent clotting of the dialysis membrane, unless patients are on systemic anticoagulation or a contraindication exists.

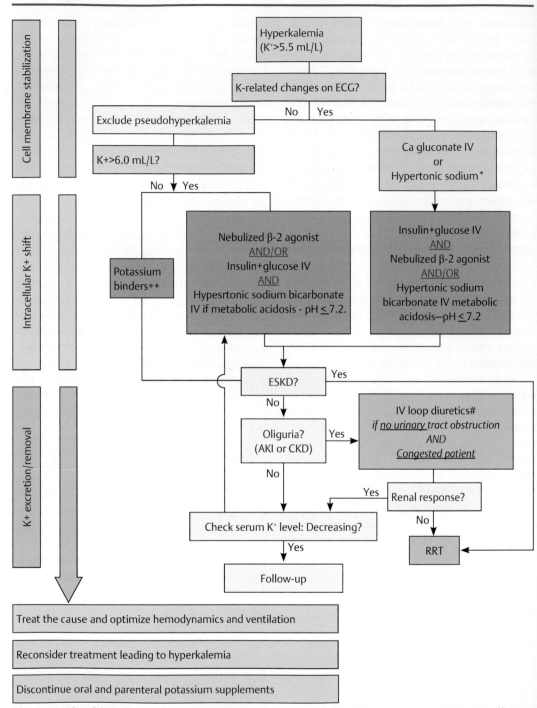

Fig. 8.4 Algorithm for management of hyperkalemia in the many cases of COVID-19 disease. Hyperkalemia is driven by factors such as academia in the setting of hypercapnia and renal failure. Medical management to induce redistribution of potassium, this may become overwhelmed as driver of potassium efflux will persist. Therefore, RRT may be initiated sooner. (Reproduced with permission from Depret et al.[103] © The Author(s) 2019. This article is distributed under the terms of the Creative Commons Attribution 4.0 International License [http://creativecommons.org/licenses/by/4.0/].)

Acute peritoneal dialysis (PD) is an option in treating COVID-19-associated AKI, depending on institutional experience in catheter placement and use of this modality. When evaluating the patient for acute PD, the same absolute contraindications for chronic PD should be considered. Caution should be taken in patients with ascites or at risk for intra-abdominal hypertension. Abdominal distension can impair the respiration of non-intubated patients with an already tenuous respiratory status.[104] Patients requiring prone ventilation may not be optimal candidates. In such cases, conventional hemodialysis or continuous forms of RRT should be considered.[104] To prevent peritoneal leakage in the first 24 to 48 hours, lower fill volumes ranging from 1,000 to 1,500 mL with dwell times of 1 hour should be employed.[104] Adequate clearance of solutes and ultrafiltration will require 8 to 24 exchanges per 24 hours, depending on the individual's catabolic state and clinical status. After 48 hours, if no peritoneal leak exists, dialysate volume, dwell time, and the number of exchanges can be adjusted.[104] It is essential to monitor electrolyte levels closely, as increased frequency, shortened dwell times, and hypertonic dialysate may result in hypokalemia and sodium sieving, leading to hyponatremia.[104]

Conclusion

In summary, AKI occurring with severe COVID-19 infection is common and is associated with an increased mortality. The development of AKI may involve multiple hits, including direct viral effects, cytokine-mediated injury, ischemic-microangiopathic events, and pulmonary–renal crosstalk. The presence of proteinuria, hematuria, Fanconi-like renal abnormalities, and electrolyte disturbances may occur early in the course of the disease and identify patients at risk for progression to more severe forms of AKI. A large percentage of patients who develop dialysis-dependent AKI do not recover renal function at the time of hospital discharge.

References

1. Nadim MK, Forni LG, Mehta RL, et al. COVID-19-associated acute kidney injury: consensus report of the 25th Acute Disease Quality Initiative (ADQI) Workgroup. Nat Rev Nephrol 2020;16(12):747–764
2. Zheng M, Gao Y, Wang G, et al. Functional exhaustion of antiviral lymphocytes in COVID-19 patients. Cell Mol Immunol 2020;17(5):533–535
3. Gagliardi I, Patella G, Michael A, Serra R, Provenzano M, Andreucci M. COVID-19 and the kidney: from epidemiology to clinical practice. J Clin Med 2020;9(8):2506
4. Kunutsor SK, Laukkanen JA. Renal complications in COVID-19: a systematic review and meta-analysis. Ann Med 2020;52(7):345–353
5. Chan L, Chaudhary K, Saha A, et al. AKI in hospitalized patients with COVID-19. J Am Soc Nephrol 2021;32(1):151–160
6. Hirsch JS, Ng JH, Ross DW, et al; Northwell COVID-19 Research Consortium; Northwell Nephrology COVID-19 Research Consortium. Acute kidney injury in patients hospitalized with COVID-19. Kidney Int 2020;98(1):209–218
7. Richardson S, Hirsch JS, Narasimhan M, et al; the Northwell COVID-19 Research Consortium. Presenting characteristics, comorbidities, and outcomes among 5700 patients hospitalized with COVID-19 in the New York city area. JAMA 2020;323(20):2052–2059
8. Paek JH, Kim Y, Park WY, et al. Severe acute kidney injury in COVID-19 patients is associated with in-hospital mortality. PLoS One 2020;15(12):e0243528
9. Kolhe NV, Fluck RJ, Selby NM, Taal MW. Acute kidney injury associated with COVID-19: a retrospective cohort study. PLoS Med 2020;17(10):e1003406
10. Cheng Y, Luo R, Wang K, et al. Kidney disease is associated with in-hospital death of patients with COVID-19. Kidney Int 2020;97(5):829–838
11. Kant S, Menez SP, Hanouneh M, et al. The COVID-19 nephrology compendium: AKI, CKD, ESKD and transplantation. BMC Nephrol 2020;21(1):449
12. See YP, Young BE, Ang LW, et al. Risk factors for development of acute kidney injury in

COVID-19 patients: a retrospective observational cohort study. Nephron 2021;145(3): 256–264

13. Na KR, Kim HR, Ham Y, et al. Acute kidney injury and kidney damage in COVID-19 patients. J Korean Med Sci 2020;35(28):e257

14. Ahmadian E, Hosseiniyan Khatibi SM, Razi Soofiyani S, et al. Covid-19 and kidney injury: pathophysiology and molecular mechanisms. Rev Med Virol 2021;31(3): e2176

15. Chaudhri I, Moffitt R, Taub E, et al. Association of proteinuria and hematuria with acute kidney injury and mortality in hospitalized patients with COVID-19. Kidney Blood Press Res 2020;45(6):1018–1032

16. Karras A, Livrozet M, Lazareth H, et al. Proteinuria and clinical outcomes in hospitalized COVID-19 patients: a retrospective single-center study. Clin J Am Soc Nephrol 2021;16(4):514–521

17. Pei G, Zhang Z, Peng J, et al. Renal involvement and early prognosis in patients with COVID-19 pneumonia. J Am Soc Nephrol 2020;31(6):1157–1165

18. Kudose S, Batal I, Santoriello D, et al. Kidney biopsy findings in patients with COVID-19. J Am Soc Nephrol 2020;31(9):1959–1968

19. Golmai P, Larsen CP, DeVita MV, et al. Histopathologic and ultrastructural findings in postmortem kidney biopsy material in 12 patients with AKI and COVID-19. J Am Soc Nephrol 2020;31(9):1944–1947

20. Farkash EA, Wilson AM, Jentzen JM. Ultrastructural evidence for direct renal infection with SARS-CoV-2. J Am Soc Nephrol 2020;31(8):1683–1687

21. Su H, Yang M, Wan C, et al. Renal histopathological analysis of 26 postmortem findings of patients with COVID-19 in China. Kidney Int 2020;98(1):219–227

22. Chen Z, Hu J, Liu L, et al. SARS-CoV-2 causes acute kidney injury by directly infecting renal tubules. Front Cell Dev Biol 2021;9: 664868

23. Sablone S, Solarino B, Ferorelli D, et al. Post-mortem persistence of SARS-CoV-2: a preliminary study. Forensic Sci Med Pathol 2021;17(3):403–410

24. Zhang L, Richards A, Barrasa MI, Hughes SH, Young RA, Jaenisch R. Reverse-transcribed SARS-CoV-2 RNA can integrate into the genome of cultured human cells and can be expressed in patient-derived tissues. Proc Natl Acad Sci U S A 2021;118(21):e2105968118

25. Kormann R, Jacquot A, Alla A, et al. Coronavirus disease 2019: acute Fanconi syndrome precedes acute kidney injury. Clin Kidney J 2020;13(3):362–370

26. Wu H, Larsen CP, Hernandez-Arroyo CF, et al. AKI and collapsing glomerulopathy associated with COVID-19 and *APOL 1* high-risk genotype. J Am Soc Nephrol 2020; 31(8):1688–1695

27. Velez JCQ, Caza T, Larsen CP. COVAN is the new HIVAN: the re-emergence of collapsing glomerulopathy with COVID-19. Nat Rev Nephrol 2020;16(10):565–567

28. Miller SE, Brealey JK. Visualization of putative coronavirus in kidney. Kidney Int 2020;98(1):231–232

29. Couturier A, Ferlicot S, Chevalier K, et al. Indirect effects of severe acute respiratory syndrome coronavirus 2 on the kidney in coronavirus disease patients. Clin Kidney J 2020;13(3):347–353

30. Diao B, Wang C, Wang R, et al. Human kidney is a target for novel severe acute respiratory syndrome coronavirus 2 infection. Nat Commun 2021;12(1):2506

31. Amraei R, Rahimi N. COVID-19, renin-angiotensin system and endothelial dysfunction. Cells 2020;9(7):E1652

32. Rajendran P, Rengarajan T, Thangavel J, et al. The vascular endothelium and human diseases. Int J Biol Sci 2013;9(10):1057–1069

33. Roberts J, Pritchard AL, Treweeke AT, et al. Why is COVID-19 more severe in patients with diabetes? The role of angiotensin-converting enzyme 2, endothelial dysfunction and the immunoinflammatory system. Front Cardiovasc Med 2021;7:629933

34. Hayashi N, Yamamoto K, Ohishi M, et al. The counterregulating role of ACE2 and ACE2-mediated angiotensin 1-7 signaling against angiotensin II stimulation in vascular cells. Hypertens Res 2010;33(11):1182–1185

35. Hall JE. The renin-angiotensin system: renal actions and blood pressure regulation. Compr Ther 1991;17(5):8–17

36. Hall JE, Guyton AC, Mizelle HL. Role of the renin-angiotensin system in control of sodium excretion and arterial pressure. Acta Physiol Scand Suppl 1990;591:48–62

37. Montezano AC, Nguyen Dinh Cat A, Rios FJ, Touyz RM. Angiotensin II and vascular injury. Curr Hypertens Rep 2014;16(6):431

38. Bhat SA, Sood A, Shukla R, Hanif K. AT2R activation prevents microglia pro-inflammatory activation in a NOX-dependent manner: inhibition of PKC activation and p47^{phox} phosphorylation by PP2A. Mol Neurobiol 2019;56(4):3005–3023

39. Varga Z, Flammer AJ, Steiger P, et al. Endothelial cell infection and endotheliitis in COVID-19. Lancet 2020;395(10234):1417–1418

40. Santos RAS, Sampaio WO, Alzamora AC, et al. The ACE2/angiotensin-(1-7)/MAS axis of the renin-angiotensin system: focus on angiotensin-(1-7). Physiol Rev 2018;98(1):505–553

41. Curran CS, Rivera DR, Kopp JB. COVID-19 usurps host regulatory networks. Front Pharmacol 2020;11:1278

42. Kurz DJ, Eberli FR. Cardiovascular aspects of COVID-19. Swiss Med Wkly 2020;150:w20417

43. Lelis DF, Freitas DF, Machado AS, Crespo TS, Santos SHS. Angiotensin-(1-7), adipokines and inflammation. Metabolism 2019;95:36–45

44. Gąsecka A, Borovac JA, Guerreiro RA, et al. Thrombotic complications in patients with COVID-19: pathophysiological mechanisms, diagnosis, and treatment. Cardiovasc Drugs Ther 2021;35(2):215–229

45. Henry BM, Vikse J, Benoit S, Favaloro EJ, Lippi G. Hyperinflammation and derangement of renin-angiotensin-aldosterone system in COVID-19: a novel hypothesis for clinically suspected hypercoagulopathy and microvascular immunothrombosis. Clin Chim Acta 2020;507:167–173

46. Kipshidze N, Dangas G, White CJ, et al. Viral coagulopathy in patients with COVID-19: treatment and care. Clin Appl Thromb Hemost 2020;26:1076029620936776

47. Magro C, Mulvey JJ, Berlin D, et al. Complement associated microvascular injury and thrombosis in the pathogenesis of severe COVID-19 infection: a report of five cases. Transl Res 2020;220:1–13

48. McFadyen JD, Stevens H, Peter K. The emerging threat of (micro)thrombosis in COVID-19 and its therapeutic implications. Circ Res 2020;127(4):571–587

49. Miesbach W, Makris M. COVID-19: coagulopathy, risk of thrombosis, and the rationale for anticoagulation. Clin Appl Thromb Hemost 2020;26:1076029620938149

50. Ackermann M, Verleden SE, Kuehnel M, et al. Pulmonary vascular endothelialitis, thrombosis, and angiogenesis in Covid-19. N Engl J Med 2020;383(2):120–128

51. Wang X, Sahu KK, Cerny J. Coagulopathy, endothelial dysfunction, thrombotic microangiopathy and complement activation: potential role of complement system inhibition in COVID-19. J Thromb Thrombolysis 2021;51(3):657–662

52. Morris G, Bortolasci CC, Puri BK, et al. The pathophysiology of SARS-CoV-2: a suggested model and therapeutic approach. Life Sci 2020;258:118166

53. Tanaka T, Narazaki M, Kishimoto T. Immunotherapeutic implications of IL-6 blockade for cytokine storm. Immunotherapy 2016;8(8):959–970

54. Chu R, van Eeden C, Suresh S, Sligl WI, Osman M, Cohen Tervaert JW. Do COVID-19 infections result in a different form of secondary hemophagocytic lymphohistiocytosis. Int J Mol Sci 2021;22(6):2967

55. Mousavi Movahed SM, Akhavizadegan H, Dolatkhani F, et al. Different incidences of acute kidney injury (AKI) and outcomes in COVID-19 patients with and without non-azithromycin antibiotics: a retrospective study. J Med Virol 2021;93(7):4411–4419

56. Moledina DG, Simonov M, Yamamoto Y, et al. The association of COVID-19 with acute kidney injury independent of severity of illness: a multicenter cohort study. Am J Kidney Dis 2021;77(4):490–499.e1

57. Cumhur Cure M, Kucuk A, Cure E. NSAIDs may increase the risk of thrombosis and acute renal failure in patients with COVID-19 infection. Therapie 2020;75(4):387–388

58. Mohamed MMB, Lukitsch I, Torres-Ortiz AE, et al. Acute kidney injury associated with coronavirus disease 2019 in urban New Orleans. Kidney360 2020;1(7):614–622

59. Jewell PD, Bramham K, Galloway J, et al. COVID-19-related acute kidney injury; temporal changes in incidence rate and outcomes in a large UK cohort. BMC Nephrol. 2021 (e-pub ahead of print). doi:10.21203/rs.3.rs-438237/v1

60. Chen J, Wang W, Tang Y, Huang X-R, Yu X, Lan H-Y. Inflammatory stress in SARS-COV-2 associated acute kidney injury. Int J Biol Sci 2021;17(6):1497–1506

61. Le Stang M-B, Desenclos J, Flamant M, Chousterman BG, Tabibzadeh N. The good treatment, the bad virus, and the ugly inflammation: pathophysiology of kidney involvement during COVID-19. Front Physiol 2021;12:613019

62. Nugent J, Aklilu A, Yamamoto Y, et al. Assessment of acute kidney injury and longitudinal kidney function after hospital discharge among patients with and without COVID-19. JAMA Netw Open 2021;4(3): e211095–e211095

63. Ahmed AR, Ebad CA, Stoneman S, Satti MM, Conlon PJ. Kidney injury in COVID-19. World J Nephrol 2020;9(2):18–32

64. Gattinoni L, Chiumello D, Caironi P, et al. COVID-19 pneumonia: different respiratory treatments for different phenotypes? Intensive Care Med 2020;46(6):1099–1102

65. Gattinoni L, Chiumello D, Rossi S. COVID-19 pneumonia: ARDS or not? Crit Care 2020; 24(1):154

66. Husain-Syed F, Slutsky AS, Ronco C. Lung-kidney cross-talk in the critically ill patient. Am J Respir Crit Care Med 2016; 194(4):402–414

67. Siddall E, Khatri M, Radhakrishnan J. Capillary leak syndrome: etiologies, pathophysiology, and management. Kidney Int 2017;92(1):37–46

68. Husain-Syed F, Gröne H-J, Assmus B, et al. Congestive nephropathy: a neglected entity? Proposal for diagnostic criteria and future perspectives. ESC Heart Fail 2021;8(1): 183–203

69. Kazory A, Ronco C, McCullough PA. SARS-CoV-2 (COVID-19) and intravascular volume management strategies in the critically ill. Proc Bayl Univ Med Cent 2020;0(0):1–6

70. Murray PT. The kidney in respiratory failure and mechanical ventilation. Contrib Nephrol 2010;165:159–165

71. Koyner JL, Murray PT. Mechanical ventilation and the kidney. Blood Purif 2010;29(1): 52–68

72. Del Vecchio L, Locatelli F. Hypoxia response and acute lung and kidney injury: possible implications for therapy of COVID-19. Clin Kidney J 2020;13(4):494–499

73. Koyner JL, Murray PT. Mechanical ventilation and lung-kidney interactions. Clin J Am Soc Nephrol 2008;3(2):562–570

74. Anderson RJ, Pluss RG, Pluss WT, Bell J, Zerbe GG. Effect of hypoxia and hypercapnic acidosis on renal autoregulation in the dog: role of renal nerves. Clin Sci (Lond) 1983; 65(5):533–538

75. Grams ME, Rabb H. The distant organ effects of acute kidney injury. Kidney Int 2012; 81(10):942–948

76. Basile DP, Anderson MD, Sutton TA. Pathophysiology of acute kidney injury. Compr Physiol 2012;2(2):1303–1353

77. Morris G, Bortolasci CC, Puri BK, et al. The cytokine storms of COVID-19, H1N1 influenza, CRS and MAS compared. Can one sized treatment fit all? Cytokine 2021; 144:155593

78. Bradley MJ, Vicente DA, Bograd BA, et al. Host responses to concurrent combined injuries in non-human primates. J Inflamm (Lond) 2017;14(1):23

79. Bautista E, Arcos M, Jimenez-Alvarez L, et al. Angiogenic and inflammatory markers in acute respiratory distress syndrome and renal injury associated to A/H1N1 virus infection. Exp Mol Pathol 2013;94(3):486–492

80. Ologunde R, Zhao H, Lu K, Ma D. Organ cross talk and remote organ damage following acute kidney injury. Int Urol Nephrol 2014;46(12):2337–2345

81. Meegada S, Muppidi V, Wilkinson DC III, Siddamreddy S, Katta SK. Coronavirus disease 2019-induced rhabdomyolysis. Cureus 2020;12(8):e10123

82. Valente-Acosta B, Moreno-Sanchez F, Fueyo-Rodriguez O, Palomar-Lever A. Rhabdomyolysis as an initial presentation in a patient diagnosed with COVID-19. BMJ Case Rep 2020;13(6):e236719

83. Tezcan ME, Dogan Gokce G, Sen N, Zorlutuna Kaymak N, Ozer RS. Baseline electrolyte abnormalities would be related to poor prognosis in hospitalized coronavirus disease 2019 patients. New Microbes New Infect 2020;37:100753

84. Chen D, Li X, Song Q, et al. Assessment of hypokalemia and clinical characteristics in patients with coronavirus disease 2019 in Wenzhou, China. JAMA Netw Open 2020;3(6):e2011122

85. Moreno-P O, Leon-Ramirez J-M, Fuertes-Kenneally L, et al; COVID19-ALC Research Group. Hypokalemia as a sensitive biomarker of disease severity and the requirement for invasive mechanical ventilation requirement in COVID-19 pneumonia: a case series of 306 Mediterranean patients. Int J Infect Dis 2020;100:449–454

86. Datta BN, Stone MD. Hyperventilation and hypophosphataemia. Ann Clin Biochem 2009;46(Pt 2):170–171

87. Kumagai A, Yamada K. Classification, symptoms, and management of hyper- and hypophosphatemia [in Japanese]. Nihon Rinsho 1982;40(12):2669–2672

88. Gennari FJ. Hypokalemia. N Engl J Med 1998;339(7):451–458

89. Gennari FJ. Disorders of potassium homeostasis. Hypokalemia and hyperkalemia. Crit Care Clin 2002;18(2):273–288, vi

90. Gerhardt LMS, Angermann CE. Hyperkalemia—pathophysiology, prognostic significance and treatment options [in German]. Dtsch Med Wochenschr 2019;144(22):1576–1584

91. Palmer BF, Clegg DJ. Diagnosis and treatment of hyperkalemia. Cleve Clin J Med 2017;84(12):934–942

92. Adrogué HJ, Madias NE. Changes in plasma potassium concentration during acute acid-base disturbances. Am J Med 1981;71(3):456–467

93. Scribner BH, Fremont-Smith K, Burnell JM. The effect of acute respiratory acidosis on the internal equilibrium of potassium. J Clin Invest 1955;34(8):1276–1285

94. Gheorghe G, Ilie M, Bungau S, Stoian AMP, Bacalbasa N, Diaconu CC. Is there a relationship between COVID-19 and hyponatremia? Medicina (Kaunas) 2021;57(1):55

95. Gregoriano C, Molitor A, Haag E, et al. Activation of vasopressin system during COVID-19 is associated with adverse clinical outcomes: an observational study. J Endocr Soc 2021;5(6):b045

96. Hu W, Lv X, Li C, et al. Disorders of sodium balance and its clinical implications in COVID-19 patients: a multicenter retrospective study. Intern Emerg Med 2021;16(4):853–862

97. Liu S, Zhang L, Weng H, et al. Association between average plasma potassium levels and 30-day mortality during hospitalization in patients with COVID-19 in Wuhan, China. Int J Med Sci 2021;18(3):736–743

98. Marik PE, Monnet X, Teboul J-L. Hemodynamic parameters to guide fluid therapy. Ann Intensive Care 2011;1(1):1–1

99. Marts LT, Kempker JA, Martin GS. Fluid management in acute respiratory distress syndrome: do we have all the FACTTs to determine the effect of race? Ann Am Thorac Soc 2017;14(9):1391–1392

100. Khan A, Milbrandt EB, Venkataraman R. Albumin and furosemide for acute lung injury. Crit Care 2007;11(5):314

101. Martin GS. Fluid balance and colloid osmotic pressure in acute respiratory failure: emerging clinical evidence. Crit Care 2000;4(2, Suppl 2):S21–S25

102. Ronco C, Reis T. Kidney involvement in COVID-19 and rationale for extracorporeal therapies. Nat Rev Nephrol 2020;16(6):308–310

103. Dépret F, Peacock WF, Liu KD, Rafique Z, Rossignol P, Legrand M. Management of hyperkalemia in the acutely ill patient. Ann Intensive Care 2019;9(1):32

104. Srivatana V, Aggarwal V, Finkelstein FO, Naljayan M, Crabtree JH, Perl J. Peritoneal dialysis for acute kidney injury treatment in the United States: brought to you by the COVID-19 pandemic. Kidney360 2020;1(5):410–415

09 Gastrointestinal Complications of COVID-19

Vinod Nookala and Priyaranjan Kata

Introduction

The pandemic of respiratory illness caused by severe acute respiratory syndrome coronavirus 2 (SARS-CoV-2) in Wuhan, China, resulted in an ongoing pandemic. The World Health Organization (WHO) named this illness "coronavirus disease 2019" (COVID-19). It is reported to cause severe illnesses in a significant proportion of infected individuals, especially in the aged and those with underlying comorbid conditions.[1-3] Infected individuals' symptoms can range from mild respiratory illness to critical illness. According to a cohort of around 44,500 patient population, 80% of individuals present with mild pulmonary symptoms. However, approximately 19% develop progressive severe disease and progressive hypoxemia requiring hospitalization and in some cases intensive care admission.[4] However, some have developed various fatal complications, including multiple organ failure, septic shock, pulmonary edema, severe pneumonia, stroke, blood coagulopathies, acute respiratory distress syndrome (ARDS), and death.[5] The case fatality ranges from 0.9% to as high as 7.0%.[6,7]

Most infected individuals develop fever, cough, dyspnea, and cold-like symptoms, indicating that the novel coronavirus commonly infects respiratory epithelium.[8,9] COVID-19 patients may also develop diarrhea, nausea, anorexia, abdominal discomfort, and dysgeusia.

The pathophysiology behind gastrointestinal (GI) manifestations is yet to be fully understood. The virus gains entry into the target cells of the host through ACE2 receptors.[10,11] These receptors are predominantly found in the respiratory tract. Abundant receptors are also present in the intestinal epithelium and other areas such as the esophagus, oral mucosa, and liver.[11-13] After the entry into the cells, RNA and proteins are produced with the help of host cell machinery. Several viral RNA copies, capsids, and proteins are synthesized and assembled to form new viral particles. These new viral particles lead to the release of various cytokines (Interleukin 2, 7, tumor necrosis factor-α, and other inflammatory mediators). These chemical mediators cause various GI manifestations. In COVID-19 patients, the viral nucleocapsid protein has been verified in the GI tract. Also, plasmacytic and lymphocytic infiltration and interstitial edema are found in various parts, including the stomach, duodenum, and rectum. Thus, the novel coronavirus may cause GI symptoms through direct invasion into the host cells and immune-mediated injury.[14]

Fecal–Oral Transmission

Respiratory transmission is the primary mode of transmission for SARS-CoV-2, and it is known to spread via the respiratory route and direct contact.[15,16] However, the novel coronavirus is known to cause various GI symptoms, and the likelihood of fecal–oral transmission warrants consideration. Several studies suggested that the virus may be viable in the feces.

Previous studies before the emergence of the COVID-19 pandemic showed that the related coronaviruses are observed in the stool. During the MERS-CoV epidemic, 14.6% of the infected patients were found to have intact virus in stool samples at low viral loads.[17] Likewise, in the SARS epidemic which occurred in 2012, individuals demonstrated viral shedding of SARS-CoV in the stool samples of infected individuals.[18] Due to the genetic similarity between the other pathogenic coronaviruses and SARS-CoV-2 and their ability to survive at low temperatures (20–30°C) for long periods, it is possible that the novel coronavirus could remain viable outside the host cell for a few days, leading to fecal–oral transmission.[19] Viral RNA has been detected in stool samples even in the clinical setting of negative nasopharyngeal PCR.[20,21] Several investigators have identified the viral shedding in the alimentary canal, and the prevalence ranged from 36 to 53% of the confirmed COVID-19 cases.[20–24] Although the presence of the viral RNA in the feces was detected, its infectivity is yet to be determined.

The tests for SARS-CoV-2 virus in stool samples were positive even after a negative throat swab test in some individuals.[25] Thus, stool sample testing may be used as an alternative and an additional test for diagnosing COVID-19 infection. Furthermore, a study showed active viral replication in the stool samples of infected patients.[22,26] Interestingly, another study revealed that the SARS-CoV-2 virus could remain viable in an external environment such as stainless steel and plastic materials.[27] The detection of the viral RNA in the feces does not confirm the infectivity, but viral spreading through the fecal–oral route is possible. A few studies have attempted to determine the infectivity of the fecal–oral route, but the evidence is weak. Therefore, more evidence is required to confirm this hypothesis.[22,28]

Gastrointestinal Manifestations

GI manifestations are common in a substantial percentage of individuals. Around 10 to 30% of COVID-19 patients may present with GI symptoms.[29,30] Most frequently presented symptoms are diarrhea, abdominal pain, anorexia, and nausea/vomiting[31] (**Fig. 9.1**).

Characteristics of Diarrhea

Diarrhea is a commonly presented symptom in COVID-19 patients.[32] In most cases, it is not severe and is self-limiting.[32] As it is subjective, the presentation is heterogeneous, and the estimates may vary. In most cases, patients present with watery diarrhea, but rarely, a few patients may present with bloody diarrhea. The presence of occult blood in the stool can be because of other underlying conditions like diverticulosis. Thus, other causes of GI bleeding such as hemorrhoids, inflammatory bowel disease (IBD), and medications must be ruled out before attributing the symptoms to COVID-related manifestations. Usually, the stools are without blood or WBC and are accompanied by nausea/vomiting. Diarrhea is associated with an increase in fecal calprotectin concentrations levels. From these findings, it is assumed that the diarrhea

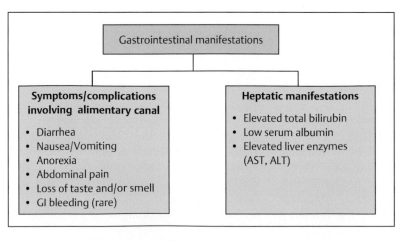

Fig. 9.1 Gastrointestinal manifestations of COVID-19. GI, gastrointestinal; AST, aspartate aminotransferase; ALT, alanine aminotransferase.

is mainly because of the secretory abnormal reabsorption of the fluid and electrolytes in conjunction with mild inflammatory colitis. Fecal calprotectin concentrations were elevated in COVID-19 patients with diarrhea than in those without diarrhea and have a tendency to be higher in patients with severe COVID-19 than in those with mild/moderate COVID-19.[29,31]

Nausea and anorexia are also very commonly reported GI symptoms in COVID-19 patients. However, nausea and anorexia can develop because of cytokine-mediated responses in inflammatory or infectious conditions. Thus, these symptoms may not be specific to the disease.[33,34] Some patients can also present with GI bleeding, anosmia, and dysgeusia.[30,35] Ageusia and dysgeusia are common symptoms. The prevalence of dysgeusia in COVID-19 patients can be as high as 70 to 80% and may persist throughout the disease course.[36,37] Smell and taste disturbances can sometimes present as initial symptoms in some patients.[36,37]

In many patients, GI symptoms can portend COVID-19 as they may appear several days prior to admission, with a significant variability of symptoms appearing up to 20 days before admission. Data from one of the studies support the inclusion of GI symptoms among the COVID-19 features, allowing for earlier diagnosis and care particularly in individuals who do not have respiratory symptoms.[38] This could be especially important given the high rate of transmission among close contacts, linked to GI viral infection and possible oral–fecal transmission, which could last even after nasopharyngeal and pulmonary viral clearance.[11,39]

Hepatic Manifestations

Hepatic injury is common in COVID-19 patients, and is associated with poor outcomes.[40] Elevation of serum aminotransferases and impaired hepatic biomarkers were observed in greater than 50% of the patients with severe COVID-19.[41-44] Injury is thought to be because of several mechanisms.

It is observed that ACE-2 receptors are abundant in cholangiocytes compared to hepatocytes.[45] Thus, viral infection impairs hepatic function by a cytopathic effect due to the intracellular replication of viral particles cells. The cytotoxicity induces apoptosis, pyroptosis, or necrosis in the host cell. Thus, hepatic manifestations are thought to be because of direct liver injury due to viral toxicity and viral entry through the hepatobiliary system due to the abundance of ACE-2 receptors. Interestingly, a recent study revealed that the peroxisome proliferator activated receptor signaling pathway and the renin-angiotensin system could enhance the infection. In addition, hypoxic injury due to compromised respiratory function and thrombosis may aggravate the ongoing disease process. Several experts suggested that bile duct cells are an important driver in hepatic immune dysregulation and inflammation.[10] The antibiotics, antipyretics, and antiviral medications used in the treatment of COVID-19 may also cause liver injury.[46]

In Patients with Pre-Existing Liver Conditions

To date, there is a paucity of evidence on the impact of chronic liver disease on the clinical outcome of COVID-19. Based on few studies, it is understood that chronic liver diseases and on-admission liver-associated laboratory results predicted a worse clinical outcome in COVID-19 disease.[47] It remains to be seen if COVID-19 disease exacerbates cholestasis in those with chronic cholestatic hepatobiliary disease with or without cirrhosis.[6] One of the studies aimed to evaluate whether there is any association between metabolic dysfunction-associated fatty liver disease (MAFLD) and COVID-19 outcomes identified MAFLD is associated with a 2.6-fold increased risk of severe COVID-19 compared to those without MAFLD.[48] One study demonstrated that in patients with MAFLD, a proinflammatory state potentially exacerbates the viral-induced cytokine storm.[49] ICU utilization rate was increased in MAFLD when compared to non-MAFLD patients.[50] However, the difference was statistically nonsignificant, but MAFLD still may adversely impact the clinical course of COVID-19. COVID-19 patients with MAFLD had a worse prognosis, twofold higher prevalence of deteriorating clinical disease course, increased viral shedding time, and more hepatic failure.[50] The link between MAFLD and COVID-19 severity is undoubtedly multifactorial. Metabolic syndrome and its elements have already been linked to worse clinical outcomes in COVID-19.[51] The presence of fibrosis in MAFLD patients is a superimposed risk factor for the severity of COVID-19, independently of metabolic syndrome comorbidities. The severity disease is substantially augmented with the extensiveness of liver fibrosis. Individuals with a FIB-4 score higher than 2.67 had the highest risk of developing severe COVID-19.[52] Another interesting point was reported in a multicenter preliminary study, where patients with MAFLD under 60 years demonstrated a more than fourfold risk of severe COVID-19 compared to those without MAFLD suggesting younger patients with MAFLD are at increased risk of severe COVID-19.[53] Neutrophil-to-lymphocyte ratio (NLR) is noted to be a recognized and commonly assessable prognostic marker in the early stage of viral infection.[54] Superimposed MAFLD in conjunction with an NLR higher than 2.8 is associated with a higher risk of severe COVID-19 compared to patients without MAFLD and with normal NLR.[49] Currently, there is no definitive data on COVID-19 and its effects on decompensated cirrhosis or those awaiting liver transplantation (LT).[55]

Colitis in the Setting of COVID-19

Colitis in COVID-19 patients has been reported in a patient who, during recovery from SARS-CoV-2 pneumonia, developed diarrhea abdominal pain and marked distension.[56] CT scan demonstrated pneumoperitoneum and almost entire distension of the large bowel, with perforation of the ascending colon. Intraoperative findings included a profuse amount of free air, distension of the entire colon, and cecal distension accompanied with cecal perforation. Neither obstruction was documented nor etiology of marked colonic distension was demonstrated.[56] The physiopathology of an acute overdistension of the entire colon, without evidence of obstruction leading to diastatic colonic perforation, is unknown. It is presumed to be due to viral cytopathic injury to colonic cells. ACE2 has been located in many cell types in the GI system, suggesting the possible viral tropism for the GI tract potentially explaining these GI manifestations.[11] Furthermore, viral RNA was mainly detected in the cytoplasm of GI epithelial cells indicating that the virus can infect cells of the GI tract.[57] Another hypothesis was altered colonic motility viral neuronal invasion resulting in dysautonomia of the colonic innervation of the colon.[58]

In Patients with Inflammatory Bowel Disease

IBD is a disorder of immune dysregulation in the GI tract. Most patients presenting with moderate to severe symptoms are managed with immune-suppressing or -modifying agents. Many patients with IBD are prescribed immunosuppressants or immunomodulators, and the use of such compounds may interfere with host defense mechanisms. As IBD is an immune response and the therapy involves immunosuppression, there is an increasing concern regarding patients' risk with IBD and prognosis in COVID-19 patients with IBD. However, despite the potential for increased exposure and risk, there is no current evidence to suggest an increased risk of infection with SARS-CoV-2 or the development of a severe clinical course of the COVID-19 in patients with IBD.[59] Experts recommend continuation of the ongoing treatment for the patients with IBD who do not have an infection with SARS-CoV-2.[60]

Management

The management should be individualized based on the patient's factors, the severity of the presentation, and associated COVID-19-related complications. Patients with new-onset GI symptoms should be considered for COVID-19 infection, especially in highly prevalent areas. Getting a detailed history regarding the clinical presentation, risk factors, location can help in identifying COVID-19-related GI symptoms. A thorough history of underlying GI disorders should be obtained. Clinical examination, laboratory, and imaging findings may help determine the cause of the presenting GI symptoms. In addition, assessment for volume depletion should be done (decreased skin turgor, dry mouth, postural hypotension) as diarrhea can cause fluid loss in the body. Clinicians should be aware of volume status and the risk of hypovolemia in patients presenting with GI symptoms associated with typical COVID-19 symptoms (fever and respiratory tract symptoms). Even after the COVID-19 diagnosis has been made, other entities should be ruled out. Similar conditions that overlap with the clinical spectrum of COVID-19 symptoms such as *C. difficile* infection, other viral infections, IBD should be ruled out. Additional testing may be needed based on the presentation. Stool testing for ova and parasites; stool cultures; antigen and molecular testing for the specific organism are needed to determine the pathogen.[61]

Several medications used in the management of COVID-19 are associated with GI side effects. Medications can sometimes cause several GI side effects. Diarrhea, nausea, and vomiting are noted side effects of Remdesivir, chloroquine, and hydroxychloroquine. Remdesivir has been associated with elevated transaminases.[62] Clinicians should be aware of these side effects while using these medications.[46]

Currently, other than supportive care, there are no specific guidelines for the management of COVID-19-associated GI symptoms. Fluid and electrolyte monitoring and replacement are essential. For milder cases of diarrhea, fluids and electrolytes can be maintained by a sufficient intake of juices, soups, sports drinks, and other electrolyte solutions.[63] Oral rehydration therapy is recommended for mild volume depletion. Intravenous fluids can be used in severe cases due to fluid loss.[64] In addition to maintaining supportive care, symptoms can be managed with antidiarrheal and antiemetic agents. In patients who desire symptomatic therapy, diarrhea can be managed with antimotility drugs such as loperamide after ruling out other infectious causes.[63,64] For patients who present with dysentery (bloody/mucoid stools), antimotility medications are usually avoided. Nausea and vomiting can be treated with antiemetics such as prochlorperazine and ondansetron.[63,64] Several antibiotics and antivirals are being used in the management of COVID-19. Thus, these medications can alter the gut microbiota and cause diarrhea. So, replenishing gut microbiota can be a potential therapeutic option to preserve the intestinal microbiome balance.[65] Patients should be monitored continuously for worsening symptoms like GI bleeding, severe vomiting, severe signs of dehydration, altered mental status.[66] If the clinical condition worsens, the patients might need either hospitalization or referral to a gastroenterologist.[66]

Clinical Outcomes

It is not yet determined whether GI symptoms are associated with different clinical outcomes or not. Several studies showed mixed results on the outcomes associated with GI manifestations.[38] According to Jin et al, individuals presenting with GI symptoms had a severe disease course, and more patients needed mechanical ventilation than those presented without GI symptoms (22.9 vs. 8.1).[67] Similarly, a meta-analysis showed that the patients presenting with GI symptoms tend to have a severe disease course with an increased risk of ARDS.[67] However, on the other hand, several studies showed that GI manifestations might be associated with a milder clinical course and lower mortality rate.[38,68-70] The heterogeneity of the results may be due to the differences in the geographical location, patient demographics, different viral strains, and variations in reporting.[70-72] Interestingly, patients with GI symptoms were observed to have longer times to viral clearance than patients presenting with respiratory symptoms alone.[73] Also, patients with GI symptoms tend to have a longer duration of illness.[69]

Conclusion

Due to the rapid spread in the community and lack of effective treatment options, the disease is taking a significant toll on healthcare systems. The management options are evolving rapidly through clinical trials and ongoing research. The knowledge about the pathophysiology, clinical presentation, and therapeutic management options still need to be refined. What we know about the pathophysiology of COVID-19 may be the tip of an iceberg, and there is much more to be learned as the presenting symptoms and management options are changing day by day. There have been many research studies going on to get a better understanding of COVID-19. Many more studies have to be done as it is imperative to get a comprehensive understanding of the pathophysiology, clinical presentation, and management options.

References

1. Zhou F, Yu T, Du R, et al. Clinical course and risk factors for mortality of adult inpatients with COVID-19 in Wuhan, China: a retrospective cohort study. Lancet 2020;395(10229):1054–1062

2. Chow N, Fleming-Dutra K, Gierke R, et al. Preliminary estimates of the prevalence of selected underlying health conditions among patients with coronavirus disease 2019—United States, Feb 12–Mar 28, 2020. Morbid Mortal Wkly Rep 2020;69(13):382

3. CDC COVID-19 Response Team. Severe outcomes among patients with coronavirus disease 2019 (COVID-19)—United States, Feb 12–Mar 16, 2020. Morbid Mortal Wkly Rep (MMWR) 2020;69(12):343–346

4. Wu Z, McGoogan JM. Characteristics of and important lessons from the coronavirus disease 2019 (COVID-19) outbreak in China: summary of a report of 72314 cases from the Chinese Center for Disease Control and Prevention. JAMA 2020;323(13):1239–1242

5. Colafrancesco S, Alessandri C, Conti F, Priori R. COVID-19 gone bad: a new character in the spectrum of the hyperferritinemic syndrome? Autoimmun Rev 2020;19(7):102573

6. KCDC, D.o.R.a.a.I.c., Updates on COVID-19 in Korea (as of 14 March). 2020

7. Onder G, Rezza G, Brusaferro S. Case-fatality rate and characteristics of patients dying in relation to COVID-19 in Italy. JAMA 2020;323(18):1775–1776

8. Chen J, Zhang Z-Z, Chen Y-K, et al. The clinical and immunological features of pediatric COVID-19 patients in China. Genes Dis 2020;7(4):535–541

9. Chen J, Qi T, Liu L, et al. Clinical progression of patients with COVID-19 in Shanghai, China. J Infect 2020;80(5):e1–e6

10. Hoffmann M, Kleine-Weber H, Schroeder S, et al. SARS-CoV-2 cell entry depends on ACE2 and TMPRSS2 and is blocked by a clinically proven protease inhibitor. Cell 2020;181(2):271–280.e8

11. Xiao F, Tang M, Zheng X, Liu Y, Li X, Shan H. Evidence for gastrointestinal infection of SARS-CoV-2. Gastroenterology 2020;158(6):1831–1833.e3

12. Hamming I, Timens W, Bulthuis MLC, et al. Tissue distribution of ACE2 protein, the functional receptor for SARS coronavirus. A first step in understanding SARS pathogenesis. J Pathol 2004;203(2):631–637

13. Zou X, Chen K, Zou J, Han P, Hao J, Han Z. Single-cell RNA-seq data analysis on the receptor ACE2 expression reveals the potential risk of different human organs vulnerable to 2019-nCoV infection. Front Med 2020;14(2):185–192

14. Tian Y, Rong L, Nian W, He Y. Review article: gastrointestinal features in COVID-19 and the possibility of faecal transmission. Aliment Pharmacol Ther 2020;51(9):843–851

15. Li Q, Guan X, Wu P, et al. Early transmission dynamics in Wuhan, China, of novel coronavirus–infected pneumonia. N Engl J Med 2020;382(13):1199–1207

16. Rothe C, Schunk M, Sothmann P, et al. Transmission of 2019-nCoV infection from an asymptomatic contact in Germany. N Engl J Med 2020;382(10):970–971

17. Corman VM, Albarrak AM, Omrani AS, et al. Viral shedding and antibody response in 37 patients with Middle East respiratory syndrome coronavirus infection. Clin Infect Dis 2016;62(4):477–483

18. Cheng PKC, Wong DA, Tong LKL, et al. Viral shedding patterns of coronavirus in patients with probable severe acute respiratory syndrome. Lancet 2004;363(9422):1699–1700

19. Yeo C, Kaushal S, Yeo D. Enteric involvement of coronaviruses: is faecal-oral transmission of SARS-CoV-2 possible? Lancet Gastroenterol Hepatol 2020;5(4):335–337

20. Zhang J, Wang S, Xue Y. Fecal specimen diagnosis 2019 novel coronavirus-infected pneumonia. J Med Virol 2020;92(6):680–682

21. Wu Y, Guo C, Tang L, et al. Prolonged presence of SARS-CoV-2 viral RNA in faecal samples. Lancet Gastroenterol Hepatol 2020;5(5): 434–435

22. Wang W, Xu Y, Gao R, et al. Detection of SARS-CoV-2 in different types of clinical specimens. JAMA 2020;323(18):1843–1844

23. Young BE, Ong SWX, Kalimuddin S, et al; Singapore 2019 Novel Coronavirus Outbreak Research Team. Epidemiologic features and clinical course of patients infected with SARS-CoV-2 in Singapore. JAMA 2020;323(15): 1488–1494

24. Ling Y, Xu S-B, Lin Y-X, et al. Persistence and clearance of viral RNA in 2019 novel coronavirus disease rehabilitation patients. Chin Med J (Engl) 2020;133(9):1039–1043

25. Gupta S, Parker J, Smits S, Underwood J, Dolwani S. Persistent viral shedding of SARS-CoV-2 in faeces: a rapid review. Colorectal Dis 2020;22(6):611–620

26. Leung WK, To KF, Chan PKS, et al. Enteric involvement of severe acute respiratory syndrome-associated coronavirus infection. Gastroenterology 2003;125(4):1011–1017

27. Lo IL, Lio CF, Cheong HH, et al. Evaluation of SARS-CoV-2 RNA shedding in clinical specimens and clinical characteristics of 10 patients with COVID-19 in Macau. Int J Biol Sci 2020;16(10):1698–1707

28. Wölfel R, Corman VM, Guggemos W, et al. Virological assessment of hospitalized patients with COVID-2019. Nature 2020; 581(7809):465–469

29. El Ouali S, Achkar JP, Lashner B, Regueiro M. Gastrointestinal manifestations of COVID-19. Cleve Clin J Med 2021;•••: 10.3949/CCJM.87A. CCC049

30. Kopel J, Perisetti A, Gajendran M, Boregowda U, Goyal H. Clinical insights into the gastrointestinal manifestations of COVID-19. Dig Dis Sci 2020;65(7):1932–1939

31. Patel N, Wen Q, Sayegh GF, et al. COVID-19 and the gastrointestinal system: a systematic review and metanalysis. Eur J Biomed. 2021;8(2):75–82

32. D'Amico F, Baumgart DC, Danese S, Peyrin-Biroulet L. Diarrhea during COVID-19 infection: pathogenesis, epidemiology, prevention and management. Clin Gastroenterol Hepatol 2020;18(8):1663–1672

33. Gautron L, Layé S. Neurobiology of inflammation-associated anorexia. Front Neurosci 2010;3:59

34. Vespa E, Pugliese N, Colapietro F, Aghemo A. STAY (GI) HEALTHY: COVID-19 and Gastrointestinal manifestations. Tech Innov Gastrointest Endosc. 2021

35. Chen T, Yang Q, Duan H. A severe coronavirus disease 2019 patient with high-risk predisposing factors died from massive gastrointestinal bleeding: a case report. BMC Gastroenterol 2020;20(1):318

36. Vaira LA, Hopkins C, Salzano G, et al. Olfactory and gustatory function impairment in COVID-19 patients: Italian objective multicenter-study. Head Neck 2020;42(7):1560–1569

37. Lechien JR, Chiesa-Estomba CM, De Siati DR, et al. Olfactory and gustatory dysfunctions as a clinical presentation of mild-to-moderate forms of the coronavirus disease (COVID-19): a multicenter European study. Eur Arch Otorhinolaryngol 2020;277(8):2251–2261

38. Sultan S, Altayar O, Siddique SM, et al; AGA Institute. Electronic address: ewilson@gastro.org. AGA institute rapid review of the GI and liver manifestations of COVID-19, meta-analysis of international data, and recommendations for the consultative management of patients with COVID-19. Gastroenterology 2020;159(1):320–334.e27

39. Gu J, Han B, Wang J. COVID-19: gastrointestinal manifestations and potential fecal-oral transmission. Gastroenterology 2020; 158(6):1518–1519

40. Parohan M, Yaghoubi S, Seraji A. Liver injury is associated with severe coronavirus disease 2019 (COVID-19) infection: a systematic review and meta-analysis of retrospective studies. Hepatol Res 2020;50(8):924–935

41. Gao Y, Li T, Han M, et al. Diagnostic utility of clinical laboratory data determinations for patients with the severe COVID-19. J Med Virol 2020;92(7):791–796

42. Yang X, Yu Y, Xu J, et al. Clinical course and outcomes of critically ill patients with SARS-CoV-2 pneumonia in Wuhan, China: a single-centered, retrospective, observational study. Lancet Respir Med 2020;8(5):475–481

43. Chen N, Zhou M, Dong X, et al. Epidemiological and clinical characteristics of 99 cases of 2019 novel coronavirus pneumonia in Wuhan, China: a descriptive study. Lancet 2020;395(10223):507–513

44. Wang D, Hu B, Hu C, et al. Clinical characteristics of 138 hospitalized patients with 2019 novel coronavirus-infected pneumonia in Wuhan, China. JAMA 2020;323(11):1061–1069

45. Chai X, Hu L, Zhang Y, et al. Specific ACE2 expression in cholangiocytes may cause liver damage after 2019-nCoV infection. biorxiv. 2020

46. Grein J, Ohmagari N, Shin D, et al. Compassionate use of remdesivir for patients with severe covid-19. N Engl J Med 2020; 382(24):2327–2336

47. Váncsa S, Hegyi PJ, Zádori N, et al. Pre-existing liver diseases and on-admission liver-related laboratory tests in COVID-19: a prognostic accuracy meta-analysis with systematic review. Front Med (Lausanne) 2020;7:572115

48. Hegyi PJ, Váncsa S, Ocskay K, et al. Metabolic associated fatty liver disease is associated with an increased risk of severe COVID-19: a systematic review with meta-analysis. Front Med (Lausanne) 2021;8:626425

49. Targher G, Mantovani A, Byrne CD, et al. Detrimental effects of metabolic dysfunction-associated fatty liver disease and increased neutrophil-to-lymphocyte ratio on severity of COVID-19. Diabetes Metab 2020;46(6):505–507

50. Ji D, Qin E, Xu J, et al. Non-alcoholic fatty liver diseases in patients with COVID-19: A retrospective study. J Hepatol 2020;73(2): 451–453

51. Williamson E, Walker AJ, Bhaskaran KJ, et al. OpenSAFELY: factors associated with COVID-19-related hospital death in the linked electronic health records of 17 million adult NHS patients. medRxiv [Preprint]. (2020). 10.1101/2020.05.06.20092999

52. Targher G, Mantovani A, Byrne CD, et al. Risk of severe illness from COVID-19 in patients with metabolic dysfunction-associated fatty liver disease and increased fibrosis scores. Gut 2020;69(8):1545–1547

53. Zhou Y-J, Zheng KI, Wang X-B, et al. Younger patients with MAFLD are at increased risk of severe COVID-19 illness: A multicenter preliminary analysis. J Hepatol 2020;73(3):719–721

54. Ciccullo A, Borghetti A, Zileri Dal Verme L, et al; GEMELLI AGAINST COVID Group. Neutrophil-to-lymphocyte ratio and clinical outcome in COVID-19: a report from the Italian front line. Int J Antimicrob Agents 2020;56(2):106017

55. Guan WJ, Ni ZY, Hu Y, et al; China Medical Treatment Expert Group for Covid-19. Clinical characteristics of coronavirus disease 2019 in China. N Engl J Med 2020;382(18):1708–1720

56. De Nardi P, Parolini DC, Ripa M, Racca S, Rosati R. Bowel perforation in a Covid-19 patient: case report. Int J Colorectal Dis 2020;35(9):1797–1800

57. Tian Y, Rong L, Nian W, He Y. Review article: gastrointestinal features in COVID-19 and the possibility of faecal transmission. Aliment Pharmacol Ther 2020;51(9):843–851

58. Conde G, Quintana Pájaro LD, Quintero Marzola ID, Ramos Villegas Y, Moscote Salazar YL. Neurotropism of SARS-CoV 2: mechanisms and manifestations. J Neurol Sci 2020;412:116824

59. Sultan K, Mone A, Durbin L, Khuwaja S, Swaminath A. Review of inflammatory bowel disease and COVID-19. World J Gastroenterol 2020;26(37):5534–5542

60. Rubin DT, Feuerstein JD, Wang AY, Cohen RD. AGA clinical practice update on management of inflammatory bowel disease during the COVID-19 pandemic: expert commentary. Gastroenterology 2020;159(1):350–357

61. Guerrant RL, Van Gilder T, Steiner TS, et al; Infectious Diseases Society of America. Practice guidelines for the management of

infectious diarrhea. Clin Infect Dis 2001; 32(3):331–351

62. Wang Y, Zhang D, Du G, et al. Remdesivir in adults with severe COVID-19: a randomised, double-blind, placebo-controlled, multicentre trial. Lancet 2020;395(10236):1569–1578

63. Riddle MS, DuPont HL, Connor BA. ACG clinical guideline: diagnosis, treatment, and prevention of acute diarrheal infections in adults. Am J Gastroenterol 2016;111(5):602–622

64. Shane AL, Mody RK, Crump JA, et al. 2017 Infectious Diseases Society of America clinical practice guidelines for the diagnosis and management of infectious diarrhea. Clin Infect Dis 2017;65(12):e45–e80

65. Gao QY, Chen YX, Fang JY. 2019 Novel coronavirus infection and gastrointestinal tract. J Dig Dis 2020;21(3):125–126

66. Farthing M, Salam MA, Lindberg G, et al; WGO. Acute diarrhea in adults and children: a global perspective. J Clin Gastroenterol 2013;47(1):12–20

67. Jin X, Lian J-S, Hu J-H, et al. Epidemiological, clinical and virological characteristics of 74 cases of coronavirus-infected disease 2019 (COVID-19) with gastrointestinal symptoms. Gut 2020;69(6):1002–1009

68. Aghemo A, Piovani D, Parigi TL, et al; Humanitas COVID-19 Task Force. Covid-19 digestive system involvement and clinical outcomes in a large academic hospital in Milan, Italy. Clin Gastroenterol Hepatol 2020;18(10):2366–2368.e3

69. Nobel YR, Phipps M, Zucker J, et al. Gastrointestinal symptoms and coronavirus disease 2019: a case-control study from the United States. Gastroenterology 2020; 159(1):373–375.e2

70. Redd WD, Zhou JC, Hathorn KE, et al. Prevalence and characteristics of gastrointestinal symptoms in patients with severe acute respiratory syndrome coronavirus 2 infection in the United States: a multicenter cohort study. Gastroenterology 2020;159(2):765–767.e2

71. Zhang H, Liao Y-S, Gong J, Liu J, Xia X, Zhang H. Clinical characteristics of coronavirus disease (COVID-19) patients with gastrointestinal symptoms: A report of 164 cases. Dig Liver Dis 2020;52(10):1076–1079

72. Tang X, Wu C, Li X, et al. On the origin and continuing evolution of SARS-CoV-2. Natl Sci Rev 2020;7(6):1012–1023

73. Han C, Duan C, Zhang S, et al. Digestive symptoms in COVID-19 patients with mild disease severity: clinical presentation, stool viral RNA testing, and outcomes. Am J Gastroenterol 2020;115(6):916–923

10

Surveying the Association between SARS-COV-2 (COVID-19) and Its Neurological Manifestations: An Overview

Sumul Raval and Ruchi N. Raval

Introduction

The December 2019 emergence of the now recognized SARS-CoV-2 novel coronavirus fundamentally altered the lens through which 21st-century public health, epidemiology, and medicine will be addressed.[1] With an estimated R_0 of 1.5 to 3.5, SARS-CoV-2 otherwise known as COVID-19 is considered a highly infectious agent.[2] Transmissible mainly through inhalation or contact with infected droplets, COVID-19 is responsible for a series of symptoms that range from mild to deadly. The most common symptoms are pyrexia, dyspnea, cough, anosmia, aguesia, and fatigue.[2] In some cases, the disease may progress to lower respiratory disease and respiratory failure.[3] Commonly, the aged and those with comorbid conditions are at risk to develop the catastrophic complications of the disease. Though many individuals experience symptoms, there are also COVID-19 patients that present with no symptoms. These asymptomatic individuals can also contribute to the spread of COVID-19.[3]

With a total of 179,241,734 confirmed global cases including 3,889,723 deaths as reported by the World Health Organization (WHO), the RNA virus COVID-19 has evoked considerable international comradery toward developing a solution.[4] In perhaps the most groundbreaking research campaign of the century, several vaccinations for COVID-19 have been developed and distributed to date. As of June 24, 2021, 2,624,733,776 vaccine doses have been administered to the general public with the United States accounting for

over 317 million.[4] **Fig. 10.1** depicts a population-adjusted image of the current international COVID-19 vaccination efforts.[5] Because of the aggressive international vaccination efforts, the rate of morbidity and mortality related to the virus has seemingly begun to decrease. There also seem to be several novel variants that have emerged over the past year. As of now, there is limited evidence on the effectiveness of vaccination toward all potential variants.[6]

COVID-19 and the Nervous System

Though the most common symptoms of COVID-19 are related to respiratory illness, there are also several others that suggest involvement of the nervous system. Neurological complications of SARS-CoV-2 include encephalopathy, ataxia, hypogeusia, hyposmia, neuralgia, and seizures.[7] The existence of these symptoms allows for several questions. What are both the acute and chronic neurological manifestations of COVID-19, when in COVID-19 disease progression do neurological symptoms manifest, and how long do they last? While some, like Nalbandian et al, in the journal *Nature* note that lingering or permanent neurological deficits of COVID-19 fall under the umbrella postacute COVID-19, wherein persistent complications exist beyond 4 weeks from onset of COVID-19-related symptoms, others state neurological complications appear concurrently with other symptoms.[8]

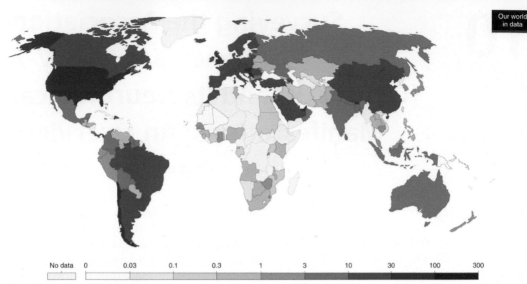

No data   0   0.03   0.1   0.3   1   3   10   30   100   300

Fig. 10.1 Cumulative vaccine doses administered per 100 individuals. Population adjustment accounts for the scale of vaccine rollout.[5] https://figshare.com/articles/software/A_global_database_of_COVID-19_vaccinations/14387702

Fig. 10.2 depicts the postulated timeline for postacute COVID-19 along with related symptoms.[8]

Understanding the timeline underlying COVID-19-related neurological manifestations further delineates whether the relationship between the two is causal. In other words, does COVID-19 directly cause neurological manifestations or are they simply a by-product? As will be discussed, research indicates that it seems to be a combination. Since December 2019, a robust amalgam of evidence has arisen that confirms the relationship between COVID-19 and nervous system involvement. Having recognized the types of symptoms and when they occur, the various potential mechanisms that allow the SARS-CoV-2 virus to infiltrate the nervous system and produce neurological symptoms will also be discussed.

COVID-19–Related Neurological Symptoms

Neurological manifestations related to SARS-CoV-2 or COVID-19 have been shown to begin as early as disease onset. As more literature related to COVID-19 is amassed, patterns indicate that the neurological manifestations can emerge in many different ways. While the manifestations can be neurological complications of the systemic disease, they can also be direct effects of the virus on the nervous system, parainfectious, or postinfectious immune-related disease.[9] Examples of parainfectious diseases include: Guillain-Barré syndrome (GBS), transverse myelitis, and acute disseminated encephalomyelitis.[10] Regardless of the mechanism, however, emergent studies demonstrate that the most frequent neurological symptoms are short term like cephalagia, muscle aches, dizziness, anosmia, and ageusia. In severe cases, other, more direct manifestations of the virus in the central nervous system (CNS) can also occur (**Fig. 10.3**).[7]

In one study, involving 214 patients, neurological manifestations occurred in 36.4% of individuals. The investigation indicated that those with more severe COVID-19 demonstrated increasing severity of neurological symptoms including acute cerebrovascular diseases, depressed levels of consciousness, and skeletal muscle injury.[11] Recently, a

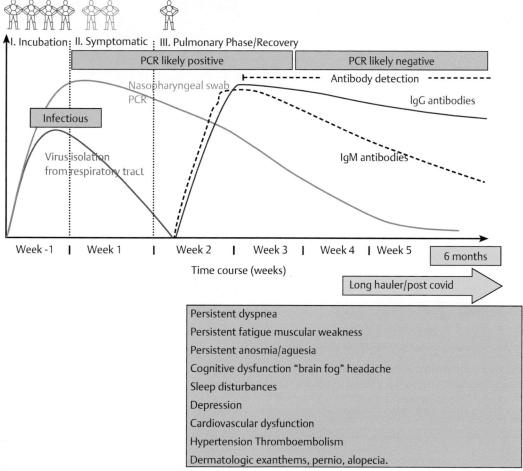

Fig. 10.2 Timeline for postacute COVID-19 defined as chronic complications ("long hauler") beyond 4 weeks of symptom onset. Permission granted by Paul Marik MD.

retrospective study of a large database containing 81 million patients of which 237,379 were diagnosed with COVID-19, 33.6% developed new-onset neuropsychiatric symptoms in the 6 months after the onset of the disease.[12,13] Interestingly, of the COVID-19 patients that were admitted to intensive care units, 46.42% diagnosed with neurological manifestations and 62.34% with encephalopathy, indicating that the more severe COVID-19 cases were, in fact, coupled with an increased incidence of neurological manifestations.[13] In the cohort of COVID-19 patients that were admitted to the ICU, the estimated incidences were as follows: 2.66% for intracranial hemorrhage, 6.92% for ischemic stroke, 0.26% for parkinsonism, 1.74% for dementia,

19.15% (17.90–20.48) for anxiety disorder, and 2.77% for psychotic disorder[13] (**Fig. 10.4**).

One of the first COVID-19 positive cases with neurological signs that was reported (April 2020) described a patient with severe cognitive impairment, bilateral ankle clonus, positive Babinski, and meningeal signs. In this patient, the computed tomography (CT) scan was unremarkable and the viral genome was not present in the patient's cerebrospinal fluid (CSF).[14]

Though COVID-19 is incredibly complex, as mentioned above, it causes considerable comprehensive risk to the entire nervous system. The manifestations can, however, be categorized by CNS involvement or peripheral nervous system (PNS) involvement.

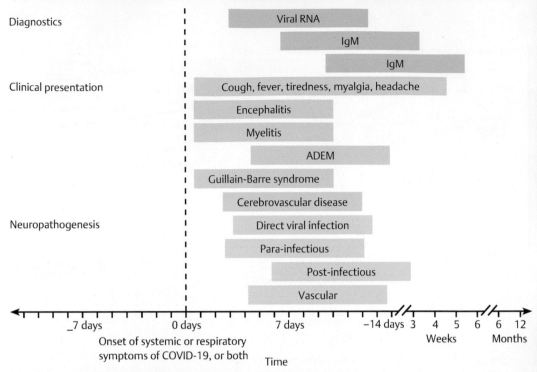

Fig. 10.3   Approximate timeline for COVID-19-related neurological symptom presentation. *Blue bars* present periods where viral RNA or antibodies can be detected via diagnostic testing. *Red bars* indicate duration of systemic and/or pulmonary symptoms. *Green bars* indicate potential neurological disease causing mechanisms.[9]   https://creativecommons.org/publicdomain/mark/1.0/

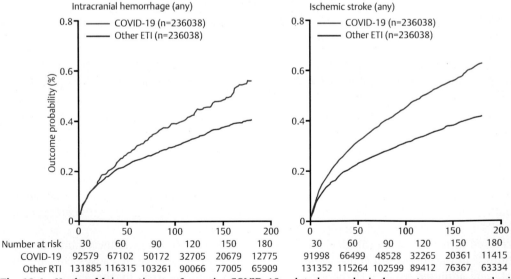

Fig. 10.4   Kaplan-Meier estimates for major COVID-19-related neurological symptoms compared with other respiratory tract infections (RTI) based symptoms.[13] http://creativecommons.org/licenses/by/4.0/ *(Continued)*

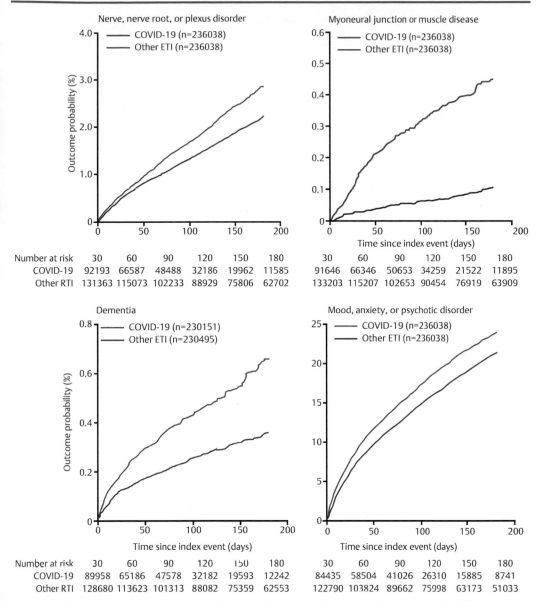

Fig. 10.4 *(Continued)* Kaplan-Meier estimates for major COVID-19-related neurological symptoms compared with other respiratory tract infections (RTI) based symptoms.[13] http://creativecommons.org/licenses/by/4.0/

Examples of COVID-19-related CNS disease include encephalopathy, acute disseminated encephalomyelitis, encephalitis, meningitis, ischemic and hemorrhagic stroke, venous sinus thrombosis, and endothelialitis.[15]

Examples of COVID-19-related PNS disease are GBS, anosmia, chemosensory dysfunction, skeletal muscle damage, neuralgia, and epilepsy among others[16] (**Fig. 10.5**).

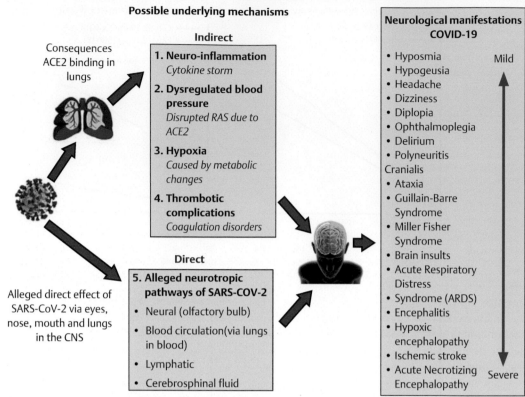

Fig. 10.5 Mechanisms of SARS-CoV-2 neuropathogenesis on the nervous system. Creative Commons License.[17]

Central Nervous System Manifestations

Encephalopathy and Neuroinflammatory Diseases (Encephalitis)

Among neurological manifestations of COVID-19, encephalopathy and encephalitis are considered to be serious.[16] Encephalopathy, collectively, is defined as alterations in mental status including disorientation, confusion, agitation, and somnolence or sleepiness.[18] These symptoms are common in elderly patients who also present with associated comorbidities or immunodeficiencies. Clinical manifestations can also include fever, headache, epilepsy, and/or impaired consciousness and is visible in magnetic resonance imaging (MRI) as altered cortical and subcortical T2/FLAIR signals.[19] In a study with 214 patients from Wuhan, China, 53 (25%) had CNS symptoms, including 36 (17%) patients with dizziness,[11] 13% with headache, and 16 (7%) with impaired consciousness.[9] In another study, a series of 58 intensive care patients were analyzed and 49 (84%) had neurological complications with 40 (69%) presenting with encephalopathy.[9]

While the vast majority of patients with encephalopathy and encephalitis do not show evidence of the presence of SARS-CoV-2 in their CSF, some patients were found to have SARS-CoV-2 in their CSF.[20] There is therefore limited evidence suggesting that entry to CSF is what causes encephalopathy and encephalitis.

Though altered mental status rarely impacts COVID-19 patients seeking care for respiratory illness, it impacts the majority of critically ill COVID-19 patients with ARDS or acute respiratory distress syndrome.[18] Importantly, the distinction between altered mental status as a result of encephalopathy caused by systemic illness or as a result of encephalitis directly caused by the SARS-CoV-2 virus itself must be made.

Encephalitis refers to inflammatory lesions caused by either pathogenic infection or the body's immune defenses.[21] Without direct brain inflammation, detection of SARS-CoV-2 in CSF does not provide definitive diagnosis of encephalitis.[9] Clinical presentation of encephalitis includes irritability, confusion, reduced consciousness, and sometimes seizures.[9]

Interestingly, SARS-CoV-2 can also promote postinfectious neurological complications. These delayed effects can impact both the CNS and the PNS. In the CNS, an example includes acute necrotizing hemorrhagic encephalopathy.[12] The first case of acute necrotizing hemorrhagic encephalopathy was reported in a 58-year-old woman with a 3-day history of cough, fever, and altered mental status (**Fig. 10.6**).[22] Though the CSF fluid showed no evidence of SARS-CoV-2, evidence of the acute necrotizing hemorrhagic encephalopathy could be observed via MRI.[1,22]

Cerebrovascular Disease or Stroke

Like other viruses, SARS-CoV-2 can also trigger acute cerebrovascular disease like acute and hemorrhagic stroke and cerebral venous sinus thrombosis.[14] Stroke incidence in patients hospitalized with COVID-19 ranges from 1 to 3% and up to 6% for those who are critically ill.[18] Even after adjustment for illness severity, this is sevenfold higher than patients with influenza. In some retrospective European and Chinese studies, stroke incidence rates were between 2.5 and 6%. Notably, critically ill SARS-CoV-2 patients often show severe platelet reduction and elevated D-dimer levels which leave the patients more susceptible to acute cerebrovascular events.[24] SARS-CoV-2 can also promote

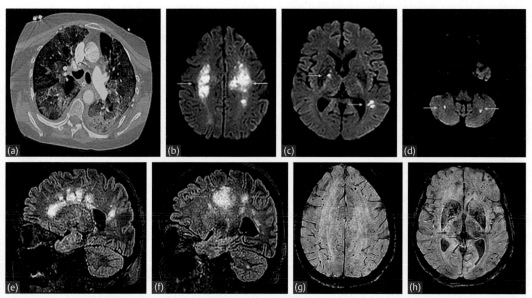

Fig. 10.6 An example of acute necrotizing hemorrhagic encephalopathy, computed tomography (CT) chest **(a)** demonstrating bilateral peripheral ground glass opacities of a 68-year-old woman who presented with severe COVID-19-associated respiratory failure. Her hospital course was complicated by coma and stupor 30 days postadmission. Magnetic resonance imaging (MRI) of the brain **(b-h)** (diffusion-weighted imaging, axial sections) showing diffuse hyperintensities in multiple areas of the brain. Creative Commons Attribution License.[23]

cytokine storm syndromes, contributing to acute cerebrovascular disease.[24,25]

While some patients having limited comorbidities experienced stroke, the majority of COVID-19 patients who experienced an acute cerebrovascular incident were elderly or had numerous vascular comorbidities.[18] The direct causal relationship therefore remains unknown. The strongest association between COVID-19 and stroke that can be made is that both share similar risk factors. SARS-CoV-2 can damage endothelial cells, thus activating thrombotic pathways and leading to vascular complications in the brain.[9,25]

Multiple Sclerosis and COVID-19

The relationship between COVID-19 and multiple sclerosis (MS) is, to date, being studied.[23] It is theorized that viral infection may contribute to pathogenesis in genetically predisposed individuals.[23] Though several human coronaviruses including CoV-OC-43 and CoV-229E have been linked to MS, the potential direct relationship of SARS-CoV-2 has not been uncovered. But, considering its structural and characteristic similarities to other beta coronaviruses, it is likely to behave similarly.[23] Thus, it is expected that SARS-CoV-2 can contribute to producing MS-like lesions as long-term consequences of COVID-19.[23] This relationship, however, is yet to be proven.[12]

Peripheral Nervous System Manifestations

Anosmia and Chemosensory Dysfunction

Anosmia and ageusia occur frequently in patients with COVID-19 and have become key diagnostic markers for disease.[9] These symptoms are more prevalent among COVID-19 patients than for any cohort of influenza patients.[9] Because the symptoms are isolated from other COVID-19-related symptoms,

there is considerable evidence of olfactory nerve involvement. The olfactory neural system is considered to be part of the PNS.

Guillain-Barré Syndrome

GBS is an acute polyradiculopathy or immune attack on peripheral nerves characterized by a rapid ascending paralysis and can include cranial nerve involvement resulting in facial muscle paralysis. Though the incidence rate is not particularly high, there have been several patients who have been diagnosed with GBS and COVID-19.[9] Symptoms of GBS typically emerge 1 week after the incidence of COVID-19-related pulmonary and/or systemic symptoms.[9] The first patient to be diagnosed with GBS and COVID-19 was a 61-year-old female in Wuhan, China, who was admitted with acute weakness of bilateral lower extremities and severe fatigue.[19] The patient recovered after treatment with antivirals.[19] Thus far, two patients have presented with the Miller Fisher variant of GBS.[9]

Other COVID-19–Related Neurological Manifestations

Long-term intensive care of critically ill patients requiring mechanical ventilation, etc., can cause related neurological manifestations.[11,18] These symptoms are not necessarily directly induced by the disease, but instead are a byproduct of therapy. Some manifestations include delirium which occurs in more than 80% of patients on mechanical ventilators in ICUs.[18] Patients who are sedated and are on neuromuscular blockade, like those with ARDS, are also at high risk of delirium.[18]

Potential SARS-CoV-2 Mechanism of Nervous System Invasion

To date, including SARS-CoV-2, there have been seven known coronaviruses that have infected humans. Of these zoonotic viruses, three have caused severe widespread illness: SARS-CoV, MERS-CoV, and most recently SARS-CoV-2 or COVID-19.[26] Characterized as a beta coronavirus, SARS-CoV-2 shares almost 80% sequence identity with SARS-CoV and MERS-CoV.[7] Similar to SARS-CoV, it acts by binding to the ACE-2 (angiotensin-converting enzyme 2) receptor on the surface of various cell types.[7] Because of strong electrostatic differences between spike protein and the ACE-2 binding interface, there seems to be more powerful interactions between these two proteins than with SARS-CoV and ACE-2. This implies a potentially higher affinity for SARS-CoV-2.[7]

To date, there have been several theories for potential neuroinvasion of SARS-CoV-2. Despite the multiple barriers protecting the CNS, some viruses can still infiltrate the system. In most cases, viral infections begin with the peripheral tissues moving into the peripheral nerves and subsequently creeping into the central nervous system. In the case of SARS-CoV-2, the existence of olfactory dysfunction as a symptom also indicates potential involvement of the cranial nerves and olfactory system.[7] In one study analyzing autopsy materials from 33 patients with fatal cases of COVID-19, researchers mapped the viral infection through olfactory nervous tracts and CNS regions.[27] By measuring viral load using RT-qPCR in the olfactory mucosa, olfactory bulb, medulla oblongata, cerebellum, and other regions, scientists demonstrated that the greatest levels of SARS-CoV-2 RNA was found in the olfactory mucosa beneath the cribriform plate.[27] Using this data, they concluded that one potential route of nervous system invasion is via the neuronal-mucosal interface in the olfactory mucosa.[27] After initial invasion and by taking advantage of close proximity to other relevant structures, SARS-CoV-2 can penetrate other neuroanatomical areas.[27]

Growing evidence indicates that the olfactory nerve is a compelling prospect for the virus gaining access to the central nervous system.[7] Due to the large amount of ACE2 in the endothelial cells of the olfactory tract, the virus can potentially invade the brain. This is known as the transcribial route.[7]

In a study administering SARS-CoV and MERS-CoV to transgenic mice, viral CNS infiltration was noted via the olfactory bulb.[7] Though the exact mechanism of access to the CNS was not fully identified, it suggested that SARS-CoV-2 may also behave similarly.[7] One possibility is the vagus nerve with pulmonary and intestinal afferent nerves that reach the brainstem. This theory is supported by the identification of SARS-CoV-2 in the feces of patients.[7] Furthermore, an in vitro study revealed the ability of the virus to infect the human intestinal epithelium.[7] Further research to support this hypothesis must still be conducted.

Another potential source of nervous system invasion is via what is known as the hematogenous route. In this mechanism, the virus, having entered the bloodstream, will go on to invade various organs including the brain. Release into the blood may increase permeability of the blood–brain barrier, thus increasing the viral entry to the brain and viral encephalitis.[24] This theory, however, is considered secondary to the olfactory nerve hypothesis as there is not as much evidence supporting the hypothesis that SARS-CoV-2 acts in this way (**Fig. 10.7**).[24]

Treatment Options

The overwhelming evidence confirming SARS-CoV-2/COVID-19-associated neurological involvement indicates a demanding pressure for developing strong treatment options and therapies for symptomatic patients. Awareness of COVID-19 mechanisms is important for this endeavor. Considering the infectious nature of the disease and the ways it altered societal norms, COVID-19 prompted, in many ways, a resurgence of telehealth technologies. According to one study by the American Epilepsy society, one-third of the patients they surveyed reported new-onset seizures after COVID-19 with no prior history.[24] Because of care delivery limitations in hospitals, clinics, etc., many patients found

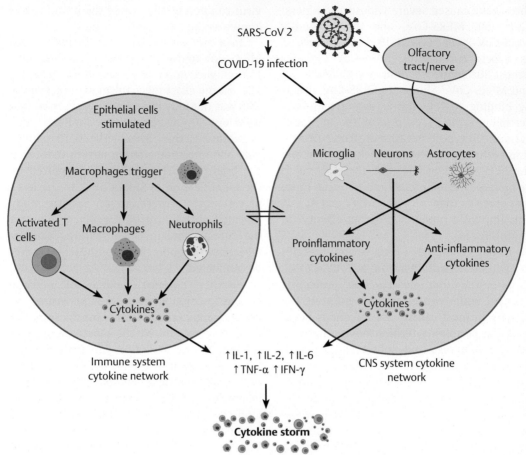

Fig. 10.7 Potential modes of SARS-CoV-2 infection causing CNS damage. As seen above, coronavirus can (1) cause direct damage via infection through blood circulation and neuronal pathways, (2) attack the lung tissue promoting hypoxia, etc., and (3) enter through the olfactory nerve.[16,35] Modified from Bhasker S. et al.[35] Creative Commons Attribution 4.0 International

value in telehealth technologies, with more than 90% indicating a willingness to use telehealth in at least some way.[24]

Stroke care and treatment protocols of patients with COVID-19 have also been evaluated since December 2019. A study with all COVID-19 patients receiving IV tPA at participating hospitals noted that despite the COVID-19 diagnosis, IV tPA continues to be safe and efficacious.[28] This study, however, only included 33 patients. A larger study would have to be conducted to produce more generalizable results.[28] A Spanish study observing 796 patients who received reperfusion therapies for stroke concluded

that during the COVID-19 pandemic, these therapies were actually less beneficial.[29] This conclusion was not because the treatment modality was less effective, but that significant hospital delays during the pandemic resulted in a decreased overall success rate.[29] Other studies also indicated prolonged stroke treatment times during the pandemic. This issue is likely a result of overcrowding. The study noted that despite "post-epidemic" conditions in some places, reperfusion times are still delayed.[30]

The care of COVID-19 patients with other chronic neurological issues that are treated via immunosuppressive therapies like multiple sclerosis (MS) and neuromyelitis optica spectrum disorder (NMOSD) must also be evaluated.[14] While some believe that clinicians should consider interrupting immunosuppressive treatment in COVID-19 patients with worsening symptoms, others have suggested that mild immunosuppression induced by MS treatment may prevent the development of more severe COVID-19 cases. The use of high-dose corticosteroids may also be halted as it could contribute to a higher risk of viral reactivation.[14]

COVID-19 patients who experience severe neurological manifestations are likely to endure intensive care stays. On the whole, most of the treatment they receive is supportive. Since December 2019, therapies like antivirals, steroids, anticoagulants, monoclonal antibodies, and antimalarial drugs have been utilized along with mechanical ventilation.[31] All these treatment protocols and therapeutic efforts are focused around addressing respiratory insufficiency, organ failure, hypercoagulable state, and immune dysregulation. These are byproducts mainly of COVID-19. To date, there are no specific therapeutic protocols for addressing the neurological manifestations of COVID-19. These are managed according to existing standard protocol.[18] For example, early therapy with antivirals has been demonstrated to be effective against viral encephalitis.[32]

Prophylaxis and Preventative Measures

The most effective way to prevent COVID-19-related neurological manifestations is to prevent COVID-19. The development of SARS-CoV-2 vaccines is considered to be one of the greatest research feats of the 21st century. To date, there are three vaccinations approved for use by the FDA in the United States. All are deemed effective preventative measures against COVID-19.[33] Because the vaccinations do not provide 100% protection against the virus, and because of the potential for mutation and creation of variants, there lies a need

for the development of other preventative therapies.

One study, utilizing human brain organoids in vitro observed that employing antibodies directed against ACE2 or administering CSF from COVID-19 patients can potentially prevent neuronal infection.[34] These results have not been applied to in vivo models.

Other studies note the potential link between environmental contaminants with neurological symptoms and neuroinflammation. Because the response of the CNS to SARS-CoV-2 may be influenced by its inflammatory state, exposure to pollution may play a role. There are, however, limited studies that analyze whether neuroinflammatory mechanisms are truly exacerbated by environmental pollutant exposure.[35] If, in fact, environmental influences are an impetus to the exacerbation of a neurological response to COVID-19, preventative measures could be imposed. In this case, limitations based on social determinants of health would be of concern. Socioeconomic differences and access to various environments could potentially impede on an individual's ability to seek the appropriate preventative measures.

Overall, besides preventing the onset of COVID-19, there are no other specific preventative techniques or therapies in the literature to directly address neurological manifestations. As was stated above, most of these symptoms are treated according to standard practice. Besides vaccinations, other standard preventative techniques include maintaining good general hygiene, wearing a mask, maintaining 6-foot social distancing, and avoiding poorly ventilated areas.[36] Notably, however, if providers encounter individuals with notable neurological manifestations, recognizing that these symptoms are potentially related to COVID-19 may lead to the appropriate diagnosis, preventing delayed diagnosis and further transmission of the disease to others.[37]

Conclusion

The overwhelming evidence indicating a strong relationship between the virus and neurological manifestations has meaningful consequences for the future of neurological care worldwide.[15] As the virus continues to pervade through all countries and civilizations, and as it continues to mutate creating variants, the paradigm of care must be adjusted accordingly.

The developing body of knowledge surrounding neurological manifestations of COVID-19 will likely grow in the coming days as more relationships between SARS-CoV-2 and cellular/immunological/neuronal pathways are uncovered. There are also several existing inquiries, like the connection between SARS-CoV-2 and MS, that have yet to be understood.

Since December 2019, COVID-19 has been the most pervasive and all-encompassing challenge facing mankind. The discussion surrounding symptoms, therapies, and, ultimately, the development of the groundbreaking vaccines has fundamentally altered the way 21st century healthcare is approached. While, as was discussed, COVID-19's correlation with neurological symptoms is undeniable, there is much left to be undiscovered. By elucidating the symptoms and underlying mechanisms, researchers and providers can begin developing more relevant and cutting edge therapies. While the fight against COVID-19 is long from over, the advances in literature that have emerged since December 2019 are a great step in the right direction.

References

1. Fauci AS, Lane HC, Redfield RR. Covid-19: navigating the uncharted. N Engl J Med 2020;382(13):1268–1269

2. Achaiah NC, Subbarajasetty SB, Shetty RM. R_0 and R_e of COVID-19: can we predict when the pandemic outbreak will be contained? Indian J Crit Care Med 2020;24(11):1125–1127

3. Singhal T. A review of Coronavirus disease-2019 (COVID-19). Indian J Pediatr 2020;87(4):281–286

4. WHO. WHO coronavirus (COVID-19) dashboard. https://covid19.who.int/. Accessed July 12, 2021

5. Mathieu E, Ritchie H, Ortiz-Ospina E, et al. A global database of COVID-19 vaccinations. Nat Hum Behav 2021;5(7):947–953

6. Rubin R. COVID-19 vaccines vs variants-determining how much immunity is enough. JAMA 2021;325(13):1241–1243

7. Reza-Zaldívar EE, Hernández-Sapiéns MA, Minjarez B, et al. Infection mechanism of SARS-COV-2 and its implication on the nervous system. Front Immunol 2021;11:621735

8. Nalbandian A, Sehgal K, Gupta A, et al. Post-acute COVID-19 syndrome. Nat Med 2021;27(4):601–615

9. Ellul MA, Benjamin L, Singh B, et al. Neurological associations of COVID-19. Lancet Neurol 2020;19(9):767–783

10. Needham EJ, Chou SH-Y, Coles AJ, Menon DK. Neurological implications of COVID-19 infections. Neurocrit Care 2020;32(3):667–671

11. Wang HY, Li XL, Yan ZR, Sun XP, Han J, Zhang BW. Potential neurological symptoms of COVID-19. Adv Neurol Disord 2020;13:1756286420917830

12. Montalvan V, Lee J, Bueso T, De Toledo J, Rivas K. Neurological manifestations of COVID-19 and other coronavirus infections: a systematic review. Clin Neurol Neurosurg 2020;194(105921):105921

13. Taquet M, Geddes JR, Husain M, Luciano S, Harrison PJ. 6-month neurological and psychiatric outcomes in 236 379 survivors of COVID-19: a retrospective cohort study using electronic health records. Lancet Psychiatry 2021;8(5):416–427

14. Orsini A, Corsi M, Santangelo A, et al. Challenges and management of neurological and psychiatric manifestations in SARS-CoV-2 (COVID-19) patients. Neurol Sci 2020;41(9):2353–2366

15. Koralnik IJ, Tyler KL. COVID-19: a global threat to the nervous system. Ann Neurol 2020;88(1):1–11

16. Poyiadji N, Shahin G, Noujaim D, Stone M, Patel S, Griffith B. COVID-19-associated acute hemorrhagic necrotizing encephalopathy: imaging features. Radiology 2020;296(2):E119–E120

17. Wenting A, Gruters A, van Os Y, et al. COVID-19 neurological manifestations and underlying mechanisms: a scoping review. Front Psychiatry 2020;11:860

18. Iadecola C, Anrather J, Kamel H. Effects of COVID-19 on the nervous system. Cell 2020;183(1):16–27.e1
19. Zhao F, Han Z, Wang R, Luo Y. Neurological manifestations of COVID-19: causality or coincidence? Aging Dis 2021;12(1):27–35
20. Ahmad I, Rathore FA. Neurological manifestations and complications of COVID-19: a literature review. J Clin Neurosci 2020;77: 8–12
21. Wu Y, Xu X, Chen Z, et al. Nervous system involvement after infection with COVID-19 and other coronaviruses. Brain Behav Immun 2020;87:18–22
22. Yachou Y, El Idrissi A, Belapasov V, Ait Benali S. Neuroinvasion, neurotropic, and neuroinflammatory events of SARS-CoV-2: understanding the neurological manifestations in COVID-19 patients. Neurol Sci 2020;41(10):2657–2669
23. Mullaguri N, Sivakumar S, Battineni A, Anand S, Vanderwerf J. COVID-19 related acute hemorrhagic necrotizing encephalitis: a report of two cases and literature review. Cureus 2021;13(4):e14236
24. Albert DVF, Das RR, Acharya JN, et al. The impact of COVID-19 on epilepsy care: a survey of the American Epilepsy Society membership. Epilepsy Curr 2020;20(5): 316–324
25. Bhaskar S, Sinha A, Banach M, et al. Cytokine storm in COVID-19-immunopathological mechanisms, clinical considerations, and therapeutic approaches: The REPROGRAM consortium position paper. Front Immunol 2020;11:1648
26. Tsivgoulis G, Palaiodimou L, Katsanos AH, et al. Neurological manifestations and implications of COVID-19 pandemic. Ther Adv Neurol Disord 2020;13:1756286420932036
27. Meinhardt J, Radke J, Dittmayer C, et al. Olfactory transmucosal SARS-CoV-2 invasion as a port of central nervous system entry in individuals with COVID-19. Nat Neurosci 2021;24(2):168–175
28. Carneiro T, Dashkoff J, Leung LY, et al. Intravenous tPA for acute ischemic stroke in patients with COVID-19. J Stroke Cerebrovasc Dis 2020;29(11):105201
29. Tejada Meza H, Lambea Gil Á, Sancho Saldaña A, et al; NORDICTUS Investigators. Impact of COVID-19 outbreak in reperfusion therapies of acute ischaemic stroke in northwest Spain. Eur J Neurol 2020;27(12):2491–2498
30. Zhang T, Chen C, Xu X, et al. Impact of the COVID-19 pandemic and post-epidemic periods on the process of endovascular treatment for acute anterior circulation ischaemic stroke. BMC Neurol 2021;21(1):238
31. Yamamoto V, Bolanos JF, Fiallos J, et al. COVID-19: review of a 21st century pandemic from etiology to neuro-psychiatric implications. J Alzheimers Dis 2020;77(2):459–504
32. Armocida D, Palmieri M, Frati A, Santoro A, Pesce A. How SARS-Cov-2 can involve the central nervous system. A systematic analysis of literature of the department of human neurosciences of Sapienza University, Italy. J Clin Neurosci 2020;79:231–236
33. Livingston EH. Necessity of 2 doses of the Pfizer and Moderna COVID-19 vaccines. JAMA 2021;325(9):898
34. Song E, Zhang C, Israelow B, et al. Neuroinvasion of SARS-CoV-2 in human and mouse brain. J Exp Med 2021;218(3):e20202135
35. Reyes MSS, Medina PMB. Environmental pollutant exposure can exacerbate COVID-19 neurologic symptoms. Med Hypotheses 2020;144(110136):110136
36. Wong SH, Teoh JYC, Leung C-H, et al. COVID 19 and public interest in face mask use. Am J Respir Crit Care Med 2020;202(3):453–455
37. Mao L, Jin H, Wang M, et al. Neurologic manifestations of hospitalized patients with Coronavirus disease 2019 in Wuhan, China. JAMA Neurol 2020;77(6):683–690

11 Cutaneous Manifestations of SARS-CoV-2

Vignesh Ravi, Alessandra Chen, Marie Donaldson, and Binh Ngo

Introduction

Severe acute respiratory syndrome coronavirus 2 (SARS-CoV-2) is a novel viral infection with dual pathogenicity that can ultimately affect multiple organ systems. It begins as a flulike infection by the SARS-CoV-2 virus. In a significant minority of patients, as the immune system overcomes the phase of viral replication, the immune response advances to an accelerating inflammatory phase, typically resulting in an organizing pneumonia.[1] A cytokine release syndrome can progress to involve multiple organ systems, including the heart and kidneys, with an associated coagulopathy that has caused thrombotic events in otherwise healthy people.[2-6] Secondary bacterial and fungal infections can occur during the inflammatory phase.[1]

The major features of the COVID-19 inflammatory phase are so severe that less attention has been devoted to associated skin problems. One large-scale study noted that 8.8% of patients positive for SARS-CoV-2 presented with cutaneous findings, in which involvement of the trunk or extremities (6.8%) was more common than that of acral surfaces (3.1%).[7] Occasionally, cutaneous symptoms were the first manifestation of COVID-19 infection (17%), and sometimes the skin rash or lesion was the only symptom (21%).[7] Notably, another study observed that significantly more patients with rash secondary to COVID-19 required invasive mechanical ventilation (60.9%) than those without rash (30.3%).[8]

Several primary patterns of cutaneous involvement in COVID-19 include eruptions consisting of macules and papules, perniosis/pseudochilblain lesions, vesicular rash, urticarial rash, and livedoid/vaso-occlusive lesions. Of these different morphologies, vesicular eruptions can appear early in the course (15% before other symptoms), and pseudochilblain lesions frequently occur late in the disease course.[9-11] The disease stage associated with each morphology may help guide appropriate treatment. However, it is also true that these different morphologies may exist concurrently, as we have seen in a single patient (**Fig. 11.1**, **Fig. 11.2**, **Fig. 11.3**, **Fig. 11.4**).

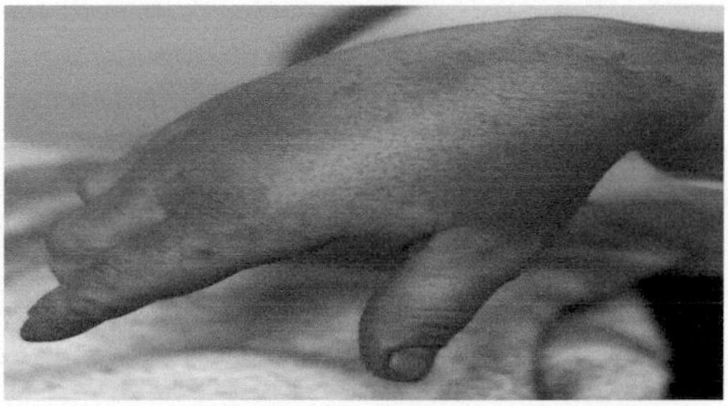

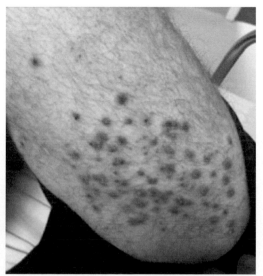

Fig. 11.1 Macular erythematous reaction in COVID-19.

Fig. 11.2 Vesicular reaction in COVID-19.

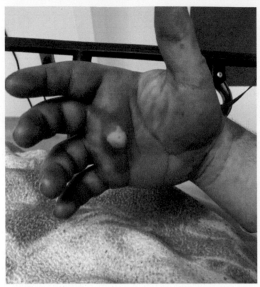

Fig. 11.3 Pernio reaction with blister in COVID-19.

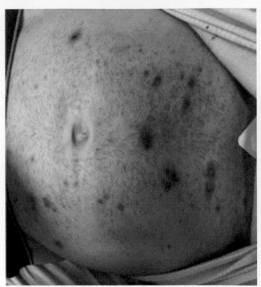

Fig. 11.4 Livedoid reaction in COVID-19.

Eruptions Composed of Macules and Papules

Several observational, large-scale studies have identified eruptions composed of macules and papules as the most commonly reported cutaneous morphology associated with SARS-CoV-2, as high a proportion as 47%.[9] These eruptions presented as a diverse array of clinical patterns, including morbilliform, purpuric, erythema multiforme–like, pityriasis rosea–like, erythema elevatum diutinum–like, and perifollicular.[9,12] The trunk was most frequently involved, followed by the neck, extremities, and buttocks.[12–14] Most patients reported pruritus and less commonly pain or burning.[9,14,15] Several cases of these eruptions co-occurring with other morphologies, including urticaria, pernio, and purpura, were reported.[9,14] Most often, the eruptions occurred at or after the onset of other COVID-19 symptoms, suggesting a viral exanthem during the phase of viral replication.[9,10,14] The average age of patients with this type of rash varied from 35.8 to 55.3 years.[9,15] A single study noted a significant female predominance among patients with morbilliform eruptions (p = 0.008).[16]

The mean length of the rash was 8 days (2 to 14 days).[17]

Regarding the different clinical morphologies observed, morbilliform eruptions were the most frequent subtype (45.5%). Most commonly, the morbilliform rash was generalized, symmetric, and confluent, starting in the trunk with centrifugal progression, and lasted 7.2 days (±4.3 days). A nonspecific pattern (20%) was recognized as localized or generalized nonconfluent erythematous macules or papules with occasional scaling, which persisted for an average of 11.8 days. Most cases were symptomatic (63.9%), primarily with pruritus. Purpuric eruptions (14.2%) were more common in males (60%), predominantly involved the trunk and upper extremities with a mean duration of 7.4 days (±4.5 days), and most often (44%) presented with pruritus. A significant proportion (88.2%) of the erythema multiforme–like eruptions (9.7%) occurred in females. These were characterized by generalized, symmetric, and confluent erythematous–violaceous macules and papules with occasional targetoid lesions that began on the trunk. Some patients had palmoplantar involvement. The mean duration of erythema multiforme–like eruptions was 9.7 days (±4.9 days). Pruritus and burning occurred in 65% of the cases. Pityriasis rosea–like eruptions (5.7%) primarily manifested as erythematous, brown, scaly, discrete annular plaques on the trunk in a generalized distribution. These lesions persisted for an average duration of 12.1 days (±4.5 days), and similar to other morphologies, symptomatic cases (50%) noted pruritus. Erythema elevatum diutinum–like eruptions (2.3%) were identified as pink to erythematous papules on the dorsum of the hands, which were present for 6 days (±4.1 days). Most cases were symptomatic (75%) with pruritus or burning. Lastly, perifollicular eruptions (2.3%) were defined as erythematous, brownish perifollicular papules mainly localized to the trunk in a symmetric and confluent distribution, lasting on average 4.5 ± 1 days. Unlike other clinical patterns, these lesions were primarily asymptomatic (75%).[18]

The most common concurrent SARS-CoV-2 symptoms in patients with an eruption consisting of macules and papules included fever, cough, dyspnea, and asthenia.[9,14] Notably, the morbilliform and erythema multiforme–like subtypes were associated with the highest rate of admission to the hospital secondary to pneumonia (80 and 76.5%, respectively), with 18.8% escalated to intensive care and 11.5% needing noninvasive mechanical ventilation.[18] Of the other morphologies consisting of macules and papules, about 44% required hospital admission due to pneumonia.[18] One study reported a 2% mortality rate in patients with SARS-CoV-2, with associated rash consisting of macules or papules.[9] The therapies these patients received were not specifically targeted for their rash; instead, the treatments was for the underlying SARS-CoV-2 infection.[17,18] There is limited evidence to suggest that topical steroids are effective.[19]

The histological features identified in these eruptions include superficial perivascular dermatitis with lymphocytic infiltrate and dilated middermal and papillary vessels with eosinophils and neutrophils. Involvement of the epidermis includes foci of hydropic changes and parakeratosis, minimal acanthosis, subcorneal pustules, spongiosis, and basal cell vacuolation.[17] Histological samples from six patients showed neither intranuclear viral inclusions nor COVID-19 positivity on in situ hybridization and immunohistochemistry.[20] These findings challenged the theory that these maculopapular rashes in SARS-CoV-2 are due to direct viral damage, postulated by other studies.[20,21] Rather, these findings suggest that these cutaneous lesions were immune mediated.

A caveat to the association between SARS-CoV-2 and maculopapular eruptions is that the etiology could be due to drug-induced hypersensitivity reactions in some cases. Certain histological features that are statistically more unique to a drug-mediated rash consisting of macules and papules would include lymphocytic exocytosis and dermal infiltrates of eosinophils, lymphocytes, and histiocytes and may assist in distinguishing an eruption due to SARS-CoV-2 infection from a drug-induced reaction.[22]

Perniosis/Pseudochilblains

Pernio- or chilblainlike lesions are another common cutaneous morphology linked to COVID-19 infection; some studies have reported as high a proportion as 46%.[23] These lesions are often referred to as pseudochilblains, given that the clinical appearance of erythematous or violaceous, occasionally ulcerated, papules favoring acral sites is similar but lacks cold exposure as the inciting event. These findings have been commonly referred to as "COVID toes" when involving the feet. Pseudochilblains usually present as erythematous or violaceous papules on acral surfaces, occasionally with vesicles or pustules.[10] The feet are affected in 94% of cases and the hands in 15%. Acrocyanosis and acral desquamation have been observed.[11,24] The majority of the cases (66%) present with pain/burning, while 43% report pruritus.[11] This cutaneous reaction is more commonly reported in white patients (89%) versus only 7.3% in Asians, 0.7% for African American, and

2.7% for Hispanic/Latino.[11] Differences in how visible inflammation manifests in various skin tones may partly account for the discrepancy in ethnicities affected. The perniolike lesions presented after the onset of COVID-19 symptoms in 35.8 to 54% of cases, and the reported median duration was 14 days (14–23).[10,11]

The perniolike rash occurred predominately in younger patients (mean age of 27.2 years) and was associated with a good prognosis (98.7% survival).[10] It was reported by a single study that 75% of these cases did not have other comorbidities, 98% were outpatients, and, of those hospitalized, 0.6% died.[11] It must be underscored that several of the patients with these pseudochilblain lesions tested negative for SARS-CoV-2. Only 29% met Centers for Disease Control and Prevention (CDC) passing criteria, a lower proportion than patients who developed morbilliform, vesicular, or urticarial eruptions.[14] Pseudochilblains may be a late-phase symptom occurring after viral clearance, as 55% of patients reported having no other symptoms of SARS-CoV-2.[11,16]

Data regarding the histopathology of these perniolike lesions of SARS-CoV-2 are limited. Reported findings include lymphoid/lymphoplasmacytic infiltrate in the dermis with a prevalent perivascular pattern, and superficial and deep dermal lymphocytic infiltrates with mild vacuolar interface dermatitis, as well as occasional basal vacuolization.[11,25] Given that vasculopathy, which is found in classic pernio, was not consistently identified on histology, it has been proposed that the pseudochilblain lesions may instead be inflammatory.[11] A study examining the histology of perniosis associated with COVID-19 infection demonstrated a superficial and deep angiocentric lymphocytic infiltrate with minimal vascular damage.[26] However, several studies of patients with pseudochilblains have shown neither positive SARS-CoV-2 polymerase chain reaction tests nor positive immunoglobulin M (IgM) or IgG antibodies to SARS-CoV-2.[24,27]

There are no dedicated studies examining treatments specifically for perniolike lesions associated with COVID-19 infection. Therapies used in treating classic chilblains, such as avoidance of cold and vasoconstrictive substances and the use of potent topical steroids, calcium channel blockers, or topical nitroglycerin, have been suggested.[25] Additionally, given that SARS-CoV-2 appears to induce a prothrombotic state, low-dose aspirin, when appropriately administered considering other comorbidities, may potentially aid in preventing the pseudochilblain lesions.[25]

Vesicular Eruption

Vesicular eruptions account for approximately 11% of cutaneous lesions secondary to SARS-CoV-2. The most commonly affected sites on the body were the chest, abdomen, upper and lower extremities, and buttocks.[14,27] Most vesicular lesions were symptomatic, as 68 to 72% experienced pruritus and 50% reported pain or burning.[9,14] The median age was 54.3 to 55 years.[9,14] The average duration of rash was 10.4 days.[9]

Studies have shown two major subtypes of vesicular eruptions, namely, a diffuse presentation and a localized presentation. The diffuse presentation, which involved more than one region of the body, was present more frequently (75%) and consisted of 7- to 8-mm papules, vesicles, and pustules, each presenting simultaneously.[27] The localized presentation (25%) appeared to favor the chest, upper abdomen, or back and consisted of 3- to 4-mm monomorphic lesions, each in the same stage of evolution.[27] Hemorrhagic vesicles were also observed.[9]

The most common noncutaneous symptoms present in association with a vesicular rash were cough, fever, asthenia, and sore throat.[9,14] The majority of these patients were treated through ambulatory care; the few hospitalized in one study did not require supplemental oxygen.[14] Akin to patients with eruptions composed of macules and papules, patients with vesicular forms of rash did not receive therapies specifically targeting the cutaneous component.[9,27] Patients with vesicular eruptions demonstrated an overall survival of 96.1 to 100%.[9,10]

A reported 29 to 79.2% of vesicular eruptions occurred after the onset of symptoms from SARS-CoV-2, 12.5 to 56% noted rash at the same time as other symptoms, and approximately 15% experienced cutaneous lesions an average of 14 days before other symptoms.[9,10,14,27]

The histology of these vesicular eruptions has been described as intraepidermal vesicles with scattered multinucleated and ballooned keratinocytes with mild acantholysis.[27] Evaluation of deeper sections showed epidermal detachment and confluent keratinocyte necrosis in addition to intravesicular fibrinoid material with acute inflammatory infiltrate.[28] Other histological findings include basket-weave hyperkeratosis, atrophic epidermis, basal vacuolization with hyperchromatic keratinocytes, and dyskeratotic cells.[29]

Urticaria

Urticaria, as characterized by erythematous and edematous transient papules and plaques associated with SARS-CoV-2, was reported to affect the trunk, buttocks, and upper and lower extremities, including the hands.[9,14] The rash was frequently associated with pruritus (74–92%); a few patients noted burning or pain.[9,14] This reaction was observed in patients aged 42 to 48.7 years, with a female predominance (64–78%).[9,14] The duration of the urticaria was, on average, 6.8 days (±7.8 days).[9]

The most frequent SARS-CoV-2 symptoms associated with urticaria were fever, cough, asthenia, headache, dyspnea, and sore throat.[9,14] Most patients (56–67%) with an urticarial rash were ambulatory.[14] A review of a national registry revealed 33 to 44% of patients required admission to the hospital, and 11 to 17.4% required intensive care with ventilatory support.[9,14] Nevertheless, patients who developed urticaria showed an overall survival rate of 97.5 to 100%.[9,10]

Urticaria was observed simultaneously (22–61%) or shortly after the onset of other

COVID-19 symptoms (33.1–67%).[9,10,14] This timing suggests that urticarial reactions possibly correspond to the viral syndrome or early inflammatory phases of infection, as the histamine- and bradykinin-induced vasodilation from uncontrolled inflammation may cause urticaria.

Cases of urticaria concurrent with SARS-CoV-2 were treated with antihistamines and steroids, with variable resolution of urticaria ranging from less than 24 hours to 2 weeks.[30] Systemic steroids likely augment the response of urticarial lesions to antihistamines through additive prevention of mast cell activation and histamine release.[31]

Histopathology of urticarial lesions showed features including interface dermatitis with lymphocytic vasculitis of the superficial plexus with foci of red cell extravasation, dilated dermal vessels, and perivascular lymphocytic and neutrophilic infiltrate with a partial compromise of the vessel wall.[32]

The mechanism of urticarial reactions associated with SARS-CoV-2 is thought to be linked to mast cell degranulation, which may occur during a systemic inflammatory response induced by infection with COVID-19. Studies have demonstrated colocalization of SARS-CoV-2 envelope glycoproteins and complement components in peripheral dermal microvessels.[33] This finding supports that activation of the complement cascade and alteration of cytokine–chemokine signaling may be responsible for the urticarial reaction in SARS-CoV-2.[30]

Livedoid/Vaso-Occlusive Lesions

Livedoid or vaso-occlusive lesions, including livedo reticularis, livedo racemosa, retiform purpura, and acral ischemia, have been described in the setting of SARS-CoV-2.[10] These vaso-occlusive lesions appeared at the time of initial infection with COVID-19 (68–86%).[9,10] In contrast to other cutaneous reactions associated with SARS-CoV-2, these livedoid lesions are primarily asymptomatic;

patients less frequently experienced pruritus (14%), burning (10%), or pain (5%).[9] Livedoid lesions are more prominent in elderly patients, affecting an average age of 63.1 years, and were reported to persist for 9.4 days (±5.4 days).[9]

Retiform purpura, a clinical pattern of livedoid vasculopathy characterized by deep red or purple patches or plaques with peripheral branching, affected the lower extremities more frequently than the upper extremities, hands, or feet and were primarily asymptomatic. These lesions occurred after the onset of other SARS-CoV-2 symptoms (91%) and demonstrated a male predominance (82%).[14] Patients with retiform purpura notably had very high rates of acute respiratory distress syndrome, thrombotic events, and infections.[14]

Noncutaneous manifestations of SARS-CoV-2 occurring with livedoid lesions were fever, cough, dyspnea, and asthenia.[9,14] Livedoid lesions were associated with more severe infection relative to other cutaneous morphologies, as 86% of patients with livedoid lesions were hospitalized, with 33% requiring intensive care.[9] Specifically with regard to retiform purpura, one study reported a 100% hospitalization rate, with 91% of patients requiring mechanical ventilation or extracorporeal membrane oxygenation.[14] Another study reported that 67% of patients with any purpuric skin lesion and 80% of patients with any necrotic skin lesion secondary to COVID-19 required mechanical ventilation.[8] Because a more significant number of patients with vaso-occlusive lesions also had more severe disease when compared to those with other cutaneous morphologies, they were more likely to be treated with systemic medications targeting COVID-19 infection such as chloroquine/hydroxychloroquine, lopinavir/ritonavir, and systemic corticosteroids.[9] The patient mortality due to SARS-CoV-2 in patients with a form of livedoid vasculopathy was 10 to 21.1%.[9,10]

Prothrombotic processes that produce the vaso-occlusive lesions may be mediated either directly by the COVID-19 virus or by the host immune response.[16] Immunohistochemical analysis of purpuric skin lesions showed pauci-inflammatory thrombotic vasculopathy with deposition of C5b-9 and C4d, with colocalization of SARS-CoV-2 spike glycoproteins.[33] Similar findings were seen in pulmonary tissue, supporting the concept that systemic activation of both the alternative and lectin-mediated complement pathways may produce microvascular damage.[10,33] Interestingly, there have been reports of the varying prevalence of vaso-occlusive lesions among different continents, suggesting that genetic causes of thrombophilia including factor V Leiden and lipoprotein A levels may influence the development of livedoid vasculopathy associated with SARS-CoV-2.[10]

It is essential to highlight that overlap in clinical presentation and nomenclature exists between acro-ischemia, a true vaso-occlusive disease, and pseudochilblains, described previously in this chapter. Observational reports published early in the pandemic initially classified acro-ischemic lesions as chilblain-like, pseudopernio, or atypical Raynaud's phenomenon.[34,35] In contrast to pseudochilblains, acro-ischemia occurs in the setting of more severe coagulopathy, specifically with elevations in D-dimer and in patients requiring hospitalization or intensive care.[32,33] Additionally, histology of these vaso-occlusive lesions revealed thrombotic vasculopathy without any additional features seen in pernio such as necrotic keratinocytes, interface vacuolization, papillary dermal edema, and dermal lymphocytic infiltrate.[14] In another study, biopsies of livedoid vasculopathy demonstrated occlusive fibrin thrombi, microvascular complement deposition, detection of SARS-CoV-2 envelope and spike proteins, and expression of interleukin 6 (IL-6) and caspase-3, a marker of cell apoptosis.[26] These findings were lacking in tissue examination of perniolike lesions associated with COVID-19 infection.

Given that these vaso-occlusive lesions appear at the onset of other SARS-CoV-2 symptoms and that IL-6 expression is found on histology, this cutaneous finding is likely linked to the early inflammatory stage of the viral symptom phase.

Pediatric Cases

It is important to mention noteworthy trends observed in the pediatric population. In contrast to adult patients with SARS-CoV-2, pediatric patients with a rash had lower rates of intensive care unit (ICU) admission and invasive mechanical ventilation, shorter duration of hospitalization, and less frequent respiratory symptoms.[36] Interestingly, mucocutaneous involvement was found in a greater proportion of patients with multisystem inflammatory syndrome in children (MIS-C) (66.8%) as compared to patients experiencing the earlier phases of viral symptom and early inflammatory response (10.2%).[37] These rash morphologies have been described as nonspecific erythema, morbilliform, retiform purpura, urticaria, targetoid lesions, and acral edema.[37] Pediatric MIS-C patients with rash also had lower rates of ICU admission, ventilatory support, and shock as well as lower levels of inflammatory markers than MIS-C patients without rash.[37]

Conclusion

SARS-CoV-2 is a novel viral infection that can affect multiple organ systems, including the skin. As highlighted in this chapter, the main cutaneous morphologies caused by the virus are eruptions composed of macules and papules, perniosis/pseudochilblains, vesicular eruptions, urticaria, and livedoid/vaso-occlusive lesions. Notably, several isolated cases of unique morphologies have been identified, including enanthemlike rashes, aphthous stomatitis, and bullous hemorrhagic vasculitis.[12,38] Other rarely reported rashes secondary to SARS-CoV-2 infection include eruptive cherry hemangiomas, acral dyshidrosis–like lesions, ecthyma, impetigo, acute generalized exanthematous pustulosis–like reactions, and the red half-moon sign.[13,39]

Prompt and accurate recognition of the cutaneous manifestation of SARS-CoV-2 has the potential to aid in categorizing the severity of and directing treatment of COVID-19. Further research is needed to elucidate the relationship between the molecular pathophysiology of COVID-19, the cutaneous findings, and their impact on disease prognosis.

References

1. Griffin DO, Brennan-Rieder D, Ngo B, et al. The importance of understanding the stages of COVID-19 in treatment and trials. AIDS Rev 2021;23(1):40–47
2. Madjid M, Safavi-Naeini P, Solomon SD, Vardeny O. Potential effects of coronaviruses on the cardiovascular system: a review. JAMA Cardiol 2020;5(7):831–840
3. Ellul MA, Benjamin L, Singh B, et al. Neurological associations of COVID-19. Lancet Neurol 2020;19(9):767–783
4. Raza A, Estepa A, Chan V, Jafar MS. Acute renal failure in critically ill COVID-19 patients with a focus on the role of renal replacement therapy: a review of what we know so far. Cureus 2020;12(6):e8429
5. Renu K, Prasanna PL, Valsala Gopalakrishnan A. Coronaviruses pathogenesis, comorbidities and multi-organ damage—a review. Life Sci 2020;255:117839
6. Jose RJ, Manuel A. COVID-19 cytokine storm: the interplay between inflammation and coagulation. Lancet Respir Med 2020;8(6): e46–e47
7. Visconti A, Bataille V, Rossi N, et al. Diagnostic value of cutaneous manifestation of SARS-CoV-2 infection. Br J Dermatol 2021;184(5): 880–887
8. Rekhtman S, Tannenbaum R, Strunk A, et al. Eruptions and related clinical course among 296 hospitalized adults with confirmed COVID-19. J Am Acad Dermatol 2021;84(4): 946–952
9. Galván Casas C, Català A, Carretero Hernández G, et al. Classification of the cutaneous manifestations of COVID-19: a rapid prospective nationwide consensus study in Spain with 375 cases. Br J Dermatol 2020;183(1):71–77

10. Tan SW, Tam YC, Oh CC. Skin manifestations of COVID-19: a worldwide review. JAAD Int 2021;2:119–133

11. Freeman EE, McMahon DE, Lipoff JB, et al; American Academy of Dermatology Ad Hoc Task Force on COVID-19. Pernio-like skin lesions associated with COVID-19: a case series of 318 patients from 8 countries. J Am Acad Dermatol 2020;83(2):486–492

12. Askin O, Altunkalem RN, Altinisik DD, Uzuncakmak TK, Tursen U, Kutlubay Z. Cutaneous manifestations in hospitalized patients diagnosed as COVID-19. Dermatol Ther (Heidelb) 2020;33(6):e13896

13. Matar S, Oulès B, Sohier P, et al. Cutaneous manifestations in SARS-CoV-2 infection (COVID-19): a French experience and a systematic review of the literature. J Eur Acad Dermatol Venereol 2020;34(11):e686–e689

14. Freeman EE, McMahon DE, Lipoff JB, et al. The spectrum of COVID-19-associated dermatologic manifestations: an international registry of 716 patients from 31 countries. J Am Acad Dermatol 2020;83(4): 1118–1129

15. Rodriguez-Cerdeira C, Uribe-Camacho BI, Silverio-Carrasco L, et al. Cutaneous manifestations in COVID-19: report on 31 cases from five countries. Biology (Basel) 2021;10(1):54

16. Lee DS, Mirmirani P, McCleskey PE, Mehrpouya M, Gorouhi F. Cutaneous manifestations of COVID-19: a systematic review and analysis of individual patient-level data. Dermatol Online J 2020;26(12):13030/qt7s34p8rw

17. Shams S, Rathore SS, Anvekar P, et al. Maculopapular skin eruptions associated with Covid-19: a systematic review. Dermatol Ther (Heidelb) 2021;34(2):e14788

18. Català A, Galván-Casas C, Carretero-Hernández G, et al. Maculopapular eruptions associated to COVID-19: a subanalysis of the COVID-Piel study. Dermatol Ther (Heidelb) 2020;33(6):e14170

19. Najarian DJ. Morbilliform exanthem associated with COVID-19. JAAD Case Rep 2020; 6(6):493–494

20. Fattori A, Cribier B, Chenard MP, Mitcov M, Mayeur S, Weingertner N. Cutaneous manifestations in patients with coronavirus disease 2019: clinical and histological findings. Hum Pathol 2021;107:39–45

21. Criado PR, Abdalla BMZ, de Assis IC, van Blarcum de Graaff Mello C, Caputo GC, Vieira IC. Are the cutaneous manifestations during or due to SARS-CoV-2 infection/COVID-19 frequent or not? Revision of possible pathophysiologic mechanisms. Inflamm Res 2020; 69(8):745–756

22. Singh S, Khandpur S, Arava S, et al. Assessment of histopathological features of maculopapular viral exanthem and drug-induced exanthem. J Cutan Pathol 2017; 44(12):1038–1048

23. Perna A, Passiatore M, Massaro A, et al. Skin manifestations in COVID-19 patients, state of the art. A systematic review. Int J Dermatol 2021;60(5):547–553

24. Herman A, Peeters C, Verroken A, et al. Evaluation of chilblains as a manifestation of the COVID-19 pandemic. JAMA Dermatol 2020;156(9):998–1003

25. Ladha MA, Luca N, Constantinescu C, Naert K, Ramien ML. Approach to Chilblains During the COVID-19 Pandemic [Formula: see text]. J Cutan Med Surg 2020;24(5):504–517

26. Magro CM, Mulvey JJ, Laurence J, et al. The differing pathophysiologies that underlie COVID-19-associated perniosis and thrombotic retiform purpura: a case series. Br J Dermatol 2021;184(1):141–150

27. Discepolo V, Catzola A, Pierri L, et al. Bilateral chilblain-like lesions of the toes characterized by microvascular remodeling in adolescents during the COVID-19 pandemic. JAMA Netw Open 2021;4(6):e2111369

28. Fernandez-Nieto D, Ortega-Quijano D, Jimenez-Cauhe J, et al. Clinical and histological characterization of vesicular COVID-19 rashes: a prospective study in a tertiary care hospital. Clin Exp Dermatol 2020;45(7): 872–875

29. Marzano AV, Genovese G, Fabbrocini G, et al. Varicella-like exanthem as a specific COVID-19-associated skin manifestation: multicenter case series of 22 patients. J Am Acad Dermatol 2020;83(1):280–285

30. Abuelgasim E, Dona ACM, Sondh RS, Harky A. Management of urticaria in COVID-19 patients: a systematic review. Dermatol Ther (Heidelb) 2021;34(1):e14328

31. Shanshal M. Low- dose systemic steroids, an emerging therapeutic option for COVID-19 related urticaria. J Dermatolog Treat. Published online July 16, 2020:1-2. doi:10.1080/09546634.2020.1795062

32. Almeida G, Arruda S, Marques E, Michalany N, Sadick N. Presentation and management of cutaneous manifestations of COVID-19. J Drugs Dermatol 2021;20(1):76–83

33. Magro C, Mulvey JJ, Berlin D, et al. Complement associated microvascular injury and thrombosis in the pathogenesis of severe COVID-19 infection: a report of five cases. Transl Res 2020;220:1–13

34. Fernandez-Nieto D, Jimenez-Cauhe J, Suarez-Valle A, et al. Characterization of acute acral skin lesions in nonhospitalized patients: a case series of 132 patients during the COVID-19 outbreak. J Am Acad Dermatol 2020; 83(1):e61–e63

35. Alonso MN, Mata-Forte T, García-León N, et al. Incidence, characteristics, laboratory findings and outcomes in acro-ischemia in covid-19 patients. Vasc Health Risk Manag 2020;16:467–478

36. Rekhtman S, Tannenbaum R, Strunk A, Birabaharan M, Wright S, Garg A. Mucocutaneous disease and related clinical characteristics in hospitalized children and adolescents with COVID-19 and multisystem inflammatory syndrome in children. J Am Acad Dermatol 2021;84(2):408–414

37. Feldstein LR, Tenforde MW, Friedman KG, et al; Overcoming COVID-19 Investigators. Characteristics and outcomes of US children and adolescents with multisystem inflammatory syndrome in children (MIS-C) compared with severe acute COVID-19. JAMA 2021;325(11):1074–1087

38. Negrini S, Guadagno A, Greco M, Parodi A, Burlando M. An unusual case of bullous haemorrhagic vasculitis in a COVID-19 patient. J Eur Acad Dermatol Venereol 2020;34(11):e675–e676

39. Neri I, Guglielmo A, Virdi A, Gaspari V, Starace M, Piraccini BM. The red half-moon nail sign: a novel manifestation of coronavirus infection. J Eur Acad Dermatol Venereol 2020;34(11):e663–e665

12 Pharmacotherapy of COVID-19

Binh Ngo and Marc Rendell

Introduction

The so-called common cold is a respiratory viral illness that has afflicted mankind for all of recorded history. Hippocrates described the "cough of Perinthus" 2,500 years ago.[1] The Chinese have been treating "wind-cold" with traditional herb remedies to relieve symptoms for thousands of years.[2] In our era, cold sufferers are offered symptomatic treatments for nasal congestion and rhinorrhea, sore throat, headache, muscle aches, and cough for the duration of the viral illness, typically several days until the body's immune system suppresses viral replication. There are well over 200 viruses that cause cold symptoms. The cold viruses have a seasonal incidence, usually surfacing when cold weather encourages people to congregate indoors, promoting person-to-person transmission, resulting in unpleasant epidemics, which usually subside without residual damage.

However, there are cold viruses that have provoked frequent epidemics of life-threatening severe illness. The influenza of 1918 was a grievous event causing death of about 50 million people worldwide.[3] Although not as catastrophic, every year there is a death toll from influenza. In the 1940s, the first inactivated influenza vaccines were developed to stimulate protective immune reactions.[4] The influenza viruses mutate rapidly, requiring annual development of new vaccines to immunize the population. The vaccinations are moderately effective, yielding reductions of influenza infections of 40 to 60% varying from year to year.[5] Several chemical agents have been used effectively to combat influenza viral replication, including amantadine, oseltamivir, peramivir, zanamivir, baloxavir, and umfenovir.[6–8] These agents are only effective if administered early

in the first few days of the influenza infection during the period of active viral replication or when used as prophylaxis among contacts of infected individuals.

The causative agent severe acute respiratory syndrome coronavirus 2 (SARS-CoV-2) is an RNA virus with high sequence similarity to other betacoronaviruses, which are responsible for perhaps 20% of common colds. The spread of COVID-19 was rapid as is typical for seasonal upper respiratory infections. The majority of individuals display no symptoms or have trifling coldlike manifestations, during a 7- to 10-day period of viral replication and immunologic response.[9] However, in up to 20% of patients, even as the viral load falls, a reactive inflammatory phase ensues characterized by rising cytokine levels and susceptibility to coagulopathy.[10–12] Clinically, this usually manifests as an organizing pneumonia with additional systemic complications. Oxygenation fails, and in perhaps 5% of patients, intubation ensues, with incipient death.[10] As of May 15, 2021, there have been 162,177,376 documented cases of COVID-19 worldwide recorded by the World Health Organization (WHO) and 3,364,178 deaths, giving a crude mortality estimate of 3.4%.[13] Given the high incidence of asymptomatic disease, this estimate is much greater than the true infection fatality ratio, but this illness has clearly changed the world. Griffin et al have called attention to the stages of COVID-19 and the necessity to provide treatment suited to each stage of the illness[14] (**Fig. 12.1**). The stages of COVID-19 so defined include: (1) the incubation stage during which virus replicates but is not yet detectable; (2) the detectable viral replication period; (3) the symptomatic stage; (4) the inflammatory stage; (5) the secondary infection stage; (6) the hyperinflammatory stage; and (7) the

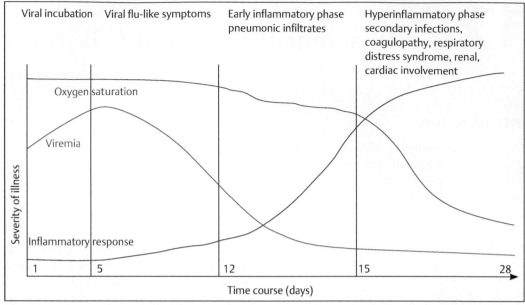

| Viral incubation | Viral flu-like symptoms | Early inflammatory phase pneumonic infiltrates | Hyperinflammatory phase secondary infections, coagulopathy, respiratory distress syndrome, renal, cardiac involvement |

Fig. 12.1 Time course of SARS-CoV-2 evolution. The phases of COVID-19 so defined include: (1) the incubation phase during which virus replicates but is not yet detectable; (2) the detectable viral replication period; (3) the viral symptom phase; (4) the early inflammatory phase; (5) the secondary infection phase; (6) the hyperinflammatory phase; and (7) the tail phase.

chronic stage, which sometimes involves a lengthy convalescence. There is significant overlap of the phases, but what is clear is that direct viral damage declines as immunologic events take hold (**Fig. 12.1**). By 10 days postinfection, viral load has dropped to near undetectable levels in most patients. Yet, this happens typically when the inflammatory phase accelerates in patients destined to severe disease. In hospitalized patients, the 28-day death rate has consistently been about 20%, although it has been as low as 6% in some centers.[15]

In China, strict control of personal interactions with isolation of all diagnosed cases was successful in limiting spread and eventually extinguishing SARS-CoV-2 transmission. Attempts were made to treat empirically with antiviral agents such as umifenovir, lopinavir/ritonavir (LPV/R), and interferons. In western developed countries, the focus of therapeutics was directed at hospitalized patients in the late stages of COVID-19. The emphasis was to carry out randomized controlled inpatient trials to prove benefit.

Patients with early disease were counseled to self-isolate for a period of 14 days until the illness ran its course. The vast majority of patients recovered but those who entered an inflammatory phase with hypoxia were then hospitalized with treatment delivered only at that late stage.

Late-Stage Therapy for Hospitalized Patients

Very few pharmacotherapeutics have proven beneficial to treat the disease in hospitalized patients, most of whom are in the inflammatory phase with significant hypoxia. Prior to COVID-19, glucocorticoids had long shown benefit to treat acute respiratory distress syndrome.[16] The RECOVERY trial confirmed a mortality reduction in hospitalized COVID-19 patients treated with glucocorticoid.[17] In this trial, randomized patients were to receive dexamethasone versus standard of care. Patient survival was greater in those individuals randomized to dexamethasone. There was a statistically significant decrease in 28-day mortality when compared to usual care. The benefit was seen predominantly in those patients requiring supplemental oxygen.

Other studies of different glucocorticoids have shown similar benefit.[18] Investigations have demonstrated that combination therapy with interleukin inhibition and glucocorticoid has yielded improved 90-day survival.[19,20]

In the RECOVERY trial, patients allocated to tocilizumab and standard of care compared to standard of care including glucocorticoids demonstrated a statistically significant survival benefit.

Antiviral Agents in Hospitalized Patients

Given that patients sick enough to be hospitalized with COVID-19 are typically at the late stage in the course of the inflammatory process with declining viral replication, antiviral treatment has been less effective at that stage of the disease.

Remdesivir

The RNA polymerase inhibitor remdesivir is an antiviral drug. It is administered intravenously for 5 days and thus it must be used only in hospitalized patients. In a preliminary double-blind, randomized trial, there was no advantage in terms of viral clearance or survival advantage.[21] In a double-blind, randomized, placebo-controlled trial of remdesivir involving moderately to severely ill patients, remdesivir-treated patients had a statistically significant median recovery time of 10 days versus 15 days in the placebo arm.[22] By 29 days following randomization, the estimates of mortality demonstrated a non–statistically significant favorable trend in mortality with remdesivir versus placebo. In a recent trial evaluating the benefits of extended therapy with remdesivir, a 5-day course of therapy demonstrated clinical improvement by day 11. However, there was no statistically significant benefit in extending therapy for 10 days.[23] The addition of baricitinib, a janus

kinase inhibitor used to treat rheumatoid arthritis, to remdesivir has shown a small improvement in time to improvement in clinical status compared to remdesivir alone.[24] For the remdesivir studies conducted in the United States, no data on virus clearance have been reported.

The WHO Solidarity trial assessed four distinct therapeutic regimens involving large numbers of hospitalized patients worldwide. The agents included: (1) remdesivir; (2) LPV/R; (3) LPV/R plus interferon β-1a; and (4) hydroxychloroquine (HCQ) and chloroquine.[25] The study found no effect of remdesivir on 28-day mortality, need for mechanical ventilation, or duration of hospitalization. Nor was there any benefit shown for any of the other agents. Similarly, the RECOVERY trial has shown no benefit for hospitalized patients in trials of agents with possible antiviral activity including LPV/R,[26] HCQ,[27] and convalescent plasma.[28] It is pertinent to note that the median duration of symptomatology for patients randomized in the RECOVERY trial was 8 to 9 days. Therefore, one would expect that the period of viral replication would be waning, reducing anticipated benefit of antiviral medication.

Interferon

There has been a positive study reported for inhaled interferon β in hospitalized patients.[29] In that trial, 51 patients receiving interferon β had greater odds of improvement on the Ordinal scale for clinical improvement (OSCI) scale on day 15 or 16 and were more likely than 50 patients receiving placebo to recover to an OSCI score of 1 (no limitation of activities) during treatment. Interferon is a standard treatment in Cuba for COVID-19, where it was demonstrated that a dual therapy with interferon α-2b and interferon γ in patients receiving antiviral therapy with LPV/R and chloroquine was successful in achieving viral clearance compared to patients receiving interferon α-2b alone.[30] Interferon is also the recommended treatment in Hong Kong.[31]

Favipiravir

This is an RNA polymerase inhibitor like remdesivir but is administered orally. There were two positive randomized, active-control clinical trials of favipiravir (FVP).[32,33] In a trial comparing patients on FVP to those on umifenovir, the 7-day clinical recovery rate was 15% greater in the FVP group.[33] A preliminary study of FVP in hospitalized patients demonstrated a reduction in viral shedding, resulting in FVP approval as a therapeutic agent in several Russian hospitals.[34] In a follow-up phase 3 study, they reported 27% clinical improvement at day 10 compared to 15% for standard care, with 98% clearance of SARS-CoV-2 compared to 79%.[35] In India, a study involving mild-to-moderate COVID-19 patients demonstrated a statistically significant difference in median time to clinical cure of 3 days for FVP versus 5 days for control.[36]

Molnupiravir is another oral RNA polymerase inhibitor. It is currently undergoing studies in outpatients after it proved ineffective in inpatient hospital studies.

Neutralizing Antibodies

Although convalescent plasma treatment is not successful as viremia wanes and the inflammatory phase of COVID-19 takes hold, early use in hospitalized patients proved beneficial.[37] Bamlanivimab, a synthetic monoclonal antibody to the SARS-CoV-2 spike protein, was not successful when administered to hospitalized patients, and inpatient studies were stopped.[38] However, studies have shown that in ambulatory patients, presumably still in the viral replication phase, bamlanivimab helps in improving the course of the illness and avoiding hospitalization in 60 to 70% of diagnosed patients.[39,40] The RECOVERY trial has recently reported that the casirivimab and imdevimab antibody cocktail lowered 28-day mortality from 30 to 24% in 3,153 seronegative patients but not in the entire cohort of 9,785 patients.[41] These antibody preparations are approved and in use for COVID-19 patients diagnosed at the early stage of viral replication.

Hydroxychloroquine

HCQ was widely used to treat COVID-19 and is still used in many countries. HCQ has an in vitro effectiveness by inhibiting viral endosomal entry due to its its action as a zinc ionophore. In addition, HCQ possesses anti-inflammatory and immune-modulating effects on the inflammatory dysregulation commonly observed in COVID-19. HCQ has a long period to reach its equilibrium drug level, making it unlikely to be of value in the acute therapy of individuals with severe disease. Certainly, the use of HCQ in hospitalized patients has not been successful. There are few studies in outpatients. In a small randomized control Spanish study with 136 HCQ-treated patients and 157 patients in the control arm, the risk of hospitalization (7.1% for control vs. 5.9% for HCQ; relative risk, 0.75 [0.32–1.77]) nor the time to complete resolution of symptoms (12 days for control vs. 10 days for HCQ; $p = 0.38$) reached significance.[42] The recent publication of a series of 10,429 patients by the Institut Hospitalo-Universitaire Méditerranée Infection group in Marseille supports combination treatment with HCQ and azithromycin (AZM). In this very large series, treatment with HCQ and AZM resulted in an infection fatality ratio of only 0.06%. Compared to other regimens received by their outpatients, treatment with HCQ+AZM was associated with a lower risk of death (0.17 [0.06–0.48]).[43]

Ivermectin

This agent is universally used for its antiparasitic properties and has a safety profile well established up to 10 times the usual antiparasitic dose. A study in Australia showed that it suppressed SARS-CoV-2 replication 5,000-fold in cell culture at a concentration thought to be 100-fold higher than typical serum levels attained at typical human dosage.[44]

However, ivermectin is taken up and concentrated in tissues including respiratory epithelium. The effect of ivermectin is broad spectrum on RNA viruses through inhibition of nuclear transport of viral components by the IMPα/β1 importer protein.[45] In clinical use, there have been many studies, including 28 randomized controlled studies, summarized in two major meta-analyses suggesting benefit of ivermectin treatment in COVID-19.[46,47] In particular, there has been evidence of 78% improvement in early treatment studies, 84% improvement in prophylaxis studies, and a 74% reduction in mortality. Almost all the ivermectin studies have occurred outside the United States and Europe. One retrospective study of hospitalized patients in the United States showed lower mortality in the ivermectin group (15 vs. 25.2%; odds ratio, 0.52; 95% confidence interval [CI], 0.29–0.96; $p = 0.03$).[48] Although results are highly positive for ivermectin early treatment and prophylaxis, there has been no urgency to begin major trials in the United States nor in Europe. In fact, the FDA and the WHO have argued against use of ivermectin to treat COVID-19 outside of randomized controlled trials.

Topical Antiviral Therapy

Several studies have shown that mouth rinses with povidone-iodine inactivate SARS-CoV-2.[49,50] In a study in Singapore among dormitory-housed migrant laborers, a povidone mouth rinse reduced the frequency of polymerase chain reaction (PCR)–positive COVID-19 diagnoses, while a single dose of ivermectin substantially decreased symptomatic COVID-19 disease.[51] There is considerable interest in the development of a slow-release nitric oxide solution from a company called SaNOtize. The solution is useable as a nasal spray, gargle, and inhaled spray. It has shown a 99% reduction in swabbed viral load. It has been granted emergency approval in Israel and New Zealand.

Outpatient Anti-Inflammatory Treatment

There is an overlapping transition between the phase of viral replication and the inception of the immune-mediated inflammatory phase of COVID-19.

Inhaled Glucocorticoid

There has been reluctance to use glucocorticoid treatment early due to concern of increased viral load and decreased viral clearance. However, clinical trials suggest that early immune suppression is beneficial. In a small trial in 146 patients in the United Kingdom, inhaled budesonide decreased the frequency of immediate care visits and hospitalizations by 91% ($p < 0.004$).[52] The mean time to recovery was 8 days in the budesonide group and 12 days in the standard care group. There was no difference in viral load at various intervals in budesonide-treated patients and controls. In a much larger trial, there were 59/692 (8.5%) COVID-19-related hospitalizations/deaths in the budesonide group versus 100/968 (10.3%) in the usual care group (estimated percentage benefit, 2.1% [95% CI, 0.7–4.8]; probability of superiority 0.928).[53]

Fluvoxamine

Fluvoxamine a selective serotonin reuptake inhibitor that has demonstrated reduction in cytokine production by inhibition of the S1 receptor in immune cells, and has shown promise as a repurposed drug for managing COVID-19.[54] In a small, randomized, placebo-controlled study, 0% of the individuals who received fluvoxamine compared to 8.3% who received placebo developed clinical deterioration measured as dyspnea, hypoxia, or hospitalization.[55] Five participants in the placebo arm and one in the fluvoxamine arm required hospitalization. In a prospective, nonrandomized observational trial of 113 participants, 65 opted to take fluvoxamine and 48 did not.[56] By 2 weeks, no patients receiving fluvoxamine required hospitalization compared to six who did not.

Colchicine

Due to colchicine's anti-inflammatory properties, the drug's potential effectiveness was evaluated in patients with COVID-19. Among 4,159 outpatients with COVID-19, there was a statistically significant decrease in hospitalization or death, which occurred in 4.6 and 6% of patients in the colchicine and placebo groups.[57] In these patients with PCR-confirmed COVID-19, the odds ratios were 0.75 (95% CI, 0.57–0.99) for hospitalization due to COVID-19, 0.50 (95% CI, 0.23–1.07) for mechanical ventilation, and 0.56 (95% CI, 0.19–1.66) for death. However, in the RECOVERY trial, which involved a large number of hospitalized patients, there was no statistically significant difference in the reduction of 28-day mortality in those allocated to receive colchicine when compared with those receiving usual care.[58] This suggests a lack of benefit of the anti-inflammatory properties of colchicine at the stage that patients are admitted to the hospital.

Pharmaceutical Management of COVID-19 in the Western World

In the United States and Europe, from the beginning of the pandemic, the plan of public health authorities was to rely on the rapid development of vaccines creating an immune reaction to the spike protein of SARS-CoV-2. The vaccines have gone through initial 3-month randomized control trials and have shown suppression of COVID-19 infection and transmission. The most impressive results have emanated from observational studies of deployment of the BNT162b2 mRNA vaccine in national populations, in particular Israel.[59] In that country, from December 20, 2020, to February 1, 2021, 596,618 vaccinated persons were matched to unvaccinated controls. At 7 or more days after the second dose of the vaccine, documented infection was reduced by 92% (95% CI, 88–95), symptomatic COVID-19 by 94% (95% CI, 87–98), and hospitalization by 87% (95% CI, 55–100). Despite the excitement over this monumental success, the full evaluation of the long-term benefits and adverse events associated with vaccination must await long-term analyses. COVID-19 has a dual pathogenicity. The initial viral phase can be blocked by the antibodies and T-cell response to vaccine production of the spike protein. What remains of concern is that some features of the inflammatory phase of COVID-19 may be caused by the spike protein produced by the vaccine.[60]

There has been little emphasis on early outpatient treatment of patients infected with SARS-CoV-2 in the western countries. Monoclonal SARS-CoV-2 antibody cocktails are a valuable option for patients, but it is not practical to immediately treat every patient with a positive SARS-CoV-2 PCR result with an antibody infusion. HCQ is a standard of treatment in Iran, Brazil, Saudi Arabia, and many other countries. The Marseille study offers a large observational cohort benefiting from HCQ combined with AZM. FVP is approved and is used in India and Russia. Ivermectin is used in many South American countries. In India, two states, Goa and Uttarakhand, are distributing ivermectin to their entire populations. Interferon preparations are standard treatment of COVID-19 in Cuba and Hong Kong. The model of treatment of influenza with concomitant vaccination and antiviral treatment early in the course appears to be a more sustainable approach than reliance on vaccination alone. We and others have strongly encouraged the parallel deployment of medications with good safety profiles for outpatient treatment of diagnosed COVID-19 while randomized clinical trials are ongoing to confirm benefit.[61-63] It is hoped that public health authorities in the United States and Europe may still invest in a belated effort to allow pharmaceutical management of the COVID-19 pandemic rather than relying exclusively on universal vaccination.

References

1. Pappas G, Kiriaze IJ, Falagas ME. Insights into infectious disease in the era of Hippocrates. Int J Infect Dis 2008;12(4):347–350

2. Hai-Long Z, Shimin C, Yalan L. Some Chinese folk prescriptions for wind-cold type common cold. J Tradit Complement Med 2015; 5(3):135–137

3. Taubenberger JK, Morens DM. 1918 Influenza: the mother of all pandemics. Emerg Infect Dis 2006;12(1):15–22

4. Barberis I, Myles P, Ault SK, Bragazzi NL, Martini M. History and evolution of influenza control through vaccination: from the first monovalent vaccine to universal vaccines. J Prev Med Hyg 2016;57(3):E115–E120

5. Dhakal S, Klein SL. Host factors impact vaccine efficacy: implications for seasonal and universal influenza vaccine programs. J Virol 2019;93(21):e00797–e19

6. Gaitonde DY, Moore FC, Morgan MK. Influenza: diagnosis and treatment. Am Fam Physician 2019;100(12):751–758

7. Ison MG, Portsmouth S, Yoshida Y, et al. Early treatment with baloxavir marboxil in high-risk adolescent and adult outpatients with uncomplicated influenza (CAPSTONE-2): a randomised, placebo-controlled, phase 3 trial. Lancet Infect Dis 2020;20(10):1204–1214

8. Leneva IA, Falynskova IN, Makhmudova NR, Poromov AA, Yatsyshina SB, Maleev VV. Umifenovir susceptibility monitoring and characterization of influenza viruses isolated during ARBITR clinical study. J Med Virol 2019;91(4):588–597

9. Wu Z, McGoogan JM. Characteristics of and important lessons from the coronavirus disease 2019 (COVID-19) outbreak in China: summary of a report of 72 314 cases from the Chinese Center for Disease Control and Prevention. JAMA 2020;323(13):1239–1242

10. Chen T, Wu D, Chen H, et al. Clinical characteristics of 113 deceased patients with coronavirus disease 2019: retrospective study. BMJ 2020;368:m1091

11. Connors JM, Levy JH. Thromboinflammation and the hypercoagulability of COVID-19. J Thromb Haemost 2020;18(7):1559–1561

12. Jose RJ, Manuel A. COVID-19 cytokine storm: the interplay between inflammation and coagulation. Lancet Respir Med 2020; 8(6):e46–e47

13. World Health Organization. WHO coronavirus disease (COVID-19) dashboard. 2021. Available at: https://covid19.who.int/

14. Griffin DO, Brennan-Rieder D, Ngo B, et al. The importance of understanding the stages of COVID-19 in treatment and trials. AIDS Rev 2021;23(1):40–47

15. Kory P, Meduri GU, Iglesias J, Varon J, Marik PE. Clinical and scientific rationale for the "MATH+" hospital treatment protocol for COVID-19. J Intensive Care Med 2021;36(2):135–156

16. Villar J, Ferrando C, Martínez D, et al; dexamethasone in ARDS network. Dexamethasone treatment for the acute respiratory distress syndrome: a multicentre, randomised controlled trial. Lancet Respir Med 2020;8(3):267–276

17. Horby P, Lim WS, Emberson JR, et al; RECOVERY Collaborative Group. Dexamethasone in hospitalized patients with Covid-19. N Engl J Med 2021;384(8):693–704

18. Salton F, Confalonieri P, Meduri GU, et al. Prolonged low-dose methylprednisolone in patients with severe COVID-19 pneumonia. Open Forum Infect Dis 2020;7(10):a421

19. Gordon AC, Mouncey PR, Al-Beidh F, et al; REMAP-CAP Investigators. Interleukin-6 receptor antagonists in critically ill patients with Covid-19. N Engl J Med 2021;384(16): 1491–1502

20. RECOVERY Collaborative Group. Tocilizumab in patients admitted to hospital with COVID-19 (RECOVERY): a randomised, controlled, open-label, platform trial. Lancet 2021; 397(10285):1637–1645

21. Wang Y, Zhang D, Du G, et al. Remdesivir in adults with severe COVID-19: a randomised, double-blind, placebo-controlled, multicentre trial. Lancet 2020;395(10236): 1569–1578

22. Beigel JH, Tomashek KM, Dodd LE, et al; ACTT-1 Study Group Members. Remdesivir for the treatment of Covid-19 - final report. N Engl J Med 2020;383(19):1813–1826

23. Spinner CD, Gottlieb RL, Criner GJ, et al; GS-US-540-5774 Investigators. Effect of remdesivir vs standard care on clinical status at 11 days in patients with moderate COVID-19: a randomized clinical trial. JAMA 2020;324(11):1048–1057

24. Kalil AC, Patterson TF, Mehta AK, et al; ACTT-2 Study Group Members. Baricitinib

plus remdesivir for hospitalized adults with Covid-19. N Engl J Med 2021;384(9):795–807

25. Pan H, Peto R, Henao-Restrepo AM, et al; WHO Solidarity Trial Consortium. Repurposed antiviral drugs for Covid-19—interim WHO Solidarity trial results. N Engl J Med 2021;384(6):497–511

26. Horby PWM, Bell JL, et al; RECOVERY Collaborative Group. Lopinavir-ritonavir in patients admitted to hospital with COVID-19 (RECOVERY): a randomised, controlled, open-label, platform trial. Lancet 2020; 396(10259):1345–1352

27. Horby P, Mafham M, Linsell L, et al; RECOVERY Collaborative Group. Effect of hydroxychloroquine in hospitalized patients with Covid-19. N Engl J Med 2020;383(21): 2030–2040

28. RECOVERY Collaborative Group. Convalescent plasma in patients admitted to hospital with COVID-19 (RECOVERY): a randomised controlled, open-label, platform trial. Lancet. 2021 May 29;397(10289):2049-2059. doi: 10.1016/S0140-6736(21)00897-7. Epub 2021 May 14. PMID: 34000257; PMCID: PMC8121538.

29. Monk PD, Marsden RJ, Tear VJ, et al; Inhaled Interferon Beta COVID-19 Study Group. Safety and efficacy of inhaled nebulised interferon beta-1a (SNG001) for treatment of SARS-CoV-2 infection: a randomised, double-blind, placebo-controlled, phase 2 trial. Lancet Respir Med 2021;9(2):196–206

30. Idelsis EM, Jésus PE, Yaquelin DR, Dania VB, Iraldo BR, et al. (2021) A combination treatment of IFN-α2b and IFN-γ accelerates viral clearance and control inflammatory response in COVID-19: Preliminary results of a randomized controlled trial. Ann Antivir Antiretrovir 5(1): 001-014. DOI: 10.17352/aaa.000010

31. Hung IFN, Lung KC, Tso EYK, et al. Triple combination of interferon beta-1b, lopinavir-ritonavir, and ribavirin in the treatment of patients admitted to hospital with COVID-19: an open-label, randomised, phase 2 trial. Lancet 2020;395(10238):1695–1704

32. Cai Q, Yang M, Liu D, et al. Experimental treatment with favipiravir for COVID-19: an open-label control study. Engineering (Beijing) 2020;6(10):1192–1198

33. Chen C, Zhang Y, Huang J, et al. Favipiravir Versus Arbidol for Clinical Recovery Rate in Moderate and Severe Adult COVID-19 Patients: A Prospective, Multicenter, Open-Label, Randomized Controlled Clinical Trial. Frontiers in Pharmacology. 2021;12:2292. doi:10.3389/fphar.2021.683296

34. Ivashchenko AA, Dmitriev KA, Vostokova NV, et al. AVIFAVIR for treatment of patients with moderate coronavirus disease 2019 (COVID-19): interim results of a phase II/III multicenter randomized clinical trial. Clin Infect Dis 2021;73(3):531–534

35. ClinicalTrials.gov. Study of favipiravir compared to standard of care in hospitalized patients with COVID-19. Available at: https://clinicaltrials.gov/ct2/show/NCT04542694

36. Udwadia ZF, Singh P, Barkate H, et al. Efficacy and safety of favipiravir, an oral RNA-dependent RNA polymerase inhibitor, in mild-to-moderate COVID-19: a randomized, comparative, open-label, multicenter, phase 3 clinical trial. Int J Infect Dis 2021;103:62–71

37. Libster R, Pérez Marc G, Wappner D, et al; Fundación INFANT–COVID-19 Group. Early high-titer plasma therapy to prevent severe Covid-19 in older adults. N Engl J Med 2021; 384(7):610–618

38. Lundgren JD, Grund B, Barkauskas CE, et al; ACTIV-3/TICO LY-CoV555 Study Group. A neutralizing monoclonal antibody for hospitalized patients with Covid-19. N Engl J Med 2021;384(10):905–914

39. Chen P, Nirula A, Heller B, et al; BLAZE-1 Investigators. SARS-CoV-2 neutralizing antibody LY-CoV555 in outpatients with Covid-19. N Engl J Med 2021;384(3):229–237

40. Weinreich DM, Sivapalasingam S, Norton T, et al; Trial Investigators. REGN-COV2, a neutralizing antibody cocktail, in outpatients with Covid-19. N Engl J Med 2021;384(3): 238–251

41. RECOVERY Collaborative Group. Casirivimab and imdevimab in patients admitted to hospital with COVID-19 (RECOVERY): a randomised, controlled, open-label, platform trial. (e-pub ahead of print). doi:https://doi.org/10.1101/2021.06.15.21258542

42. Mitjà O, Corbacho-Monné M, Ubals M, et al. Hydroxychloroquine for Early Treatment of Adults with Mild Covid-19: A Randomized-Controlled Trial. Clin Infect Dis. Published online July 16, 2020. doi:10.1093/cid/ciaa1009

43. Million M, Lagier J-C, Tissot-Dupont H, et al. Early combination therapy with hydroxychloroquine and azithromycin reduces mortality in 10,429 COVID-19 outpatients. Rev Cardiovasc Med. 2021;22(3):1063-1072. doi:10.31083/j.rcm2203116

44. Caly L, Druce JD, Catton MG, Jans DA, Wagstaff KM. The FDA-approved drug ivermectin inhibits the replication of SARS-CoV-2 in vitro. Antiviral Res 2020;178: 104787

45. Jans DA, Martin AJ, Wagstaff KM. Inhibitors of nuclear transport. Curr Opin Cell Biol 2019;58:50–60

46. Kory P, Meduri GU, Varon J, Iglesias J, Marik PE. Review of the emerging evidence demonstrating the efficacy of ivermectin in the prophylaxis and treatment of COVID-19. Am J Ther 2021;28(3):e299–e318

47. Bryant A, Lawrie TA, Dowswell T, et al. Ivermectin for Prevention and Treatment of COVID-19 Infection: A Systematic Review, Meta-analysis, and Trial Sequential Analysis to Inform Clinical Guidelines. Am J Ther. 2021;28(4):e434-e460. doi:10.1097/MJT.0000000000001402

48. Rajter JC, Sherman MS, Fatteh N, Vogel F, Sacks J, Rajter JJ. Use of ivermectin is associated with lower mortality in hospitalized patients with coronavirus disease 2019: the ivermectin in COVID nineteen study. Chest 2021;159(1):85–92

49. Davies K, Buczkowski H, Welch SR, et al. Effective *in vitro* inactivation of SARS-CoV-2 by commercially available mouthwashes. J Gen Virol 2021;102(4):001578

50. Bidra AS, Pelletier JS, Westover JB, Frank S, Brown SM, Tessema B. Comparison of in vitro inactivation of SARS CoV-2 with hydrogen peroxide and povidone-iodine oral antiseptic rinses. J Prosthodont 2020;29(7):599–603

51. Seet RCS, Quek AML, Ooi DSQ, et al. Positive impact of oral hydroxychloroquine and povidone-iodine throat spray for COVID-19 prophylaxis: an open-label randomized trial. Int J Infect Dis 2021;106:314–322

52. Ramakrishnan S, Nicolau DV Jr, Langford B, et al. Inhaled budesonide in the treatment of early COVID-19 (STOIC): a phase 2, open-label, randomised controlled trial. Lancet Respir Med 2021;9(7):763–772

53. Yu L-M, Bafadhel M, Dorward J, et al. Inhaled budesonide for COVID-19 in people at high risk of complications in the community in the UK (PRINCIPLE): a randomised, controlled, open-label, adaptive platform trial. Lancet. 2021;398(10303):843-855. doi:10.1016/S0140-6736(21)01744-X

54. Rosen DA, Seki SM, Fernández-Castañeda A, et al. Modulation of the sigma-1 receptor-IRE1 pathway is beneficial in preclinical models of inflammation and sepsis. Sci Transl Med 2019;11(478):478

55. Lenze EJ, Mattar C, Zorumski CF, et al. Fluvoxamine vs placebo and clinical deterioration in outpatients with symptomatic COVID-19: a randomized clinical trial. JAMA 2020;324(22):2292–2300

56. Seftel D, Boulware DR. Prospective cohort of fluvoxamine for early treatment of coronavirus disease 19. Open Forum Infect Dis 2021;8(2):b050

57. Tardif J-C, Bouabdallaoui N, L'Allier PL, et al. Colchicine for community-treated patients with COVID-19 (COLCORONA): a phase 3, randomised, double-blinded, adaptive, placebo-controlled, multicentre trial. Lancet Respir Med. 2021;9(8):924-932. doi:10.1016/S2213-2600(21)00222-8

58. RECOVERY Collaborative Group. Colchicine in patients admitted to hospital with COVID-19 (RECOVERY): a randomised, controlled, open-label, platform trial. (e-pub ahead of print). doi:https://doi.org/10.1101/2021.05.18.21257267

59. Dagan N, Barda N, Kepten E, et al. BNT162b2 mRNA Covid-19 vaccine in a nationwide mass vaccination setting. N Engl J Med 2021;384(15):1412–1423

60. Chung MK, Zidar DA, Bristow MR, et al. COVID-19 and cardiovascular disease: from bench to bedside. Circ Res 2021;128(8): 1214–1236

61. Risch HA. Early outpatient treatment of symptomatic, high-risk COVID-19 patients that should be ramped up immediately as key to the pandemic crisis. Am J Epidemiol 2020;189(11):1218–1226

62. Ngo BT, Marik P, Kory P, et al. The time to offer treatments for COVID-19. Expert Opin Investig Drugs 2021;30(5):505–518

63. McCullough PA, Kelly RJ, Ruocco G, et al. Pathophysiological basis and rationale for early outpatient treatment of SARS-CoV-2 (COVID-19) infection. Am J Med 2021;134(1): 16–22

13

Hospital Medicine

Eric Osgood, Steven Hamilton, Ahmed Ellkhouty, and Jose Iglesias

Introduction

The COVID-19 pandemic, which originated in Wuhan, China, likely in December 2019, has caused devastation to global human health as well as incalculable socioeconomic harms and burdens. The world faced multiple waves of infection as well as several predominant variants with seemingly increasing contagiousness. While the majority of infected individuals either are asymptomatic or experience a self-limiting viral illness, many will progress to a severity of disease requiring visits to urgent care centers and emergency departments; although the proportion of these patients who progress further and require hospitalization has been relatively low with respect to overall infections, it was enough to overwhelm entire hospital systems during waves and local surges.

While the case fatality rate of COVID-19 is low, this number rises significantly among those who are hospitalized.[1] The quality of hospital care has proven to be extremely impactful on survival—the original "supportive care only" and "early intubation" strategies recommended by public health agencies and professional medical societies resulted in unprecedentedly high inpatient mortality rates as well as ventilator dependence rates and lengths of stay. Conversely, when improved treatment protocols emerged, particularly those centered around corticosteroids, mortality rates improved markedly.

During peak community infection rates, hospitals experienced severe staffing shortages and personal protective equipment (PPE) shortages, as well as bed and equipment shortages, requiring everything from interstate staffing, to recycling N95 masks, to splitting ventilators, and other extreme measures. Hospital staff members suffered extreme physical, psychological, emotional, and spiritual hardship, as mass amounts of rapid clinical deterioration and death surrounded them, and they simultaneously feared for their own well-being and the safety of their household members. Fortunately, as the medical and scientific community accumulated increasing knowledge and understanding about the transmission dynamics of severe acute respiratory syndrome coronavirus 2 (SARS-COV-2) and pathophysiology of COVID-19, this disease became quite manageable. Sound, evidence-based hospital practice is therefore critical in reducing morbidity and mortality of patients and preserving the safety and well-being of hospital staff. Here, we will review an evidence-based approach to the hospitalized patient with COVID-19.

Evaluation and Diagnosis

Thorough history taking is the cornerstone of diagnosing COVID-19 infection and primarily categorizing the patients upon initial presentation according to the severity of their illness. Clinicians should balance the need for a thorough history with the importance of avoiding unnecessarily prolonged exposure. The patient should be wearing a surgical or well-fitted mask during the interview and exam. Proper hand sanitizing, donning and doffing of protective equipment, and proper N95 respirator fit test and use are also critical in order to protect the clinician, colleagues, patients, and the community. A clinician may consider obtaining a portion of the history by calling into the room and discussing by telephone or video telemedicine, and limiting the in-person encounter to the physical examination and possibly key portions of history, if the necessary setup is in place and the patient is capable of participating.

A focused history needs to be meticulously obtained with attention to recent travel, contact with suspicious or confirmed cases of COVID-19, and the duration of symptoms, if any. Wide ranges of symptoms have been identified with COVID-19 infection, ranging from asymptomatic to severe multiorgan failure. Common generalized symptoms include fatigue, muscle and body aches, fever and/or chills, and malaise. Upper respiratory symptoms vary between dry and/or productive cough, shortness of breath, rhinorrhea, and sore throat with or without respiratory distress. Approximately 15% of patients will present with purely gastrointestinal (GI) symptoms including anorexia, nausea, vomiting, diarrhea, and abdominal pain. Neurological symptoms include headaches, anosmia/dysgeusia, and confusion. Less frequently, acute lower motor neuropathies such as facial palsy and Guillain–Barré syndrome have been causally linked to COVID-19 infection. Onset of symptoms has ranged between 2 days and 2 weeks after confirmed exposure to SARS-CoV-2. A study in Wuhan, China, reported that the mean incubation period was 5.1 days and that 97.5% of individuals who developed symptoms did so within 11.5 days of being infected.[2]

Detailed past medical history must be obtained; underlying lung diseases, diabetes, hypertension, chronic corticosteroids, or immunosuppressant usage may predispose patients to severe COVID-19 pneumonia and can worsen the outcome. A meta-analysis of eight studies including 46,248 infected patients found that the most prevalent comorbidities were hypertension and diabetes, followed by cardiovascular diseases and respiratory system disease.[3] Aggressive treatment from the beginning of the onset should be considered for these patients. Relevant social history needs to be addressed; patients of low socioeconomic classes living in overcrowded households must be isolated and other members of their families tested for possible infection.

It is of utmost importance that patients with suspected and/or confirmed cases of COVID-19 be reported to the local or state health department. Caution should be exercised while caring for suspected/confirmed cases; Centers for Disease Control and Prevention (CDC) guidelines call for practicing airborne and contact precautions with such cases. Airborne and contact precautions must be practiced with all patients with suspected/confirmed diagnoses as per the CDC to protect health care providers and limit the spread of the virus. Physical examination of COVID-19 patients should include proper general physical, cardiopulmonary, neurological, and other systems examination as relevant and should ideally be done in isolated designated areas within the health care facilities. Similar to history taking, a clinician must find a proper balance between a sufficiently thorough examination and avoidance of unnecessarily prolonged exposure.

Clinicians should carefully evaluate vital signs and any deviations from normal range or concerning trends. Fever, tachycardia, tachypnea, and reduction in oxygen saturation (SpO_2) are common.

In performing a general examination, the clinician should assess whether the patient appears distressed or toxic. Other findings may transiently appear normal—the clinician must be able to recognize impending deterioration, as it occurs rapidly and is difficult to mitigate once it becomes severe, whereas patients will respond much more favorably to prompt treatment.

Examination of the head, ears, eyes, nose, and throat should assess for signs of sinusitis as well as pharyngitis. Extraocular muscle examination is important as patients are at risk of stroke. Examination of mucosal membranes may reveal dehydration and need for resuscitative fluids. Examination of the neck should assess for tracheal tugging as well as lymphadenopathy. A careful cardiac examination may detect tachycardia, arrhythmia, or signs of heart failure. Patients are also at risk for myocardial infarction and myocarditis.

Pulmonary examination poses a challenge, as lung auscultation has limited concordance with severity of lung injury in

COVID-19. Course crackles and dullness to percussion could indicate a secondary bacterial lobar pneumonia. Clinicians must recognize signs of hypoxia, such as increased work of breathing, accessory muscle use, and cyanosis. In some cases, the phenomenon of "happy hypoxia" has been described, in which patients, despite low oxygen saturation and/or low PaO_2, do not experience respiratory distress and do not seem to experience sequelae such as end-organ ischemic injury.

Examination of the extremities and skin may reveal rashes or decreased skin turgor in the case of dehydration. Edema can be a manifestation of edema. The extremities should be evaluated for edema as patients are at risk for pathologies that can cause right heart failure (left heart failure, pulmonary embolism, and pulmonary vasoconstriction). The clinician should also assess for signs of vascular occlusive disease, such as decreased pulse, decreased skin temperature, and decreased sensation, as well as small vessel vaso-occlusive distal skin lesions ("COVID toes").

Neurological examination is highly important, as a patient in respiratory failure who may otherwise respond well to noninvasive respiratory support may become confused or encephalopathic and require airway protection. A full neurological examination is important as patients are at risk for cerebral ischemia as well as inflammatory neuropathies.

Laboratory tests to detect the viral nucleic acids or antigens are obtained on initial presentation to confirm the viral infection using nucleic acid amplification tests (NAATs) such as real-time reverse transcription–polymerase chain reaction test of a nasopharyngeal specimen obtained with a swab. Immunoassay tests (antigen tests) may also be used, yet with less sensitivity than most NAATs.[4]

Arterial blood gases (ABG) test should be obtained to characterize the patients' oxygen partial pressure in the blood and the degree of hypoxia that may necessitate different types of assisted ventilation. In addition, ABG test will enable physicians to calculate the A-a gradient, which provides an insight into the extent of alveolar damage. Inflammatory markers including C-reactive protein (CRP), D-dimer, lactate dehydrogenase, and ferritin levels can play a role in both diagnostic and prognostic workup. Observing the trend of these inflammatory markers is helpful in either reinforcing or modifying the treatment plan. Rising acute-phase reactants may indicate the need for increased corticosteroid dosing. Markedly rising fibrin split product may indicate the need to transition from prophylactic to intermediate or full anticoagulation, although the literature has been mixed.

Complete blood count can reveal leucopenia, leukocytosis, and lymphopenia. According to a meta-analysis of 3,062 COVID-19 patients, normal leucocyte count, lymphopenia, and elevated levels of CRP and erythrocyte sedimentation rate were found to be the most prevalent laboratory findings in these patients.[5]

Hepatic injury is common, and liver transaminases along with bilirubin should be monitored. Marked elevations in transaminases, hypertriglyceridemia, and hyperferritinemia suggest the development of hemophagocytic lymphohistiocytic syndrome/macrophage activation syndrome. Of 417 hospitalized patients, over 75% were found to have abnormal liver tests and 21.5% had hepatic injury, according to a study by Bai et al.[6] Bai et al concluded that patients with abnormal liver tests were at a significantly increased odds of developing severe pneumonia.

Acute kidney injury in COVID-19 patients may be causally related to the direct damage of the renal tubules by the virus or as a result of the heightened inflammatory response by the immune response. Monitoring renal function and applying renal supportive measures can prevent lifelong renal damage to these patients.[7] If the patient presents with abdominal pain, nausea, vomiting, or diarrhea, obtaining a lipase level should be considered, as the patient could be experiencing acute pancreatitis.

Due to the nonspecificity of findings on chest imaging and to minimize the risk of airborne transmission of the virus in fixed radiography or computed tomography (CT) scanner rooms, the CDC does not recommend chest X-ray or CT to diagnose COVID-19 infection. In addition, the current American College of Radiology (ACR) Appropriateness Criteria statement on Acute Respiratory Illness states that chest CT is "usually not appropriate."[8] The ACR recommends frugal use of CT chest, only for hospitalized, symptomatic patients with specific clinical indications for CT and stresses on the importance of practicing proper infection control in order to limit any potential transmission of infection.[9]

COVID-19 pneumonia presents with several possible changes in the CT chest: ground-glass opacities with consolidation and infiltrates affecting (commonly) both lungs, which may have a peripheral distribution. Compared with non-COVID-19 pneumonia, COVID-19 pneumonia was less likely to have a central and peripheral distribution, pleural effusion, or lymphadenopathy.[6]

A 12-lead electrocardiogram should be performed to assess for any arrhythmia, ischemia, conduction disturbance, or sign of right ventricular strain, which, in turn, could raise suspicion of pulmonary embolism.

Once admitted to the hospital, complete blood counts, metabolic profile, hepatic profile, and acute-phase reactants should be monitored closely. Electrolytes must be repleted appropriately, anemia must be evaluated, and the etiology identified. Patients may be at risk for GI bleeding as well as microangiopathy. Hemodilution from aggressive hydration must also be considered. Platelet count must also be evaluated and monitored. It has been proposed that the viral spike protein may bind to the CD147 receptor expressed on the surface of leukocytes and erythrocytes, which in turn behaves as a platelet activator, and may result in a "catch-and-clump" mechanism of intravascular thrombosis.[10] Also, the use of heparin products, along with other pharmacological agents, may be associated with thrombocytopenia. Offending agents should be discontinued or changed when possible.

Management

A number of nonpharmacologic (high-flow oxygen support, noninvasive ventilatory support, permissive hypoxia, and awake prone positioning) and pharmacologic interventions have been utilized with mixed results in terms of outcomes data. Pharmacologic modalities have included antiviral therapy (remdesivir), targeted immunomodulatory therapy (tocilizumab), passive immunization therapy (convalescent plasma, monoclonal antibodies), antithrombotic therapy (heparin, direct anticoagulants, aspirin [ASA]), and micronutrient supplementation (ascorbic acid, zinc, cholecalciferol, thiamine) as well as repurposed use of various medications with putative angioprotective, immunomodulatory, and/or antiviral activity (statins, hydroxychloroquine [HCQ], ivermectin, colchicine, famotidine, melatonin). However, the pharmacologic modality universally recognized to have resulted in a marked reduction in hospital mortality, and therefore emerged as global standard of care for hospitalized patients with COVID-19 pneumonia, is corticosteroid therapy.

Patients requiring hospital admission are likely experiencing the pulmonary–inflammatory phases of COVID-19. At this stage, little to no viral replication persists, and the patient is experiencing a maladaptive host response to the presence of RNA viral material, which is highly reactogenic. The most common form of lung injury appears to be organizing pneumonia, whereas chest radiography consistent with viral pneumonia is less frequent.[11] Additionally, lung biopsy findings have not been consistent with an invasive viral disease, with few viral cytopathic changes noted.

In addition to parenchymal and interstitial lung involvement, patients experience a multifaceted vascular disease as well.

This includes a vasculitic component, a microangiopathic thrombotic component, and a pulmonary vasoconstrictive component, likely driven by excessive serotonergic activity driven by activated platelets.

In order to counteract these mechanisms of disease, various pharmacological interventions have been included in hospital protocols.

As with any patient presenting with bacterial or viral sepsis, airway, breathing and circulation (ABC) must be assessed and patients must be triaged, stabilized, and appropriately dispositioned. If the patient is suitable for the medical wards and does not require step-down or intensive care, he or she should be placed on telemetry and admitted to an appropriate COVID-19 treatment unit. Large-bore intravenous (IV) access should be obtained in the emergency department, appropriate IV crystalloid should be administered, and oxygen therapy should be titrated ideally to SpO_2 92% or higher; however, if a patient with lower oxygen saturation is comfortable and tolerating high-flow oxygen, increasing to more advanced modalities, especially endotracheal intubation and invasive ventilation, should be avoided, as these modalities may increase transpulmonary pressures and pulmonary inflammation, in addition to increasing intrathoracic pressure and impairing venous return, whereas end-organ injury has not been observed among patients with "happy hypoxia."

Nonpharmacological

When patients progress to more severe states of illness despite basic supportive measures, a number of nonpharmacological techniques can be applied to mitigate clinical deterioration. In patients with severe acute respiratory distress syndrome (ARDS) supported by invasive mechanical ventilation (MV), prone positioning is considered standard management. However, prior to the COVID-19 pandemic, proning was not considered usual practice for nonintubated awake individuals in respiratory failure. The applicability of proning to both MV and nonventilated patients has yielded positive results with improved oxygenation. In addition, prone positioning has been observed in nonintubated patients.

Prone positioning results in physiological and anatomic modifications that decrease ventilation and perfusion mismatch, thus improving oxygenation. In addition, pronation of patients facilitates improved expansion of posterior lung segments, resulting in improvement of airway secretions, decreases in alveolar collapse, and improvement of atelectasis. The prone positioning may potentially decrease lung injury. Typically, a six-member team is required for proning. Typical proning teams consists of critical care nurses, respiratory therapists, physicians, and physical therapists. Most patients during the COVID-19 pandemic spend 16 to 18 hours prone and then 6 to 8 hours supine. In one small study, involving 25 patients undergoing awake proning, over 75% patients (19 patients) demonstrated an improvement in oxygenation, with oxygen saturation levels above 95%; thus, they did not need to be intubated, at least immediately. Of those 19 patients, only 7 subsequently required intubation.[12] There was a decrease in the immediate need to proceed to MV in many patients. In those patients who did not respond to proning, 83% required MV.[12] During proning, expansion of the anterior chest wall is limited. This results in increased uniformity of chest wall compliance. The gravitational changes induced by proning improve alveolar recruitment in the posterior lung zones, allowing for an increased number of alveoli to engage in gas exchange. In both awake nonintubated patients and those on MV, changes in diaphragmatic excursion result in equalization of stress dynamics, thereby attenuating lung injury and improving recruitability in posterior lung zones and thus relieving atelectatic changes.[13] Furthermore, the posterior lung zone is highly perfused and thus recruitment of alveoli in this zone will result in improved V/Q matching.[13]

The presence of the SARS-CoV-2 in patients who develop severe COVID-19 disease generates a dysregulated immune response, resulting in hypercytokinemia, capillary leak migration of inflammatory cells, monocytes, and polymorphonuclear leukocytes. This occurs both in the lung and systemically. The pulmonary manifestations are alveolar injury, organizing pneumonia, and ARDS response. As the inflammations escalate, disruption of the alveolar capillary units occurs and progressive severe hypoxemic respiratory failure ensues. The maximization of oxygen delivery via by ancillary therapies such as high-flow nasal cannula (HFNC) and noninvasive ventilation has proven to be beneficial in many patients who have not undergone invasive MV. The overall goal is to safely delay or abate MV as long as possible.

During the pandemic, HFNC, which is able to provide warm humidified concentrations of 21 to 100% oxygen, was used with increasing frequency. HFNC is able to deliver flow rates of up to 60 L/min and provide some degree of PEEP. The benefits of this mode of oxygenation are potential for improvement in mucous clearance and prevention of atelectasis. In the management of hypoxemic respiratory failure, HFNC can be employed as a bridge to MV or in the prevention of early intubation. Although the use of this ancillary method of oxygenation did not decrease mortality, it was effective in decreasing intensive care unit (ICU) length of stay and increased ventilator-free days.[14,15]

There has been a concern for dispersion of SARS-CoV-2 particles or airborne transmission from patients with noninvasive positive-pressure ventilation (NIPPV) devices. The risk of viral transmission with NIPPV can be significantly reduced with the use of a filter on the expiratory circuit and the automatic measurement and quantification of a leak at the interface (which allows prompt leak correction and reduction of virus dispersion).

NIPPV includes continuous positive airway pressure and bilevel positive airway pressure. In the initial management of severe hypoxemic respiratory failure not immediately requiring endotracheal intubation and MV, several representative bodies such as the Society of Critical Care Medicine, the National Institutes of Health (NIH), and the European Society of Intensive Care Medicine as well as the World Health Organization (WHO) recommend the use of HFNC over NIPPV. In settings where HFNC is unavailable, NIPPV should be employed with close monitoring of respiratory and oxygenation status.[16-18]

A recent analysis of the HOPE COVID-19 registry demonstrated that in patients with respiratory failure 20% were managed with NIPPV, with 50% of these patients not ever requiring MV.[19] Failure of NIPPV in preventing MV was associated with a poor prognosis and increased mortality. Thus, NIPPV with close monitoring of patient is a viable strategy in preserving resource utilization and reducing the need for MV.[19] Noninvasive ventilation may represent a viable strategy particularly in cases of overcrowded and limited intensive care resources in this setting, but prompt identification of those failing is mandatory to avoid harm.[19]

Recommendations and guidelines vary on the use of NIPPV, as currently there is insufficient evidence regarding true effectiveness of NIPPV in acute viral pneumonia with hypoxia. However, we have enough data to support clinically guided use of NIPPV in some patients in order to abate and thus reduce the need for MV.

It is pertinent to note that patients on HFNC and NIPPV due to possible encumbrance of using the oropharyngeal route of nutrition can go days without oral intake and are at risk for the development of malnutrition. The increased catabolic state due to infection easily throws off the patients' metabolism. Oral diet or enteral nutrition (EN) in patients with pre-existing GI conditions (e.g., inflammatory bowel disease) has been the preferred route for nutrition to allow patients to benefit from gut nutrition. Nasogastric tube insertion and any other nutrition access procedures should be done as soon as possible in eligible patients to avoid further malnutrition. Switching to parenteral nutrition can be considered in patients intolerant to EN and in more critical cases.[20]

The psychological stress on both hospitalized critical and noncritical COVID-19 patients and their families adds further hindrance to the successful treatment of patients. The social distancing, isolation, and sense of impending doom are all contributing factors to patients' anxiety and worsening psychological stress. Hence, implementing psychological support in the patients' treatment regimen is essential. Continued social support from relatives and friends can be achieved through texts, phone, and video calls and should be encouraged.[21] When it comes to end-of-life care and more severe states of illness, policies should be flexible and allow families the proper autonomy to make informed risk-based decisions, as opposed to potentially depriving them from seeing their loved ones again. Proper protective measures should be maintained, and family members should be encouraged to isolate, if feasible, and to follow all state and local public health guidelines to avoid promoting community spread after a hospital visit. If there is very high local community transmission, a more conservative and restrictive approach may be warranted. These matters should be the subject of debate and discussion involving patient advocacy service, ethics committee members, infection control officers, nursing management, and hospital upper management.

Pharmacologic Therapy

Corticosteroid Therapy

The pathologic hallmarks of COVID-19 are a dysregulated hyperinflammatory state, endothelial activation, and injury with ensuing coagulopathy.[22,23] The pathogenesis of COVID-19 illness appears to be induced by dysregulated systemic and pulmonary inflammation, along with endothelial injury, hypercoagulability, and thrombosis.[22,23] Clinical evidence and autopsy studies evaluating the pulmonary parenchyma and vasculature

demonstrated the presence of microvascular and macrovascular thrombosis.[22-24] In part, recent evidence supports that the coagulopathy occurring in these patients is mediated by uncontrolled release of neutrophil extracellular traps (NETs). Emerging data indicate that hypercoagulability in COVID-19 is induced by dysregulated release of NETs.[25] Glucocorticoid therapy may decrease NET formation and may in part explain the therapeutic benefit observed by implementing corticoid therapy in severe COVID-19.[25]

It is worth noting that early guidelines cautioned against using systemic glucocorticoids because of concerns about deteriorating clinical state, delayed virus clearance, and adverse effects.[26-28] Currently, the data do not support the use of systemic glucocorticoids in individuals who do not require supplementary oxygen.[28,29] In the RECOVERY trial, a subgroup analysis demonstrated no improvement in outcome and a trend toward harm in individuals not requiring oxygen therapy.[28]

A cohort study conducted at Montefiore Medical Center in New York demonstrated that patients with CRP of 20 or greater benefitted from steroids, while patients with CRP below 10 showed nonstatistically significant trends toward harm.[29]

The choice, dose, and duration of corticosteroid also remain a matter of controversy. While a fixed dose of 6-mg dexamethasone emerged from the RECOVERY trial, multiple trials have compared this regimen to higher doses of methylprednisolone, a steroid with a much longer track record of effectiveness in lung disease. A dose of 1 to 2 mg/kg/day has been proposed, with several head-to-head studies demonstrating substantively beneficial effect sizes over dexamethasone 6 mg, based on important outcomes (mortality, duration of ICU stay), and in more severe refractory cases, pulse dose methylprednisolone has been demonstrated to be more effective.[28,30,31]

Methylprednisolone achieves higher lung tissue concentrations than dexamethasone, which raises questions about whether it would be more effective.

In a recent prospective triple-blinded randomized controlled trial, 2 mg/kg of methylprednisolone was found to be superior to fixed-dose dexamethasone employed in the RECOVERY trial (6 mg/day) in terms of hospital length of stay, need for MV, and improved clinical status.[31]

Remdesivir

Remdesivir is an inhibitor of the SARS-CoV-2 RNA-dependent RNA polymerase (RdRp), which is essential for viral replication. At present, it is the position of the WHO that there are insufficient data to recommend for or against the use of remdesivir.[18] We suggest that clinicians make the judgment about which patients may be appropriate recipients of remdesivir based on their risk of clinical deterioration.

The Adaptive COVID-19 Treatment Trial (ACTT-1), a randomized controlled trial that compared remdesivir to placebo in hospitalized individuals, demonstrated no significant benefit in patients with mild-to-moderate disease.[32] In an open-label randomized trial involving individuals with moderate disease, individuals treated with remdesivir for 5 days demonstrated improvement in clinical symptoms by day 11. The results of this trial are of questionable benefit.[33]

The Solidarity trial, a large, multinational, open-label randomized controlled trial in which a 10-day course of remdesivir was compared to standard of care, demonstrated no difference between groups in the primary end point of in-hospital mortality.[34] These trials have conflicting results and as such there is a paucity of data to advise for or against establishing remdesivir as routine therapy for hospitalized patients with moderate COVID-19. In light of this, the NIH panel recognizes that there may be situations in which a clinician judges that remdesivir is an appropriate treatment for a hospitalized patient with moderate disease (e.g., a person who is at a particularly high risk for clinical deterioration).

Ascorbic Acid

The coronavirus elicits a cytokine storm with subsequent lung damage including oxidative damage from reactive oxygen and nitrogen species. There is ongoing inflammation and pulmonary injury in that setting, which may lead to subsequent respiratory failure. It has been theorized that large dosages of an antioxidant such as ascorbic acid may blunt the oxidative stress induced by the coronavirus. Additionally, during states of increased oxidative stress, ascorbic acid may be rapidly depleted and as such mega dosages may be required.

A proof-of-concept trial 1 randomized adults in the ICU to receive parenteral vitamin C 24 g per day or placebo for 7 days. Unfortunately, due to the case of COVID-19 dropping in China, the study was terminated early due to lack of enrollment. Overall, the study found no differences between the arms in mortality, the duration of MV, or the change in median sequential organ failure assessment (SOFA) scores. The investigators did observe a significantly improved PaO_2/F_iO_2 ratio from baseline to day 7 in the treatment arm when compared to placebo.[35]

The COVID A to Z study investigated whether high-dose zinc and/or high-dose ascorbic acid decreased the severity or duration of symptoms compared with usual care among ambulatory patients with COVID-19. The investigators observed no statistically significant difference in duration or severity of symptoms between the treatment and the control groups.[36]

The NIH COVID-19 Treatment Guidelines Panel states that there are insufficient data to recommend for or against the use of ascorbic acid for COVID-19.

We recommend that ascorbic acid be given in the following doses: for non-ICU patients with O_2 level less than 4 L on hospital ward, 2,000 to 4,000 mg oral in divided doses daily as tolerated until discharge; for those in ICU or with O_2 level more than 4 L, 50 mg/kg IV every 6 hours up to 7 days or until discharge from ICU and then transitioning to oral dose as mentioned previously. If in ICU and not improving, consider mega-doses: 25 g IV twice daily for 3 days.[37]

Vitamin D

B lymphocytes, T lymphocytes, and other antigen-presenting cells express vitamin D receptors on their cell surface and thus play a role in regulating the immune response.[38] Vitamin D supplementation has been shown to enhance the number of T regulatory cells in both healthy people and those with autoimmune disorders.[39] The rationale for using vitamin D is based largely on immunomodulatory effects that could potentially protect against COVID-19 infection or decrease the severity of illness. A trial involving the effect of a single high dose of vitamin D_3 on hospital length of stay in patients with moderate-to-severe COVID-19 did not demonstrate a significant difference in hospital length of stay in patients administered a single high dose of vitamin D compared to placebo.[40]

It was observed that individuals with severe disease have coexistent decreased vitamin D levels. It, however, remains unclear whether there is a causal link between low vitamin D levels and severity of disease. Further studies are necessary to understand the role that vitamin D plays in COVID-19.

We recommend calcifediol (if available) at a dose of 0.5 mg orally on day 1, then 0.2 mg orally day 2, and weekly thereafter, or cholecalciferol at a dose of 20,000 to 60,000 IU single dose orally and then 20,000 IU weekly until discharge.[37]

Thiamine

Thiamine is a cornerstone in the concept of "metabolic resuscitation," an approach based on the concept that once severe or critical illness develops, multiple deficiencies in key vitamins and hormones are created via "consumption" induced via the body's attempts to fight off the insult or invader. Immediate and aggressive repletion of such substances is critical to strengthening the immune system's ability to maintain balance and prevent the onset of multiorgan failure.[37]

Thiamine is involved in adaptive immunity, and antibody formation is important in eliminating the SARS-CoV-2 virus; as such, thiamine deficiency may predispose a patient to inadequate antibody response and as a consequence increased severity of symptoms. Adequate thiamine levels are necessary for the synthesis of essential coenzymes thiamine pyrophosphate and pyruvate dehydrogenase required for glucose metabolism and proper immune cell and neurologic function. Thus, thiamine supplementation may play a role in reducing the risk of developing several diseases.[41] A retrospective observational propensity-matched study comprising 738 ICU patients with severe disease demonstrated a statistically significant link between thiamine usage and reduction in thrombosis and in-hospital mortality.[42] Further randomized trials are needed to corroborate this study. However, from a pathophysiologic basis with little downside risk, we recommend thiamine 200 mg IV twice daily for up to 7 days or until discharge.[37]

Zinc

The link between zinc and COVID-19 is presently being investigated, specifically how zinc deficiency impacts the severity of disease and if zinc supplementation can improve patient outcomes. When employed in vitro with a zinc ionophore, zinc has been demonstrated to increase cytotoxicity and cause apoptosis (e.g., chloroquine). Chloroquine has also been found to increase zinc uptake inside cells.[43]

An open-label, outpatient randomized trial of zinc against ascorbic acid versus zinc plus ascorbic acid versus standard of care demonstrated that therapy with high-dose zinc gluconate, ascorbic acid, or a combination of the two supplements did not substantially reduce the number of days necessary to achieve a 50% reduction in symptom severity of disease in outpatients when compared to placebo.[36]

A retrospective analysis included 242 hospitalized patients. A total of 196 patients

(81.0%) got a total daily dosage of 440-mg zinc sulfate (100-mg elemental zinc), with 191 patients (97%) receiving HCQ as well. There were 46 patients who did not receive zinc therapy and 70% of these received HCQ. Overall, this complicated study, undertaken to evaluate the causal relationship of zinc therapy and the clinical outcome of 28-day mortality, failed to demonstrate any significant mortality benefit.[44] From a pathophysiological standpoint, the confluence of recognized risk factors for zinc deficiency in acute illness and the link between deficiency and severe disease has been demonstrated.[45] Zinc supplementation may inhibit viral cellular penetration and decrease replication. In addition, zinc is important in supporting the host's antiviral response. Zinc plays a critical role in the formation and function of immune cells.[45] It is important to note that zinc's effects are not always defined as activating or inhibiting, since zinc can help to regulate overactive immune responses and balance the ratios of different immune effector.[45] However, from a clinical standpoint, there has been very little supportive evidence. Given very little evidence for any toxic effects during short-term therapy and the known propensity of zinc deficiency in acute illness, we recommend zinc 75 to 100 mg orally daily until discharge.[37]

Anticoagulants

One of the earliest and most profound insights into the pathophysiology of COVID-19 disease was that of its extreme "hypercoagulability," found in the most severely ill patients suffering severe inflammation. Nonetheless, the use of anticoagulation for prophylaxis or treatment of COVID-19 is controversial.

The employment of systemic anticoagulation versus prophylactic-dose anticoagulation has been complex. Data demonstrate that systemic treatment-dose anticoagulation may be beneficial in certain subgroups of patients, despite limitations such as unobserved confounding, unclear reason for anticoagulation, lack of metrics to further

categorize disease severity in the mechanically ventilated cohort, and indication bias.[46]

The ACTION trial was multicenter, randomized controlled trial comparing therapeutic (systemic) with prophylactic anticoagulation for patients admitted to hospital with COVID-19 risk stratified by a high D-dimer concentration.

In patients with COVID-19 and increased D-dimer concentrations who were admitted to the hospital, therapeutic anticoagulation with unfractionated heparin or enoxaparin followed by transition rivaroxaban to day 30 compared with prophylactic-dose heparin, systemic anticoagulation did not demonstrate improvement in clinical outcomes.[47] In addition, there was ans associated with an increased risk of bleeding complications.

Vaughn et al and the Mi-COVID19 consortium evaluated the Mi-COVID19 database involving a large number of patients from multiple centers and assessed the frequency and diversity, among hospitals, and modifications of strategies over time in venous thromboembolism prevention and treatment-dose anticoagulation in patients. In addition, the relationship between anticoagulation methods and in-hospital and 60-day mortality was evaluated. This study demonstrated that hospitals rapidly deployed anticoagulation and prophylactic-dose heparin protocols. However, only prophylactic-dose heparin protocols were associated with an improved 60-day mortality outcome.[48]

Observational studies have demonstrated that therapeutic anticoagulation was associated with survival, and a longer duration of anticoagulation was associated with a survival benefit in patients with COVID-19-associated acute respiratory distress syndrome (CARDS) on MV. Interim analysis of the ATTACC, ACTIVE IV-1, and REMAP-CAP trial revealed that in critically ill COVID-19 patients with CARDS on organ support, therapeutic anticoagulation did not improve survival compared to thromboprophylaxis doses of heparin.[49] In contrast, regardless of D-dimer levels, in patients with moderate disease not in the ICU, full-dose anticoagulation resulted in a significant survival benefit.[49]

Based on the varying recommendations, the use of anticoagulation is best left to a clinician-guided decision.

For patients on the general medical floor, enoxaparin 1 mg/kg is given twice daily—monitor anti-Ax levels, target 0.6 to 1.1 IU/mL. For patients in the ICU, enoxaparin 0.5 mg/kg is given twice daily—monitor anti-Ax levels, target 0.2 to 0.5 IU/mL. For both regimens, one continues throughout hospitalization. Upon discharge start a direct oral anticoagulant at half dose and complete 4 weeks of therapy.[37] Attention in renal function is essential as enoxaparin dose needs to be adjusted according to creatinine clearance. In patients with marked renal impairment or those on dialysis, unfractionated heparin should be used.

Famotidine

Famotidine is a type 2 antihistaminergic drug typically used in the management of gastroesophageal reflux disease, as a second-line agent in upper GI bleed, or as an adjunctive agent in the management of allergy and anaphylaxis. However, there is evidence that famotidine exerts antiviral effects.[50,51] It has been proposed as a useful adjunctive agent in the hospital management of COVID-19.[50,51]

Additionally, there are observational studies suggesting a link between proton pump inhibitors and worsened outcomes in COVID-19, although a causal relationship has not been conclusively identified. As such, in COVID-19, clinicians should consider the use of famotidine as opposed to pantoprazole or other PPIs for GI prophylaxis if needed, and should be considered as an adjunctive agent in the management of COVID-19 irrespective of whether it is needed for GI purposes, based on its putative antiviral effects and favorable safety profile.

Statins

HMG-CoA reductase inhibitors (also known as statins) have known anti-inflammatory effects and are protective against vascular injury. They have also been shown to increase thrombus permeability and may play an antithrombotic role in the management of COVID-19. Studies have shown an association between statins and improved outcomes in the hospital management of COVID-19, and should be considered as an adjunctive agent in the absence of a contraindication.[52,53]

Fenofibrate

Similar to statins, fibrates are known to increase thrombus permeability, and may serve a vasculoprotective role in COVID-19. It has also been proposed that pulmonary lipotoxic fatty acid formation during the severe hypermetabolic state in patients hospitalized with COVID-19 may be inhibited by fibrate therapy.[54,55]

Convalescent Plasma

Convalescent plasma's role in the hospital management of COVID-19 remains controversial, and studies have been mixed. This is a modality that has been used for a century in severe viral illnesses, with a favorable safety profile. It was believed that if only high-titer samples were utilized, and administered very early in hospitalization, there were improved outcomes. To date, the largest and most well-designed randomized controlled trial conducted in the United Kingdom, using high-titer samples administered early in hospitalization, did not show clinical benefit.[56–58]

Tocilizumab

Interleukin 6 (IL-6) is well known for promoting the inflammatory cascade and the cytokine storm, a not uncommon feature in severe disease resulting in vascular leak, the accumulation of immune effector cells and macrophages in the pulmonary and systemic microcirculation. This cascade leads to endotheliitis, thrombotic events, and organ failure.[59] Elevated IL-6 levels and evidence of hyperinflammation have increased rates of more severe disease.[60,61] Tocilizumab is an IL-6 receptor alpha-monoclonal antibody that has been used to treat select rheumatological diseases and as part of CAR-T cell therapy. Inhibition of IL-16 receptors by tocilizumab leads to reduction in cytokines and acute-phase reactant production. The use of tocilizumab in treating COVID-19 is aimed at mitigating the hyperinflammatory state.[62-64]

Both RECOVERY and REMAP CAP (the two tocilizumab trials that reported a benefit) initiated treatment early (randomization at median of 2 days of hospitalization in RECOVERY; <24 hours in the ICU for REMAP-CAP), suggesting tocilizumab may be more beneficial in people with early rapidly progressive disease.[62-64] Furthermore, a mortality benefit was observed when tocilizumab is administered in conjunction with glucocorticoids.[62-64]

Based on existing meta-analyses and systematic reviews, there appears to be cumulative moderate certainty evidence of reduced mortality.[64]

Antibiotics

Antibiotics are not generally recommended as empiric therapy for COVID-19 pneumonia, but should be used judiciously at the discretion of the physician if secondary bacterial pneumonia is suspected. Choice and duration of therapy should reflect usual care for the management of community acquired, or nosocomial, if appropriate, pneumonia; however, the clinician should consider the use of antibiotics with putative anti-inflammatory or antiviral properties, such as doxycycline or azithromycin. Both of these agents will cover atypical bacterial organisms as well.

Aspirin

From a pathophysiologic standpoint, the use of ASA is ideal due to its antithrombotic and anti-inflammatory properties. A large retrospective propensity-matched trial demonstrated in-hospital use of ASA along with intermediate-dose heparin anticoagulation was associated with a decrease in hospital mortality.[65] Chow et al, in a retrospective analysis of hospitalized patients, after adjusting for confounding variables, observed that the use of ASA was associated with a decrease need for MV.[66] However, recently, the

RECOVERY trial demonstrated that the use of ASA was not linked with a decrease in 28-day mortality or the likelihood of progressing to invasive MV or death in hospitalized patients, although it was associated with a modest increase in the chance of being released alive within 28 days.[67]

Baricitinib

Recently, baricitinib, a Janus kinase inhibitor, has shown some promise in improving clinical severity outcomes in patients with severe disease who require HFNC or noninvasive ventilation particularly when used in conjunction with remdesivir.[68] When employed without remdesivir, the COV-BARRIER trial demonstrated a nonstatistically significant trend in abating escalation of oxygen requirements, noninvasive ventilation, MV, and mortality.[69]

Conclusion

Patients with COVID-19 infection represent a subgroup of patients at increased risk for clinical deterioration. Early aggressive pharmacologic and nonpharmacologic aspects of patient management are essential in improving and assuring patient outcome. Although early in the phase of disease antiviral therapy may be effective, the inflammatory and coagulopathic nature of this disease is best managed with multimodal therapy, including anti-inflammatory agents, which modulate the dysregulated immune response. In addition, appropriate anticoagulation therapy in the proper clinical setting should be employed to decrease the risk and prevent thrombotic complications.

References

1. CDC. 2019 novel coronavirus, Wuhan, China. CDC. Available at: https://www.cdc.gov/coronavirus/2019-ncov/symptoms-testing/symptoms.html
2. Lauer SA, Grantz KH, Bi Q, et al. The incubation period of coronavirus disease 2019 (COVID-19) from publicly reported confirmed cases:

estimation and application. Ann Intern Med 2020;172(9):577–582

3. Yang J, Zheng Y, Gou X, et al. Prevalence of comorbidities and its effects in patients infected with SARS-CoV-2: a systematic review and meta-analysis. Int J Infect Dis 2020;94:91–95

4. CDC. Overview of testing for SARS-CoV-2 (COVID-19). Available at: https://www.cdc.gov/coronavirus/2019-ncov/hcp/testing-overview.html

5. Zhu J, Ji P, Pang J, et al. Clinical characteristics of 3062 COVID-19 patients: a meta-analysis. J Med Virol 2020;92(10):1902–1914

6. Cai Q, Huang D, Yu H, et al. COVID-19: Abnormal liver function tests. Journal of Hepatology.2020;73(3):566-574.doi:https://doi.org/10.1016/j.jhep.2020.04.006

7. Li Z, Wu M, Yao J, et al. Caution on kidney dysfunctions of COVID-19 patients. medRxiv 2020 (e-pub ahead of print). doi:10.1101/2020.02.08.20021212

8. Kirsch J, Ramirez J, Mohammed TL, et al. ACR Appropriateness Criteria® acute respiratory illness in immunocompetent patients. J Thorac Imaging 2011;26(2):W42–W44

9. ACR. ACR recommendations for the use of chest radiography and computed tomography (CT) for suspected COVID-19 infection. Available at: https://www.acr.org/Advocacy-and-Economics/ACR-Position-Statements/Recommendations-for-Chest-Radiography-and-CT-for-Suspected-COVID19-Infection

10. Chung MK, Zidar DA, Bristow MR, et al. COVID-19 and cardiovascular disease: from bench to bedside. Circ Res 2021;128(8):1214–1236

11. Kory P, Kanne JP. SARS-CoV-2 organising pneumonia: 'Has there been a widespread failure to identify and treat this prevalent condition in COVID-19?'. BMJ Open Respir Res 2020;7(1):e000724

12. Thompson AE, Ranard BL, Wei Y, Jelic S. Prone positioning in awake, nonintubated patients with COVID-19 hypoxemic respiratory failure. JAMA Intern Med 2020;180(11):1537–1539

13. Venus K, Munshi L, Fralick M. Prone positioning for patients with hypoxic respiratory failure related to COVID-19. CMAJ 2020;192(47):E1532–E1537

14. Mellado-Artigas R, Ferreyro BL, Angriman F, et al; COVID-19 Spanish ICU Network. High-flow nasal oxygen in patients with COVID-19-associated acute respiratory failure. Crit Care 2021;25(1):58

15. Bonnet N, Martin O, Boubaya M, et al. High flow nasal oxygen therapy to avoid invasive mechanical ventilation in SARS-CoV-2 pneumonia: a retrospective study. Ann Intensive Care 2021;11(1):37

16. Alhazzani W, Møller MH, Arabi YM, et al. Surviving sepsis campaign: guidelines on the management of critically ill adults with coronavirus disease 2019 (COVID-19). Crit Care Med 2020;48(6):e440–e469

17. Tran K, Cimon K, Severn M, Pessoa-Silva C, Conly J. Aerosol-generating procedures and risk of transmission of acute respiratory infections: a systematic review. CADTH Technol Overv 2013;3(1):e3201

18. WHO. Clinical management of severe acute respiratory infection (SARI) when COVID-19 disease is suspected. Interim guidance. March 13, 2020. Available at: https://www.who.int/publications/i/item/clinical-management-of-covid-19

19. Bertaina M, Nuñez-Gil IJ, Franchin L, et al; HOPE COVID-19 investigators. Non-invasive ventilation for SARS-CoV-2 acute respiratory failure: a subanalysis from the HOPE COVID-19 registry. Emerg Med J 2021;38(5):359–365

20. Stachowska E, Folwarski M, Jamioł-Milc D, Maciejewska D, Skonieczna-Żydecka K. Nutritional support in coronavirus 2019 disease. Medicina (Kaunas) 2020;56(6):E289

21. Passavanti M, Argentieri A, Barbieri DM, et al. The psychological impact of COVID-19 and restrictive measures in the world. J Affect Disord 2021;283:36–51

22. Joly BS, Siguret V, Veyradier A. Understanding pathophysiology of hemostasis disorders in critically ill patients with COVID-19. Intensive Care Med 2020;46(8):1603–1606

23. Helms J, Tacquard C, Severac F, et al; CRICS TRIGGERSEP Group (Clinical Research in Intensive Care and Sepsis Trial Group for Global Evaluation and Research in Sepsis). High risk of thrombosis in patients with severe SARS-CoV-2 infection: a multicenter prospective cohort study. Intensive Care Med 2020;46(6):1089–1098

24. Carsana L, Sonzogni A, Nasr A, et al. Pulmonary post-mortem findings in a series of COVID-19 cases from northern Italy: a two-centre descriptive study. Lancet Infect Dis 2020;20(10):1135–1140

25. Ackermann M, Anders H-J, Bilyy R, et al. Patients with COVID-19: in the dark-NETs of neutrophils. Cell Death & Differentiation. Published online May 24, 2021. doi:10.1038/s41418-021-00805-z

26. Arabi YM, Mandourah Y, Al-Hameed F, et al; Saudi Critical Care Trial Group. Corticosteroid therapy for critically ill patients with Middle East respiratory syndrome. Am J Respir Crit Care Med 2018;197(6):757–767

27. Lee N, Allen Chan KC, Hui DS, et al. Effects of early corticosteroid treatment on plasma SARS-associated coronavirus RNA concentrations in adult patients. J Clin Virol 2004;31(4):304–309

28. Horby P, Lim WS, Emberson JR, et al; RECOVERY Collaborative Group. Dexamethasone in hospitalized patients with Covid-19. N Engl J Med 2021;384(8):693–704

29. Cui Z, Merritt Z, Assa A, et al. Early and significant reduction in C-reactive protein levels after corticosteroid therapy is associated with reduced mortality in patients with COVID-19. J Hosp Med 2021;16(3):142–148

30. Ko JJ, Wu C, Mehta N, Wald-Dickler N, Yang W, Qiao R. A comparison of methylprednisolone and dexamethasone in intensive care patients with COVID-19. J Intensive Care Med 2021;36(6):673–680

31. Ranjbar K, Moghadami M, Mirahmadizadeh A, et al. Methylprednisolone or dexamethasone, which one is superior corticosteroid in the treatment of hospitalized COVID-19 patients: a triple-blinded randomized controlled trial. BMC Infect Dis 2021;21(1):337

32. Beigel JH, Tomashek KM, Dodd LE, et al; ACTT-1 Study Group Members. Remdesivir for the treatment of Covid-19 - final report. N Engl J Med 2020;383(19):1813–1826

33. Spinner CD, Gottlieb RL, Criner GJ, et al; GS-US-540-5774 Investigators. Effect of remdesivir vs standard care on clinical status at 11 days in patients with moderate COVID-19: a randomized clinical trial. JAMA 2020;324(11):1048–1057

34. Pan H, Peto R, Henao-Restrepo AM, et al; WHO Solidarity Trial Consortium. Repurposed antiviral drugs for Covid-19 - interim WHO Solidarity trial results. N Engl J Med 2021;384(6):497–511

35. Zhang J, Rao X, Li Y, et al. Pilot trial of high-dose vitamin C in critically ill COVID-19 patients. Ann Intensive Care 2021;11(1):5

36. Thomas S, Patel D, Bittel B, et al. Effect of high-dose zinc and ascorbic acid supplementation vs usual care on symptom length and reduction among ambulatory patients with SARS-CoV-2 infection: the COVID A to Z randomized clinical trial. JAMA Netw Open 2021;4(2):e210369

37. MATH+ Protocol | FLCCC | Front Line COVID-19 Critical Care Alliance (covid19criticalcare.com) Home | FLCCC | Front Line COVID-19 Critical Care Alliance. Available at: covid19criticalcare.com

38. Aranow C. Vitamin D and the immune system. J Investig Med 2011;59(6):881–886

39. Fisher SA, Rahimzadeh M, Brierley C, et al. The role of vitamin D in increasing circulating T regulatory cell numbers and modulating T regulatory cell phenotypes in patients with inflammatory disease or in healthy volunteers: a systematic review. PLoS One 2019;14(9):e0222313

40. Murai IH, Fernandes AL, Sales LP, et al. Effect of a single high dose of vitamin D3 on hospital length of stay in patients with moderate to severe COVID-19: a randomized clinical trial. JAMA 2021;325(11):1053–1060

41. Amrein K, Oudemans-van Straaten HM, Berger MM. Vitamin therapy in critically ill patients: focus on thiamine, vitamin C, and vitamin D. Intensive Care Med 2018;44(11):1940–1944

42. Al Sulaiman K, Aljuhani O, Al Dossari M, et al. Evaluation of thiamine as adjunctive therapy in COVID-19 critically ill patients: a two-center propensity score matched study. Crit Care 2021;25(1):223

43. Xue J, Moyer A, Peng B, Wu J, Hannafon BN, Ding WQ. Chloroquine is a zinc ionophore. PLoS One 2014;9(10):e109180

44. Yao JS, Paguio JA, Dee EC, et al. The minimal effect of zinc on the survival of hospitalized patients with COVID-19: an observational study. Chest 2021;159(1):108–111

45. Wessels I, Rolles B, Rink L. The potential impact of zinc supplementation on COVID-19 pathogenesis. Front Immunol 2020;11:1712

46. Paranjpe I, Fuster V, Lala A, et al. Association of treatment dose anticoagulation with in-hospital survival among hospitalized patients with COVID-19. J Am Coll Cardiol 2020;76(1):122–124

47. Lopes RD, de Barros E Silva PGM, Furtado RHM, et al; ACTION Coalition COVID-19

Brazil IV Investigators. Therapeutic versus prophylactic anticoagulation for patients admitted to hospital with COVID-19 and elevated D-dimer concentration (ACTION): an open-label, multicentre, randomised, controlled trial. Lancet 2021;397(10291): 2253–2263

48. Vaughn VM, Yost M, Abshire C, et al. Trends in venous thromboembolism anticoagulation in patients hospitalized with COVID-19. JAMA Netw Open 2021;4(6):e2111788

49. ATTACC, ACTIV-4a and REMAP-CAP Investigators. ATTACC, ACTIV-4a and REMAP-CAP. Results of interim analysis. January 28, 2021. Available at: https://static1.squarespace.com/static/5cde3c7d9a69340001d79ffe/t/6013892709de942b53f6e3da/1611893037749/mpRCT+interim+presentation_v21-slides+22+and+23+corrected.pdf (accessed March 26, 2021)

50. Malone RW, Tisdall P, Fremont-Smith P, et al. COVID-19: famotidine, histamine, mast cells, and mechanisms. Front Pharmacol 2021;12:633680

51. Mather JF, Seip RL, McKay RG. Impact of famotidine use on clinical outcomes of hospitalized patients with COVID-19. Am J Gastroenterol 2020;115(10):1617–1623

52. Daniels LB, Sitapati AM, Zhang J, et al. Relation of statin use prior to admission to severity and recovery among COVID-19 inpatients. Am J Cardiol 2020;136:149–155

53. Diaz-Arocutipa C, Melgar-Talavera B, Alvarado-Yarasca Á, et al. Statins reduce mortality in patients with COVID-19: an updated meta-analysis of 147 824 patients. Int J Infect Dis 2021;110:374–381

54. Davies SP, Mycroft-West CJ, Pagani I, et al. The hyperlipidaemic drug fenofibrate significantly reduces infection by SARS-CoV-2 in cell culture models. Front Pharmacol 2021;12:660490

55. New study suggests COVID-19 lung damage reduced in patients prescribed fenofibrate. Clin OMICs 2021;8(1). https://doi.org/10.1089/clinomi.08.01.16

56. Klassen SA, Senefeld JW, Senese KA, et al. Convalescent plasma therapy for COVID-19: a graphical mosaic of the worldwide evidence. Front Med (Lausanne) 2021;8:684151

57. Korley FK, Durkalski-Mauldin V, Yeatts SD, et al. Early Convalescent Plasma for High-Risk Outpatients with Covid-19. N Engl J Med. Published online August 18, 2021. doi:10.1056/NEJMoa2103784

58. Piechotta V, Iannizzi C, Chai KL, et al. Convalescent plasma or hyperimmune immunoglobulin for people with COVID-19: a living systematic review. Cochrane Database Syst Rev 2021;5(5):CD013600

59. Rosas IO, Bräu N, Waters M, et al. Tocilizumab in hospitalized patients with severe Covid-19 pneumonia. N Engl J Med 2021;384(16):1503–1516

60. Chen G, Wu D, Guo W, et al. Clinical and immunological features of severe and moderate coronavirus disease 2019. J Clin Invest 2020;130(5):2620–2629

61. Kalikshteĭn DB, Levantovskaia OM, Vyshenpol'skiĭ Iula, Ol'shanskiĭ Ala. Svertyvaiushchaia i protivosvertyvaiushdhaia sistemy krovi pri allergicheskikh zabolevaniiakh [Coagulation and anticoagulation systems of the blood in allergic diseases]. Sov Med 1988;(9):104–106

62. RECOVERY Collaborative Group. Tocilizumab in patients admitted to hospital with COVID-19 (RECOVERY): a randomised, controlled, open-label, platform trial. Lancet 2021;397(10285):1637–1645

63. Gordon AC, Mouncey PR, Al-Beidh F, et al; REMAP-CAP Investigators. Interleukin-6 receptor antagonists in critically ill patients with Covid-19. N Engl J Med 2021;384(16):1491–1502

64. Tleyjeh IM, Kashour Z, Riaz M, Hassett L, Veiga VC, Kashour T. Efficacy and safety of tocilizumab in COVID-19 patients: a living systematic review and meta-analysis, first update. Clin Microbiol Infect 2021;27(8):1076–1082

65. Meizlish ML, Goshua G, Liu Y, et al. Intermediate-dose anticoagulation, aspirin, and in-hospital mortality in COVID-19: a propensity score-matched analysis. Am J Hematol 2021;96(4):471–479

66. Chow JH, Khanna AK, Kethireddy S, et al. Aspirin use is associated with decreased mechanical ventilation, intensive care unit admission, and in-hospital mortality in hospitalized patients with coronavirus disease 2019. Anesth Analg 2021;132(4):930–941

67. RECOVERY Collaborative Group, Horby PW, Pessoa-Amorim G, et al. Aspirin in patients

admitted to hospital with COVID-19 (RECOVERY): a randomised, controlled, open-label, platform trial. medRxiv 2021 (e-pub ahead of print). doi:10.1101/2021.06.08.21258132

68. Goletti D, Cantini F. Baricitinib therapy in Covid-19 pneumonia - an unmet need fulfilled. N Engl J Med 2021;384(9):867–869

69. Marconi VC, Ramanan AV, de Bono S, et al. Efficacy and safety of baricitinib for the treatment of hospitalised adults with COVID-19 (COV-BARRIER): a randomised, double-blind, parallel-group, placebo-controlled phase 3 trial. Lancet Respir Med. Published online August 31, 2021. doi:10.1016/S2213-2600(21)00331-3

14 COVID-19 and Emergency Medicine

William Dalsey, Nicole Maguire, Danielle Biggs, Joslyn Joseph, and Lisa Armstrong

Introduction

COVID-19 has and continues to transform the house of medicine and has had a significant impact on the field of Emergency Medicine (EM). There is not an aspect of EM from patient demographics and volume to emergency medicine services, clinical care, staffing, education, research, and safety and quality initiatives that the pandemic has not affected. During the height of the pandemic, Emergency Department (ED) volumes across the United States dropped by 50% and even by April 2021 volumes remained 20% below pre-COVID levels.[1] The greatest reductions in volume have been in the pediatric population and minor illness and injury presentations.[2] During the height of the pandemic there was a significant reduction in all types of ED patients including stroke and acute myocardial infarctions thereby leading to higher than normal prehospital deaths and higher acuity presentation volumes to the ED. Many of these changes are likely to permanently alter the role of EM in the healthcare system.

When COVID-19 began, the healthcare community underestimated its severity and responded using plans built for a Flu pandemic (US Department of Health and Human Services Pandemic Flu Plan/CDC Response Framework).[3] Stockpiles of personal protective equipment (PPE) that were accumulated during the Ebola presentation, years before, were depleted or out of date. There was great difficulty purchasing PPE, and producers were hampered by disruptions in supply chains which created limited access of respirator masks and gowns. This made access to PPE for frontline workers very difficult and often individual groups and persons began to rely on a privatized access to PPE.

The healthcare community did not recognize or act on many aspects of COVID-19, including the role of asymptomatic spread, the mortality rate to high-risk patients, or the route of transmission, and thereby the appropriate PPE, to prevent contraction. Early in the pandemic the country was without adequate testing capabilities, contact tracing, and other public health interventions which lead to wide, fast spread of the disease. Initial guidance by the CDC was focused on droplet transmission of COVID-19 and in fact it was not until March of 2021 that the CDC recognized the risk of aerosol transmission. It was also not until March 2021 that the CDC revised its position and stated that fomites were a rare risk of transmission and deep cleaning was not necessary to ensure safety.[4] For a year the concerns related to cleaning and ensuring safety created logistical delays for patients needing admission and at time even increased waiting times in the ED secondary to lack of available rooms.

Many EDs have reported significant increases in overdoses, alcohol-related illness, and psychiatric conditions including suicidal ideation, anxiety, and depression. Stress on ED personnel working with COVID patients led to burnout, staffing difficulties, posttraumatic stress disorder, anxiety, and depression. The closing of schools added to this burden for many healthcare workers trying to care for ED patients and their families. Witnessing the volume of deaths, and the impersonal nature of such events since family and friends were not allowed to visit or be present, further added to the mental strain on all of us.

In this chapter we aim to review the major key aspects of COVID-19 as well as specifically addressing its affects and developments on Emergency Medical Services (EMSs), Pediatrics, and our Obstetric populations.

Emergency Department Facilities and PPE

Most EDs have limited numbers of negative pressure rooms and designated areas for infectious disease. These areas in many facilities were rapidly overwhelmed, and EDs explored opportunities to add additional rooms, created negative pressure or positive pressure areas of departments, and, in some cases, were able to turn the entire ED into a negative pressure environment. Open bay bed designs created challenges to minimize the risk of transmission for COVID patients in the ED. As cases increased the entire ED in most facilities was considered a high-risk area and all patients were treated as potential COVID patients regardless of their presenting complaints. This was embraced as we learned of the numbers of asymptomatic COVID patients and the delay in symptoms despite active COVID infection.

The risk of exposure and lack of understanding of the transmission of the disease challenged all of us. There were severe shortages of PPE in many EDs. Concerns about transmission and frequently changing CDC recommendations forced us to adjust accordingly. Recommended N95 respirators were in such limited supply that they were rationed and used for up to a week. Subsequent studies have shown they degrade and should not be used for more than 2 to 3 days.[5] Extending the use of N95 masks included sterilization with UV light systems which initially was thought to allow use for up to 30 days but subsequent studies have disproven this.[6] Sterilization with hydrogen peroxide systems were given emergency use authorization (EUA) but later studies showed degradation of the integrity of masks and the EUA was rescinded a year later in May 2021.

Recommendations for "deep cleaning" of surfaces and rooms challenged the ED in many ways. Rooms required hours of cleaning

by environmental services that were already strained with the challenges of cleaning inpatient rooms. ED rooms were not able to be efficiently utilized due to this slow turnover. This was exacerbated by prolonged holding of patients in the ED while waiting for inpatient rooms to be cleaned.

Intensive care units (ICUs) were overwhelmed and this forced EDs to provide prolonged ICU care for many patients being held in the ED waiting for inpatient rooms. ICUs were greatly expanded and in many institutions ED personnel were utilized to support this expansion. This was also true for non-ICU patients and hospitalist services. Multiple EDs utilized their clinicians to create inpatient teams for patients that were holding to assure they would receive adequate care.

Since we could not ensure a safe environment and provide appropriate PPE for all of our normal ED personnel and visitors, attempts were made to mitigate these issues. Visitation at most hospitals were restricted or eliminated. This created great challenges in communication with the patient's family and friends. Telephones, IPad, internet, and many other technologic solutions were employed to help with these challenges.

Nonessential personnel were removed from the ED or performed their jobs remotely. Students were not allowed to rotate in the ED clinical areas. Secretaries and scribes were often able to perform their jobs remotely. Many consultants were reluctant to come to the ED which resulted in the expansion of the ED physicians' authority and decision-making abilities. Routine and nonemergent consultations were greatly reduced. Consultants used telemedicine and technology to provide input by assessing patients remotely.

Work as a frontline clinician came with significant risk: healthcare workers were three times more likely to be infected with COVID-19 compared to the general public. This high infectivity rate was likely exacerbated by PPE shortages during the initial phases of the pandemic, with many healthcare workers either having inadequate PPE or being forced to reuse their equipment well beyond its intended use. Emergency providers and ICU critical care providers had the highest rate of COVID illness.[7]

COVID-19 and Emergency Department Expansion and Triage

As more COVID hotspots burned throughout the world and the manufacturing and supply chain of PPE, life-saving supplies, cleaning products, ventilators, and availability of hospital beds were stressed to a breaking point, it became essential to implement new triage systems to spread these scarce resources throughout the hospitals in these communities. Though overall ED volume was down across the world, there became an obvious need to find space to treat COVID positive and patients under investigation (PUIs) safely. A separation between PUI and Co-COVID (+) patients and "clean" patients allowed providers to wear continuous PPE and thereby decreased waste, as well as decreased exposure to patients that presented to the ED for non-COVID complaints. Screening questions initially focused on travel to endemic areas, exposure risk, and signs and symptoms of COVID. As the pandemic progressed and community spread became rampant, travel history, and exposure often became irrelevant and difficult to track. Even symptomology became unreliable, as it was determined by the CDC that the virus may take 2 weeks to present symptomatically. Thus, in addition to the prehospital telephone triage systems, to attempt to keep worried well patients at home, EDs revamped physical structures, triage operations, and even staffing models to continue providing care.

One of the most notorious COVID hotspots early in the COVID pandemic was New York City. New York Presbyterian Hospital–Weill Cornell Medical Center (NYP-WCMC), an urban academic level 1 trauma center, reconfigured both physical structures and their triage process to expand the number of adult COVID patients they could see on a daily basis. Like many other hospitals, NYP-WCMC utilized the precipitous drop-off in pediatric ED volume to reconfigure professional emergency management (PEM)-designated areas into adult COVID areas. Pediatric-designated resuscitation bays and negative pressure rooms were turned into treatment and holding areas for adult COVID patients awaiting beds. With this additional space and additional PEM providers available to staff them, a triage nurse would assign adult patients up to their 35th birthday to be evaluated by PEM providers in pediatric areas. Patients who were intoxicated, incarcerated, critically ill, or in respiratory failure were excluded and triaged to the adult ED to be evaluated by an adult ED provider. Pediatric patients continued to also be managed by these PEM providers.[8]

Many hospitals acted in a similar manner to divide their existing EDs into COVID spaces and "clean" areas and implemented triage processes to determine which patients would be seen in each area. The Sheba Medical Center in Tel Hashomer, Israel divided their existing ED into both an advanced Biologic ED and a regular non-COVID ED, and then created a novel triage system to determine which of the EDs a patient would be evaluated in.[9] A professional triage nurse in full PPE would evaluate a patient at the door and directed patients to each ED section based on epidemiology, medical history, and clinical manifestations. The biologic ED was subdivided further based on the presence of symptomology and severity of illness. Many other institutions have devised similar severity of illness triage models (**Fig. 14.1**).[110]

Hospitals without the physical space to subdivide into COVID EDs were forced to create temporary structures to accommodate this. These structures varied from army-style disaster tents to hospital cafeterias, and even covered parking garages. EDs utilized these facilities differently with some using them for triage, or as screening and testing facilities, or as additional treatment areas for less sick patients. In many cases, these areas were an

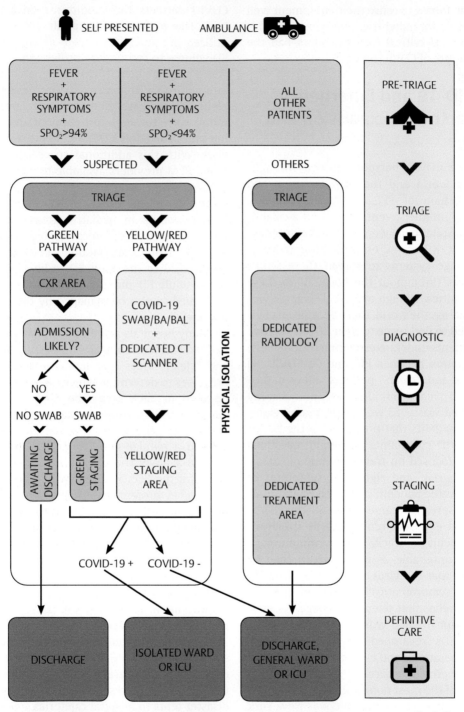

Fig. 14.1 Patient flow within the hospitals from presentation through assessment to final disposition. Disposition based on risk factors and clinical presentation, Green (minor), yellow (moderate) and red (immediate) triage codes based on local emergency department triage protocol. Abbreviations. CXR, chest X-ray; BA bronchial aspirate; BAL, bronchoalveolar lavage; CT, computed tomography; ICU, intensive care unit.[110]

integral part of a new extended triage process such as that developed in Israel. The Robert Wood Johnson Barnabas Hospital system in New Jersey utilized a series of tents at each individual hospital site to perform medical screening and evaluations on potential COVID patients. Patients that were extremely hypoxic, critically ill, or requiring admission were immediately transferred to internal COVID areas in the ED. Most were screened and discharged to quarantine with or without testing. Tents allowed faster movement of patients in and out of one-way screening areas with decreased wait times in a safe, climate-controlled area outside of the waiting rooms. All staff in the tent areas remained in full PPE and would be decontaminated with wipes upon leaving the tent. Wheelchairs and one stretcher were also available inside these tents in case a patient decompensated or needed to be moved into the main ED.

Vanderbilt University Medical Center in Nashville, Tennessee converted a covered parking garage into an additional treatment pod, called an "E-Pod," where COVID patients were sent to have medical work-ups performed.[10] In E-Pod, like a tent, COVID patients were most often tested and discharged to home, allowing decreased exposure to other patients and staff. Both examples required power, oxygen, and integration with the electronic medical record (EMR) to be developed for both charting and visibility of patients in these areas. Vanderbilt also developed an extended triage program prior to assigning patients to the E-Pod in an attempt to capture specific high-risk patients with chest pain, hypoxia, or tachypnea from presenting to that area (**Fig. 14.2**).[10]

Signs, Symptoms, and Testing

The signs and symptoms of COVID-19 varied widely on presentations to the ED from asymptomatic to mild headaches to severe respiratory failure and cardiac collapse. Since COVID-19 symptoms overlap with many other illnesses, it is important to have specific testing that is rapid and reliable for ED patients. This is also true because up to 40% of COVID patients are asymptomatic and all ED patients being admitted need to be screened.[11] Early in the pandemic, the availability of testing was scarce and turnaround time for results was extensive. Therefore, the clinician's judgement was relied upon to consider each patient as low risk or high risk for having the disease based upon their presentations and other diagnostics. Those at high risk were, and still, are termed patients under investigation (PUI) for COVID-19 and were placed on airborne and contact isolation, assumed to have and treated for the disease until definitive testing could be obtained (**Table 14.1**).

Directly testing for COVID was not widely available for several months in the early portions of the pandemic. Results were often delayed for more than a week which did not help in contact tracing or the management of patients in our hospitals. After several months, point of care (POC) polymerase chain reaction (PCR) testing for COVID became the standard but limits of tests and reagents meant that this was not readily available for most EDs for several months.[12]

Currently, there are point of care (POC) COVID PCR tests that can determine if there is an active infection by identifying the presence of COVID RNA in 15 to 20 minutes. These tests provide answers with acceptable sensitivity and specificity to be routinely used to help diagnose and appropriately place or disposition patients in the ED (**Table 14.2**).

Other basic types of COVID tests less commonly ordered in EDs include viral antigen detection which also indicates active infection, and the detection of antibodies to the virus. Antibody tests provide evidence of prior infection with SARS-CoV-2 (**Table 14.2**). The CDC and FDA advise against the use of antibody tests for the diagnosis of acute infection.[12] Antigen tests are less sensitive than RNA detection with a meta-analysis showing the average sensitivity as 56.2%.[13, 14]

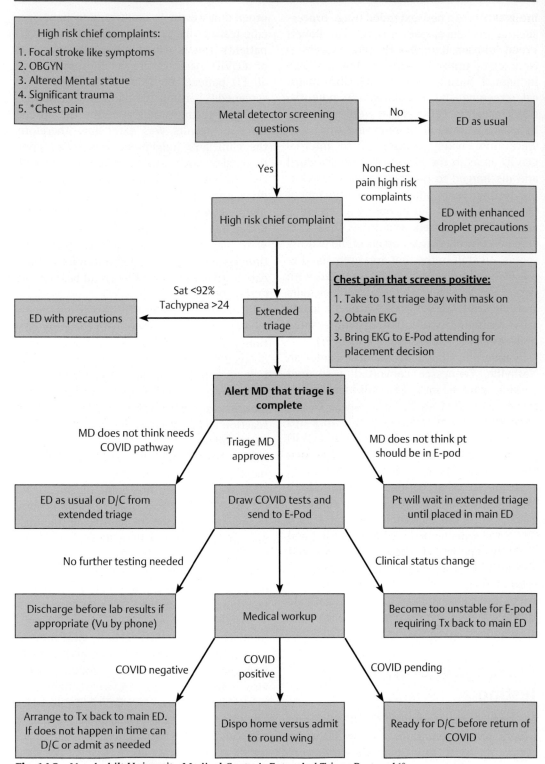

Fig. 14.2 Vanderbilt University Medical Center's Extended Triage Protocol.[10]

Table 14.1 CDC updated February 22, 2021

Mild symptoms and signs of COVID-19	Emergent warning signs for COVID-19
Fever or chills	Troubled breathing
Cough	Persistent pain or pressure in the chest
Shortness of breath or difficulty breathing	New confusion
Fatigue	Inability to wake or stay awake
Muscle or body aches	Pale, ray, or blue-colored skin, lips, or nail beds, depending on skin tone
Headache	
New loss of taste or smell	
Sore throat	
Congestion or runny nose	
Nausea or vomiting	
Diarrhea	

Laboratory diagnostics routinely ordered expanded to include signs of inflammatory response, coagulopathies, and organ failure. Studies routinely ordered included CBC, chemistry panel, liver enzymes, blood urea nitrogen (BUN), creatinine, troponin, d-dimer, fibrinogen, and C-reactive protein (CRP).

The findings associated with COVID infection included high or low white blood cells (WBCs), lymphocytosis, elevated creatinine, elevated liver enzymes, as well as elevated troponin, d-dimer, and CRP. Clinically, these findings increased the likelihood of active infection. Many of these tests also seemed associated with the severity of disease and in many hospitals help to direct treatment utilization of steroids and anticoagulation.

Chest X-ray findings for COVID were typically multifocal and ground-glass opacities and consolidations with peripheral and basal predominance. However, the diagnosis based off chest X-ray (CXR) was limited and found to only have a sensitivity of 69%.[14, 15]

Computed tomography (CT) scanning also displayed bilateral and peripheral ground-glass and consolidative pulmonary opacities. They were more sensitive than CXR but the time, logistics, and risks of transmission to further personnel and patients all limited routine adoption of CT scan to confirm COVID illness. Additionally, early in the disease process (3–5 days) up to 56% of patients had no findings on CT scan.[16] computed tomographic angiography (CATs) were routinely used to identify pulmonary emboli which occurred as a complication of COVID illness.

Ultrasound findings at the bedside showed B lines and added to the sensitivity of clinical assessment and CXR findings. US was frequently used by Emergency Physicians (EPs) to assist in the evaluation of patients. Combining US with clinical assessment showed improved sensitivity and negative predictive value 94.4% vs. 80.4% for PCR testing alone.[17]

Treatment

Early in the pandemic, there were no specific treatments available for patients who were diagnosed with COVID-19 infections. EM physicians provided supportive care and were given the responsibility of identifying which patients were safe to go home, which may decompensate, and which were sick enough to require hospitalization. One of the first methods used to identify which patients needed to be hospitalized was

Table 14.2 Sensitivity and specificity of COVID testing[13–14]

SARS-CoV-2 detection tests								
Test	Type	Intended use	Detects	Average specificity	Average sensitivity	NPV	PPV	Turnaround time
Nucleic acid amplification Tests (NAATs)	RT-PCR	Detect active infection	RNA	99.5% (95% CI, 97–100%)	84.6% (95% CI 69.5–94.4%)	96.8% (CI 93.5–98.4%)	97.1% (CI 82.3–99.6%)	1–3 d
Antigen detection tests	Immunoassay	Detect active infection	Viral antigens	99.5% (95% CI 98.1–99.9%)	56.2%, (95% CI 29.5–79.8%)			15–20 min
Point of care NAATs	RT-PCR	Detect active infection	RNA	98.9% (95% CI 97.3–99.5%)	95.2% (95% CI 86.7–98.3%)	99%	90%	15–20 min
Serology	Antibody assay	Detective active or prior infection	Antibodies	>98%	Days 1–7: 30.1% (95% CI 21.4–40.7)			1–2 d
					Days 8–14: 72.2% (95% CI 63.5–79.5			
					Days 15–21: 91.4% (95% CI 87.0–94.4)			

Abbreviations: CI, confidence interval; NPV, negative predictive value; PPV, positive predictive value; RNA, ribonucleic acid; RT-PCR, reverse transcriptase polymerase chain reaction.

their oxygenation saturation. Patients with oxygen saturation levels of 92 to 94% on room air required supplemental oxygen and therefore were admitted to the hospital.[18] As the number of patients meeting this criteria increased, many hospitals developed coordinated care systems to provide oxygen and pulse oximetry at home to decrease the number of patients requiring admission. These patients were followed closely with Telehealth or paramedicine. Another hurdle early on was that aerosolized viral particles via nebulizers, bilevel positive airway pressure (BIPAP), continuous positive airway pressure (CPAP), and noninvasive ventilation were thought to greatly increase the risk of transmission of COVID-19 to healthcare providers. Therefore, many EDs were not utilizing these means of oxygenation in patients who were high risk or confirmed cases of COVID-19. This led to many more patients being treated with mechanical ventilation and managed similar to acute respiratory distress syndrome (ARDS). As a result, there was an increased need for ICU beds, a shortage of ventilators, and intensivists. This management was also found to be associated with a higher mortality rate.[19]

As the pandemic continued and more and more data was collected and analyzed, it was found that the risks of aerosolization through methods of oxygenation such as nebulizers and BIPAP were exaggerated. As long as the patient care team wore appropriate PPE there was no increased risk of transmission of viral particles. Once the successfulness of PPE was demonstrated, strategies changed to try to avoid intubation in these patients and utilize other methods of oxygenation. Interventions such as supplemental oxygen, high flow oxygen, BIPAP, and proning, in conjunction with supportive care, were shown to have better outcomes.[20] If tolerated, proning patients became routine as patients were better able to maintain oxygenation. In addition to avoiding aggressive, early intubation, aggressive fluid resuscitation was also associated with poorer outcomes. In terms of treating fever and the severe body aches

commonly accompanying COVID-19 infection, nonsteroidal anti-inflammatory drugs (NSAIDs) were implicated early by the French Health Ministry and therefore avoided whenever possible. However, later research found that the use of NSAIDs did not result in worse outcomes. After adjusting for confounders, in-hospital mortality for patients who were taking NSAIDs prior to admission was no different from those who were not (matched OR 0.95, 95% CI 0.84–1.07).[21] NSAID use was also not associated with critical care admission (matched OR 0.96, 95% CI 0.80–1.17) or noninvasive ventilation (matched OR 1.12, 95% CI 0.96–1.32).[21]

Disposition decisions evolved throughout the pandemic. Initially, many patients with suspected COVID were admitted for supportive care. As facilities were overwhelmed, physicians were forced to become more selective when determining who should be admitted for hospitalization. Risk factors for progression to severe disease were used to stratify these patients and included age, obesity, comorbidities, such as hypertension, coronary artery disease, diabetes mellitus, as well as lab abnormalities (**Fig. 14.3**). American College of Emergency Physicians (ACEP) developed an evidence-based tool to help assess the risk of developing severe disease in order to aid in this complex decision-making process.[24] Once intravenous (IV) treatments became available, the decision to admit was also determined based on whether or not the patient met criteria for these IV therapies. These treatments included IV steroids, remdesevir, tocilizumab, as well as anticoagulation. The cornerstone of treatment of hospitalized COVID patients focused on maintaining oxygenation in the face of hyperinflammatory respiratory failure.[23]

In the beginning of the pandemic, there was great uncertainty in regard to treatment modalities. Some of the medical community adhered to evidence-based strategies until studies could provide adequate information to direct treatment. Studies for treatments embraced adaptive study designs to accelerate information and guidance for clinicians.

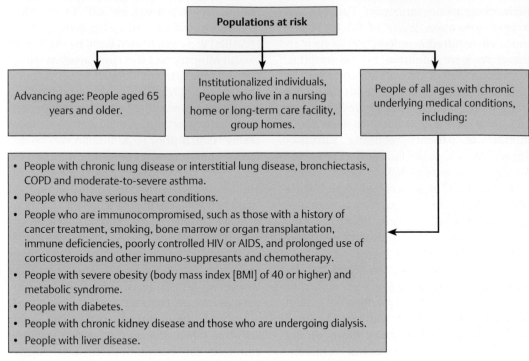

Fig. 14.3 Populations at risk– modified from the American College of Emergency Physicians (ACEP) COVID-19 field guide.[24]

Other providers embraced treatment modalities that were based on the ever-evolving understanding of the pathophysiology of the disease process and extrapolation of possible treatments for critically ill patients. Despite numerous studies investigating potential treatments, there has not been a single agent or combination therapy that has been shown to be a cure for COVID-19. However, there continues to be incremental progress and an evolution of our understanding of the disease and how to treat it effectively. With the continued research and development of treatment strategies, it seems inevitable that we will be using newer, more effective agents and strategies over the next few years.

The first attempts at treating patients with COVID-19 infection used existing antiviral therapies in hopes of reducing the severity of infection and in some cases lower risk of becoming infected. These antivirals included drugs such as hydroxychloroquine, ivermectin, colchicine, remdesivir, and a few others used in cancer treatment.[26] There was never any strong evidence to support utilization of these drugs unless it was in a select patient population or very early in the course of the illness. However, even under those circumstances, it remained controversial and under further investigation. Remdesivir was approved in October 2020 under an EUA by the FDA. Remdesivir became and remains routinely used in hospitalized patients as it has demonstrated benefits in patients requiring supplemental oxygen, especially when used in conjunction with dexamethasone. It has not shown significant benefit in critically ill patients requiring mechanical ventilation or in mild disease.[25]

The hyperinflammatory respiratory failure caused by COVID-19 infection led to the investigation of many anti-inflammatory drugs. The most severely ill COVID-19 patients had progressive hyperinflammatory responses with cytokine storm. Dexamethasone and other steroid treatments were some of the first treatments to demonstrate a significant impact on outcome for patients with moderate-to-severe disease. Dexamethasone was the first treatment that showed significant clinical benefit in improving severity of illness and mortality in hospitalized patients requiring supplemental oxygen.[25] The use of dexamethasone was widely adopted by EPs and is routinely administered in the ED. Dexamethasone is recommended in conjunction with remdesevir in patients requiring supplemental oxygenation. If remdesivir is unavailable at a facility, dexamethasone is recommended to be given alone. If dexamethasone is unavailable, other glucocorticoids may be used. The RECOVERY trial demonstrated that dexamethasone decreased mortality by 35% in patients requiring mechanical ventilation. Incidence of death was significantly lower for patients in the dexamethasone group who received mechanical ventilation versus those receiving usual care (29.3% vs. 41.4%, RR 0.64, 95% CI 0.51–0.81) and those receiving supplemental oxygen without mechanical ventilation (23.3% vs. 26.2%, RR 0.82, 95% CI 0.72–0.94).[25] Mortality decreased for all hospitalized patients who were treated with dexamethasone.[25] The use of these medications in the ED is determined at a local level and coordinated with physicians that will manage these patients once they are hospitalized. Some institutions have developed clinical pathways or guidelines to integrate care and determine which treatments will be initiated in the ED and which will be started by the admitting physicians.

In addition to corticosteroids, the national institutes of health (NIH) does recommend the use of other anti-inflammatory agents under certain conditions. Tocilizumab (Actrema), an IL-6 inhibitor, is an anti-inflammatory agent that is recommended for use in conjunction with dexamethasone in hospitalized patients showing rapid respiratory decompensation.[25] However, it is rarely administered in the

ED and should be coordinated with the admission team when its use is being considered. Tocilizumab should be avoided in immunocompromised patients. Other anti-inflammatory agents such as baricitinib, a JAK-inhibitor, were found to be beneficial when used in conjunction with remdesivir. The NIH recommends remdesivir be used in conjunction with baricitinib, if other corticosteroids cannot be used.[26]

Another approach initiated early on in the treatment of COVID-19 included passive immunization using neutralizing antibodies in convalescent serum. Convalescent plasma received an EUA from the FDA to treat hospitalized patients with COVID-19 infection. However, this approach was limited by availability and the difficulty in determining the appropriate concentration of neutralizing antibodies. Clinicians were rarely able to determine if the plasma available had a high enough titer with adequate antibodies to be effective against the disease. When there were adequate antibodies, effectiveness was demonstrated; however, it appeared to be more effective when it was administered to patients earlier in the disease process. The EUA was narrowed in February to specify the use of only high-titer plasma. The development of monoclonal antibodies allowed for much higher doses of effective antibodies to be used, and therefore convalescent serum is rarely used anymore. The NIH guidelines recommend against the use of convalescent plasma for hospitalized patients without impaired immunity, who are mechanically ventilated.[26] These guidelines also recommend against the use of high-titer plasma for hospitalized, nonvented patients, unless they are enrolled in a clinical trial.[26] The NIH states that there is insufficient data to recommend for or against the treatment with convalescent plasma in patients with impaired immunity. The NIH also states there is insufficient evidence to make recommendations regarding the use of plasma in nonhospitalized patients.[28]

Monoclonal antibodies are administered intravenously and recommended in patients with mild-to-moderate disease with risk factors for progression to severe disease or at high risk for the development of complications from COVID-19. Monoclonal antibodies effectively block the replication cycle of COVID-19 and are most effective early in the course of infection when viral particles are replicating, during the first 10 days of symptoms. The BLAZE-1 trial showed an 87% reduction in hospitalization or death when selected patients at high risk for disease progression were given bamlanivimab.[29] Initially, the FDA gave an EUA for the use of bamlanivimab for outpatients with mild-to-moderate illness who did not require supplemental oxygen or hospitalization. The development of SARS-CoV-2 variants decreased the efficacy of using a single monoclonal antibody and increased the risks of further mutations. On April 16, 2021, the FDA removed the EUA for single antibody use, but continues to recommend the use of bamlanivimab in combination with a second antibody such as etesevimab, which was given an EUA in February 2021.[30] The FDA also recommends the combination of casirivimab and imdevimab (REGEN-COV), which was given an EUA in November 2020. A study showed that REGEN-COV provided 72% protection against symptomatic infections in the first week and 93% protection in the following weeks. In patients who had moderate disease, REGEN-COV was shown to help clear the infection faster. Patients with symptomatic COVID-19 recovered in 1 week as compared to 3 weeks in patients who did not receive this antibody combination.[31] In the study, none of the patients who received REGEN-COV were hospitalized over the course of 29 days. Adverse events were reported in 29% of patients receiving the placebo and in 20% of patients who received the actual treatment.[31] There are other monoclonal antibodies and combinations of antibodies under development. In June 2021, the FDA authorized the monoclonal antibody, sotrovimab, for emergency use. In terms of administering monoclonal antibodies, most EDs try to identify patients that qualify for treatment and

coordinate care with an outpatient infusion center. However, some EDs administer treatments in the ED or in observation areas and then discharge patients home. The patients are identified if they meet certain criteria based on age and comorbidities, do not require supplemental oxygen, and are stable to be discharged home after administration. RWJBarnabas Health instituted one such system in their EDs utilizing specific criteria.

COVID-19 disease has shown to be a hypercoagulable state and the associated thrombosis in hospitalized patients includes deep venous vein thrombosis (DVT), pulmonary embolus (PE), acute myocardial infarction (AMI), stroke, and more unusual blood clots. Many EPs consider initiating anticoagulation for high-risk hospitalized COVID-19 patients. The NIH recommends prophylactic anticoagulation for all hospitalized, non-pregnant, adult patients.[26] Some trials have shown that full anticoagulation does not improve clinical outcomes and mortality in ICU patients and those on mechanical ventilation without evidence of acute thromboembolic disease, leading to bleeding events and inferior outcomes.[32] However, other studies have associated systemic anticoagulation with heparin with better outcomes. There remains controversy over the use of full anticoagulation versus prophylaxis for hospitalized patients.[33] Many EPs administer lovenox in the ED for high-risk patients. Choosing full anticoagulation versus prophylaxis is usually coordinated with the admitting physicians. NIH recommends against anticoagulation in the outpatient setting.[26] The development of platelet-laden clots in the microcirculation of patients infected with COVID-19 has led some clinicians to recommend aspirin therapy in the outpatient setting. One study by Chow showed that patients treated with aspirin were less likely to need mechanical ventilation (35.7% vs. 48.4%) and ICU admission (38.8% vs. 41%) than patients who did not receive aspirin.[34] Furthermore, after multivariable adjustment for nine confounding variables, aspirin was independently associated with a reduced risk of mechanical ventilation,

ICU admission, and in-hospital mortality. The use of aspirin should depend on a clinical decision made by EPs based on a risk versus benefit analysis. The NIH has not made any recommendations regarding this yet.

EPs frequently have to decide what outpatient treatment, if any, they would recommend in patients with mild-to-moderate COVID-19 infection. Given the lack of strong evidence, some physicians are uncomfortable with making such recommendations. When recommendations are made, it should be part of the standard shared decision-making that physicians use when there is significant uncertainty. Most physicians also incorporate the current practices of their medical community and attempt to coordinate care with patients' primary care physicians. Hydroxychloroquine was one of the first drugs that was being considered for treatment early on in the pandemic. The FDA granted an EUA in March 2020, but rescinded it in June following studies that showed no benefit. The RECOVERY trial showed that the use of hydroxychloroquine did not reduce mortality in hospitalized patients.[37] Another clinical trial in the NEJM found that hydroxychloroquine with or without azithromycin did not improve outcomes for hospitalized patients with mild to moderate COVID-19 infection after 15 days.[111] A retrospective cohort study demonstrated improved survival rates among patients treated with hydroxychloroquine, but the study did not account for confounding variables including ICU admission differences and dexamethasone use.[36] Many of the negative clinical trials enrolled hospitalized patients later in the course of disease when an antiviral therapy would not be expected to be effective. There have been prospective trials that have shown benefit if used very early on in the course of the disease and when used at the appropriate dose. Both the WHO and the NIH recommend against the use of hydroxychloroquine, with or without azithromycin. It is rarely prescribed by EPs. Ivermectin is an antiparasitic drug that inhibits SARS-CoV-2 replication cell cultures. However, according

to the NIH, achieving the plasma concentrations necessary to achieve antiviral efficacy against the virus may require doses much higher than the dose approved for use in humans.[26] The NIH changed its recommendation from "against" use in COVID-19 to there is "insufficient data" to recommend for or against use in January 2021. Ivermectin has been used as an antiviral early in the disease process and when there has been COVID-19 exposures in many areas of the world.[26,35] There is emerging evidence of its efficacy when used in this manner. It is occasionally prescribed by EPs.[35]

Vitamins and supplements have been used in the treatment of COVID-19 infection with the rationale of providing supportive and therapeutic levels to support a patient's immune system. This included vitamin C, D, and other agents such as zinc, which were associated with improved outcomes. There are several ongoing clinical trials evaluating the efficacy of vitamin C (ascorbic acid) in COVID-19; however, the NIH currently states that there is insufficient data to recommend for or against its use.[26] The NIH also states that there is insufficient data to recommend for or against the use of vitamin D in COVID-19. In regards to zinc, the NIH states that there is insufficient data to recommend for or against its use, and it also recommends against supplementation above the recommended dietary allowed for prevention of COVID-19, except if in a clinical trial.[26]

Other drugs of various classes have been considered in the outpatient treatment of COVID-19. Protease inhibitors such as lopinavir/ritonavir and other HIV protease inhibitors are not recommended by the NIH as clinical trials have not shown benefit. These drugs were studied in both the RECOVERY trial and the WHO Solidarity Trial and did not demonstrate efficacy in either.[36-38] As of April 2021, the NIH recommends against the use of colchicine in the treatment of COVID-19. However, the COLCORONA trial showed improved outcomes in patients with mild illness who were treated with colchicine.[39] Fluvoxamine, an selective serotonin reuptake inhibitor (SSRI), has gained some attention based on two recent studies that showed lower clinical deterioration and hospitalization in patients who were treated with it.[40] One of the studies was a small, randomized controlled trial of 152 patients, published in the *Journal of the American Medical Association*, which showed that none of the patients taking fluvoxamine reached the primary end point of clinical deterioration compared with 8.3% of those on the placebo, and only one patient required hospitalization as compared to five patients in the placebo group.[40] In a pragmatic British trial, budesonide, an inhaled corticosteroid, showed to shorten the duration of illness in patients at risk for severe disease as well as diminish rates of hospitalization or death in the outpatient setting. The NIH is yet to weigh in on this therapy.[41]

Ultimately, like many aspects of COVID, treatment has been variable and uncertain (**Table 14.3**). As clinical trials continue, treatment plans that are effective will be developed.

Vaccinations

The development of several effective vaccinations and the treatment of enough of the population have greatly reduced the number of COVID patients presenting to EDs. It has also made the ED a much safer environment for healthcare workers and other patients. In the short term, it appears that all of the vaccinations have a high safety profile. We have, however, become familiar with some of the complications of COVID vaccinations including allergic reactions, postvaccination symptoms, and unusual coagulopathies, including central venous occlusion. The healthcare system and government have worked to immunize as many people as possible and a few EDs have even participated in distributing vaccinations, especially aimed at vulnerable populations. Many of our personnel have volunteered at vaccination distribution centers and have contributed to the campaign to vaccinate patients.

COVID-19 and Emergency Medical Services and Prehospital Care

Like many other specialties in the House of Medicine, Emergency Medical Services (EMS) and Prehospital Care was greatly affected by the COVID-19 pandemic. EMS, the frontline of the frontline, saw huge changes and played a vital role in combating the COVID-19 pandemic in all parts of the world. Not only will we discuss the changes that the COVID-19 pandemic had on EMS and Prehospital Care, but we will also discuss how these changes affected the mental health and well-being of the professionals who served in these roles.

In the United States, a large portion of the data on types of emergency responses can be obtained through the National Emergency Medical Services Information System (NEMSIS) database. Several studies queried this database to make conclusions on how the types and volumes of prehospital emergencies changed in response to the declaration of the COVID-19 pandemic.

Since little had been studied on EMS call type and volume during a pandemic prior to 2020, Lerner performed a 3-year retrospective cohort analysis of NEMSIS data to quantify the general trends in EMS incidents as well as the incidence in prehospital death. The National Syndromic Surveillance Program found that from the 11th to 14th week of the year 2020, ED visits across the United States dropped from 2.5 million to 1.2 million, and anecdotally, acuity sharply increased. In places where COVID was rampant at the time (New York, New Jersey, and Puerto Rico), volumes still dropped from 223,489 to 144,249 with an increase in acuity.[43] This information, combined with preliminary media reports that out-of-hospital cardiac arrest rates at the time were soaring, painted a dismal scene. It appeared that the most critically ill were avoiding emergency medical care due to the "stay at home" order or fear of exposure to the virus in an ambulance or in the hospital. Furthermore, this combination could indicate

Table 14.3 Summary of CDC recommendations for treatment of acute COVID-19 infection[26, 42]

Therapy	Outpatient	Inpatient	Critically ill
Monoclonal antibodies	Recommended for patients with mild-to-moderate disease with high risk of clinical progression	Not recommended for hospitalized patients	Not recommended for hospitalized patients
Hydroxychloro-quine +/– Azithromycin	Recommends against	Recommends against	Recommends against
Dexamethasone/ systemic glucocorticoids	Recommends against	Recommended in conjunction with remdesivir in patients requiring supplemental oxygen; other glucocorticoids may be used if dexamethasone is unavailable; may be given alone if remdesivir not available	Recommended in conjunction with remdesivir in patients requiring supplemental oxygen; other glucocorticoids may be used if dexamethasone is unavailable; may be given alone if remdesivir not available
Antibacterial therapy	Recommends against in absence of other indication	Recommends against in absence of other indications	Recommends against in absence of other indications
Remdesivir	Not indicated for outpatient therapy	Recommended in patients requiring supplemental oxygen; recommended to be given in conjunction with dexamethasone in patients requiring increasing amounts of oxygen	Recommended in patients requiring supplemental oxygen; recommended to be given in conjunction with dexamethasone in patients requiring increasing amounts of oxygen
Antithrombotic therapy	Recommends against	Recommended in all nonpregnant adults	Recommended in all nonpregnant adults
tocilizumab	Recommends against	Recommends against	Recommended in conjunction with dexamethasone for rapidly decompensating patients
Baricitinib	Recommends against	Recommended in conjunction with remdesivir when corticosteroids cannot be used and patient's supplemental oxygen requirements are increasing	Recommended in conjunction with remdesivir when corticosteroids cannot be used and patient's supplemental oxygen requirements are increasing

that COVID was much more prevalent in the community, resulting in an increased number of deaths faster than cases could be reported due to lack of testing availability.

PCRs between October 2–8, 2021 and May 18–24, 2021 were studied to simulate responses during flu seasons from 2017 to 2020. Results showed that overall the numbers of EMS activations from 2019 to 2020 increased from the 2017–2018 year.[42] Beginning in the 10th week of 2020 (March 2–8), however, there was a sharp decrease in 9-1-1 EMS call activations compared to previous years. The weekly call volume decreased by approximately 26.1% at this time. In addition, at the 11th week (March 9–15, 2020) scene deaths nearly doubled from 1.49 to 2.77%. Conversely, EMS calls for trauma patients dropped from 18.43 to 15.27% from week 10 to week 13.[42] These findings support the hypothesis that individuals during this time did not access the EMS system as frequently as they have in the past, and that those who did access the EMS system did not do so in a timely manner.[3] Similar trends were noted in other countries such as Portugal and Italy, indicating that the number of prehospital cardiac arrests were increasing, but were not fully explained by COVID-positive tests alone.[42-45]

A similar NEMSIS study focused on the above critical patients with emergent time-sensitive cardiovascular complaints. The database was queried for cardiac rhythms suggestive of STEMI, cardiac calls, out-of-hospital cardiac arrest (ventricular tachycardia/ventricular fibrillation), asystole, and stroke alerts during the time period of January 2020 to April 2020.[46] Overall, the EMS call volume decreased by 21.95% at this time. Cardiac calls, ST-segment elevation myocardial infarction (STEMI) alerts, and stroke alerts decreased significantly during this time at a higher rate than call volume did. Interestingly, EMS responses in the United States for VT/VF initially decreased from January to March but increased from March to April by 3.04% and responses for asystole increased by 27.34%.[46] This trend was not

noted seasonally in years prior. This supports the conclusion from the previous study that during the time of the initial "stay at home" quarantine order, individuals with acute cardiovascular conditions accessed the EMS and healthcare system less frequently, presumably from fear of exposure to COVID-19. This combined with the possibility of a pathophysiological effect on the body as a result of COVID-19 infection resulted in higher incidences of on-scene death and less favorable outcomes.[46]

Prior to the COVID-19 pandemic, the United States suffered from an opioid epidemic. Since 1999, 841,000 people have died from a drug overdose. In 2019, 70,630 drug overdose deaths occurred in the United States. The age-adjusted rate of overdose deaths increased by over 4% during the pandemic.[47-48] Social isolation during quarantine during the COVID-19 pandemic seemed to affect not only the decision to seek timely healthcare, but also the mental health of our nation. In addition to this, those suffering from opioid use disorder may have had increased strain on their well-being due to economic distress and disruption of treatment with many opioid recovery and mental health services unavailable.

Multiple studies of EMS call volume during the COVID-19 pandemic observed an increase in both opioid overdoses and cardiac arrests from overdoses.[44-48] One study was performed to determine the number of EMS responses for opioid overdoses in the 52 days before and after the initial COVID-19 state of emergency declaration in Kentucky between January 14, 2020 and April 26, 2020. There was a 17% increase in the number of EMS opioid overdose runs with transportation to an ED, and a 71% increase in overall runs with refused transportation.[48]

Most concerning was an increase in runs for suspected opioid overdoses, with deaths at the scene increasing by 50% during the postdeclaration period.[49]

The mental health of the first responders facing this increased burden of death and disease while putting their own lives at risk to interface with the public should not be ignored. Researchers out of Turkey conducted a two-part voluntary survey to determine the anxiety level of frontline EMS workers.[49] After completing one part of the survey for sociodemographic information, EMS professionals completed the State Anxiety Inventory, a 20-question validated tool. Results showed that anxiety scores were significantly elevated in females and those with family members at high risk of COVID-19 infection at home. They also found that the majority of those who had family members at risk were not living in their homes and were most worried about transmitting COVID to their family.[49]

As EM physicians became the default experts to the COVID-19 response inside of the hospital, EMS physicians took on the unique role of coordinating community response efforts and integrating public health interests with healthcare and government stakeholders. National agencies across the country helped to support EMS physicians accomplish these goals. The National Association of EMS Physicians (NAEMSP), as well as the ACEPs all created a simple online repository of COVID-19 resources including protocols, data, and how to navigate national CARES Act relief programs that EMS physicians could easily access. NAEMSP hosted multiple virtual Town Hall meetings on ZOOM to bring cutting edge resources and data to EMS physicians in real time. ACEP also helped EMS physicians by creating Amazon Business accounts for members to have access to ordering PPE for field physicians and field staff that were in short supply. Specifically, EMS physicians took on roles of occupational health experts, EMS system resource managers, clinical practice modifications, public health response experts, and advocates.[4, 50, 52]

EMS physicians and EMS medical directors have always played an important role in occupational health ensuring fitness for duty and proper PPE. However, occupational health took on a primary role during the COVID-19 pandemic to keep the frontline of the frontline safe. In Seattle, a retrospective cohort investigation of laboratory positive COVID-19 patients from February 14, 2020 to March 26, 2020 showed that by instituting a program to EMS operations that identified high-risk patients and a PPE program, including masks, eye protection, gown, and gloves (MEGG), decreased documented exposures from 94 to 6%. Furthermore, less than 0.5% of EMS providers experienced a COVID-19 illness within 14 days of treating a COVID-19 positive patient. Of those that tested positive, none were directly linked to a known exposure while in full MEGG.[51] EMS medical directors spent many hours developing safety protocols, including educational programs on hand-washing, decontamination, and preventing occupational exposures. As news outlets and social media continued to sensationalize COVID-19 and as information changed daily, EMS physicians played an important role in deciphering fact from fiction and distilling evolving medical knowledge and guidelines down to concise recommendations that all levels of EMS providers can implement and follow.

EMS resource managers, medical directors, and EMS physicians implemented processes to identify the likelihood of COVID exposure for first responders from the time an emergency call was made to 9-1-1 and PSAP (Public Service Answering Point) centers. This was accomplished in agencies across the country by screening questions to determine whether the patient was a PUI for COVID. This allowed responding crews to make informed decisions on PPE and the type or units of personnel responding. In addition, it was a resource to the community to allow for retrospective case tracking and exposure identification. EMS physicians had to ensure situational awareness during responses via specific dispatch protocols. In some cases, this meant drastically altering response configuration and even adjusting community standards of care when call volume overwhelmed available EMS units. Liaisons with local healthcare institutions such as group homes, nursing facilities, as well as transport destinations, such as ED directors, were crucial to determine COVID hotspots in the community and to ensure that the final destinations had the capability to care for these patients once they arrived at the hospital.[50, 52]

As clinical guidance from the Centers for Disease Control and Prevention (CDC) rapidly changed for EMS and fire services, EMS physicians were tasked with implementing new infection control practices and PPE protocols to protect personnel and patients alike. Some of these policies included drastic changes from standards of care and decontamination between patients. Prior to COVID, standard PPE for a cardiac arrest requiring chest compressions and intubation would include only gloves and perhaps a surgical mask with a splash shield for the provider managing the patient's airway. This evolved into full gown or jumpsuit with an N95/P100 respirator, face shield, or Powered Air Purifying Respirator (PAPR) for aerosolizing procedures such as chest compressions or intubation.[50–52]

In New York state and other areas where cases and acuity overwhelmed EMS demand and availability of PPE for rescuers, clinical practice morphed from standard care to triage Crisis Standards of Care.[53] In April 2020, the AMA released guidance on Crisis Standards of Care which stated that physicians have the responsibility to evaluate the risks of providing care to individual patients versus the need to be available to provide care in the future in public health emergencies. Furthermore, the AMA stated that when CPR is unlikely to provide the intended clinical benefit, and participating in resuscitation significantly increases already higher than usual risk for healthcare professionals, it may be ethically justifiable to withhold Cardio pulmonary resuscitation (CPR) without the patient's consent.[54] Translated to EMS, this meant that when responding to an out-of-hospital cardiac arrest (OHCA), CPR could be withheld or discontinued en route to the hospital by paramedics by Termination of Resuscitation Efforts (TRE). Though many EMS agencies have already been doing this for years, many more EMS agencies began to pronounce cardiac arrest patients in the field in asystole, or when efforts were deemed futile by protocols, or via Online Medical Control (OLMC), where a physician directly provides orders for paramedics to execute in the field.

Other states, such as New Jersey, adjusted both their resources and clinical practice through the use of waivers and executive orders where the standards of care and clinical practice of EMS rests in state law. As the pandemic progressed, PPE and personnel were scarce secondary to illness, exposure, and/or quarantine. This prompted many important waivers to state law to compensate for the shortage in EMS workers and included allowing any licensed emergency medical technician (EMT) or paramedic from other states to practice in the state of New Jersey.[55-56] The configuration of response units was also waivered, from initially mandating 9-1-1 paramedic units to have two paramedics to a one paramedic one EMT model. The state of New Jersey also allowed expired EMTs and paramedics to re-enter the work force to expand the labor pool. A third waiver involved the "Triage to Home" protocol, which allowed paramedics to follow a stepwise path in order to refuse transport to the ED if COVID patients met certain criteria and could safely be treated at home to quarantine and convalesce (**Fig. 14.4**). Though several EMS agencies adopted this protocol, rarely did patients qualify to be triaged to home.[55]

In addition to 9-1-1 EMS units being affected, clinical practices of interfacility transport SCTU (Specialty Care Transport Units) changed as well. Interfacility transports across the country were often delayed due to the decreased availability of specialty care for nonemergent surgical procedures and treatments as well as bed availability due to the high volume of COVID patients admitted to the hospital for oxygen and ventilator support. In many areas of the country, where COVID volume was extremely heavy, many inpatient units, beds, and even cafeterias and parking lots were converted to COVID units

This protocol is applicable for patients presenting with symptoms of suspected influenza-like illness or viral syndrome including fever (measured or subjective), chills, cough, sore throat, body aches, malaise, fatigue, or are asymptomatic/ or seeking testing/guidance.

This protocol DOES NOT APPLY if patient meets criteria for any state or local guidelines for treatment by ALS, (e.g., suspected cardiac chest pain, wheezing due to bronchoconstriction, etc.)

All criteria Met?

YES	NO	
☐	☐	**Criteria #1: Medical History** • Age between 13 and 64 • **NOT** pregnant • **NOT** immunocompromised/suppressed (including cancer with active chemo/radiation therapy, history of organ transplant, HIV, autoimmune or rheumatological disorders, or taking immunosuppresive medications including high dose steroids • **NO** heart disease, chronic lung disease (COPD, pulmonary fibrosis), uncontrolled DM, chronic renal disease (ESRD on HD)
YES	NO	
☐	☐	**Criteria #2: Physical Assessment and Vital Signs** • Heart rate less than or equal to 120 bpm: • Systolic blood pressure greater than or equal to 100 mm Hg • For pediatric patients greater than or equal to 90 mmHg or consult with appropriate medical direction • Oxygen saturation at least or greater than 94% on room air • Respiratory rate between 8–22 breaths per minute • **NO** respiratory difficulty/distress on exam • **NO** drop in pulse oximetry to < 94% on movement/walking (if capable at baseline) • **NO** alteration in mentation or new confusion
YES	NO	
☐	☐	**Criteria #3: Capability for Home Care** • Patient (or caregiver) has capacity, has access to caregiver (s) and/or healthcare, and is agreeable to Home Care • Patient or caregiver has access to food, water, medications, and other basic necessities (shelter, heat/cooling)
Home	Transport	
☐	☐	**Triage to Home Eligible?** • If all three criteria marked YES, then patient is eligible for Triage to Home after medical command contact • If any criteria are marked as NO then follow standard BLS and ALS EMS treatment protocols and Transport

For Triage to Home eligible patients, contact your designated medical direction for confirmation and approval. Provide patient and/or caregiver(s) with Home Care Instructions.

Fig. 14.4 The New Jersey Triage to Home Protocol. Put into place by waivers, this protocol allowed patients who met criteria to be triaged to home to convalesce instead of being transported to the Emergency Department in order to decrease exposure to Emergency Medical Service (EMS) providers and preserve limited resources when New Jersey was a hotspot for COVID-19.[55-56]

and ICUs. Furthermore, due to the decreased volume of patients seeking care for illnesses in the ED for routine time-sensitive emergencies such as strokes, STEMI, and pediatric and adult surgical emergencies such as appendicitis, bowel perforations, and ovarian and testicular torsions, the volume of these potential emergent transfer cases decreased significantly. New protocols were put in place to determine the safety of moving one patient from one facility to another. If specific services were available and the patient was accepted for transfer, patients faced the new requirement of securing COVID testing prior to transport. This not only determined whether an appropriate bed was available at the receiving facility to avoid accidental exposure and infection but also ensured a proper unit could respond with appropriate PPE and decontamination services. In many locations, a shortage of available COVID tests made it extremely difficult if not impossible to secure a timely, emergent transfer. When testing was first available, it could take days and often involved a courier process to specialty state or county run labs at first. As more testing became available and finally, rapid testing became widespread, the logistics of transferring patients became easier.

Across the country and the world, EMS agencies developed new protocols, processes, and functions in the interest of Public Health as COVID spread to their communities through the use of community paramedicine. Community paramedicine is a fairly new and evolving concept that allows paramedics and EMTs to operate in expanded roles by assisting with public health and primary healthcare and preventive services to underserved populations in the community. The goals are to improve access to care and to avoid duplicating existing services.[57]

Outside of China, one of the first and largest major COVID-19 outbreaks occurred in Milan, Italy. The EMS system of the Lombardy region, where Milan is located, was the first to respond to emergency calls. The system not only handled calls for symptomatic patients but also developed protocols to adopt containment measures, and address population concerns. The Lombardy region Public-Safety Answering Point (PSAP), which typically functioned to serve the EMS systems of the area, now took on the new role of becoming COVID information call centers.[58-59] The Metropolitan EMS system of Milan in this area formed a COVID-19 Response Team, made up of ten healthcare professionals and two technicians that were active around the clock. The COVID-19 Response Team developed a procedural algorithm for COVID-19 detection and community needs based on call intake to their PSAP Center (**Fig. 14.5**).[58-59] PSAPs provided counseling to the "worried well" callers who did not meet screening criteria and were very unlikely to have COVID-19. Next, call takers would triage those symptomatic or likely infected callers to determine the appropriate prehospital response. Callers assessed the clinical conditions of those who screened positive. For those with severe respiratory or life-threatening symptoms, an ambulance was dispatched to the caller for transport. If the caller could safely quarantine at home with only mild symptoms, the caller was ordered to quarantine at home and a public health officer visited the caller's domicile for testing. Finally, the COVID-19 Response Team handled issues as they arose regarding patient flow and transport to different facilities and would also facilitate transfers between facilities as hospitals became more crowded. Creating a COVID-19 team in their EMS system allowed Milan to track cases and outcomes of COVID-19 as well as appropriately direct care to prevent overburdening their healthcare system.[58]

The Israeli Ministry of Health and Magen David Adom (MDA), Israel's national EMS system, partnered to develop a similar COVID-19 tele-triage center and utilized community paramedicine in Tel Aviv, Israel to combat the spread of COVID-19 in their community. Three days after the first COVID-19 case in Israel was diagnosed, a special call center was opened to handle all issues related to COVID-19 as a subsidiary of Israel's

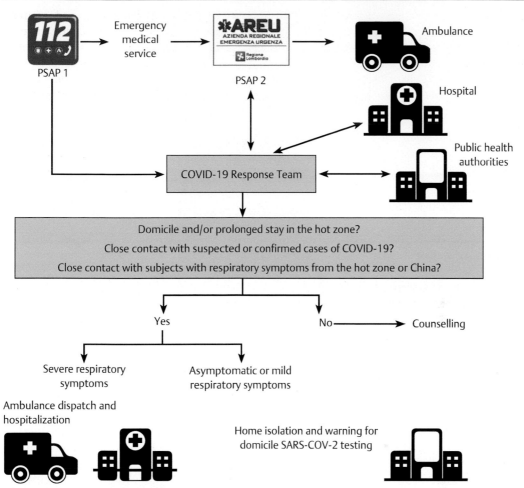

Fig. 14.5 Milan, Italy's prehospital COVID-19 Response Team assisted in providing telephone triage and support expanding the basic emergency call system (112) to track community spread of COVID-19 and guide members of their community through the medical system to either an Emergency Medical Service (EMS) response or to isolate at home and receive home-based COVID-19 testing through the help of Community Paramedicine.[58-59]

National Medical Emergency Dispatch Center (NMEDC). It was staffed 24/7 with approximately 300 MDA call takers and dispatchers trained to conduct triage for suspected COVID-19 cases to prevent the spread of COVID-19 and to identify and test suspected cases. MDA would first rule an active medical emergency requiring an ambulance dispatch. A flowchart algorithm was developed and then utilized for call takers to follow to determine whether a case required quarantine at home and then should be referred to a paramedic to perform home testing (**Fig. 14.6**).

The call center was also synced with a "MyMDA" phone app where "callers" could follow the same algorithm to determine if they required home quarantine or testing. A retrospective analysis was performed on the call center during its inception on February 23, 2020 to March 15, 2020 to describe the nature of calls. During the study period 28,454 (8.5%) of all emergency calls were routed to the COVID-19 call center and 8,390 calls

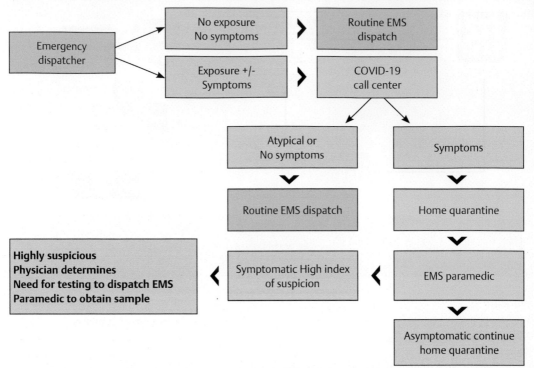

Fig. 14.6 Schematic work flow from emergency call from the emergency hotline (101) to a novel COVID-19 call center. The work flow above determines whether to dispatch a trained paramedic to perform home testing or have patient quarantine at home based on levels of exposure and symptomology.[60,61]

(29.49%), or an average of 381 calls per day, required the dispatch of a dedicated vehicle with a paramedic in PPE to collect samples for testing. This was a significant burden taken off of NMEDC call centers, as well as hospitals and healthcare systems that may have otherwise presented inappropriately for management of asymptomatic or minimally symptomatic disease and exposures.[60,61]

During the COVID-19 pandemic, EMS physicians and EMS providers both played new and important roles and expanded their knowledge and function to serve their communities. As quarantine and stay-at-home orders were implemented around the world, less people felt safe calling 9-1-1 and engaging in the EMS and healthcare system. As a result, many time-sensitive emergencies such as strokes and STEMI went undetected, resulting in an increased number of EMS responses for prehospital cardiac arrests

and death. Furthermore, another side effect along with the mental and economic strains of quarantine life was an increase in opioid overdoses and deaths from opioid overdoses. EMS physicians responded to the COVID-19 pandemic all around the world by focusing on precise occupational health and education of EMS providers, overseeing EMS resource management, developing new and sometimes controversial protocols in response to constantly changing CDC and local EMS guidance, and utilizing community paramedicine to improve the public health of their communities. As the entire House of Medicine was affected by COVID-19, EMS Physicians and EMS providers performed a vital role at the intersection of the healthcare system, public health system, and individuals of the community to manage scarce resources and to decrease the incidence of exposure to COVID-19. In the ED, creativity, flexibility, and strong leadership allowed EDs to develop new triage protocols and create space to conserve resources and prevent exposing staff and healthy patients to COVID. These functions were vital to ensuring the continued care of both COVID and non-COVID patients in hotspots all around the world.

Pediatrics

The global pandemic of COVID-19 has affected and impacted all aspects of children's lives. From school closures, to home quarantines, many of the social support mechanisms for children were disrupted. So many children depend on school for not only educational support, but also meals, and a social structure. School is often also a source of childcare for those with parents who work out of the home. This especially affected foster children, as some saw their family placement be absolved once schools were no longer in session. Older children were faced with nowhere to go when universities closed dormitories. Overall, the stress of home quarantine led to an increased potential for abuse and neglect. This stress has also caused increased rates of mental health concerns, a problem that is compounded by limited in-person visits during the pandemic. Furthermore, those with chronic and complex medical conditions saw their care compromised as they had limited access to their care network, in particular home services.[62,63] These examples are just a small fraction of the way this pandemic has affected the lives of children.

Risk Stratification

Compared to adults, children tend to have a milder course of illness, with reports of 76 to 90% having mild-to-moderate disease and another large percentage (4.4–21%) being asymptomatic.[62–65] Despite this, 1 to 6% of cases were reported to have critical course of illness. Young children (under 1 year of age) appear to be especially at risk, with some reports saying that they can account for >10% of severe cases.[66,67] Other conditions that appear to place children at a higher risk include asthma, underlying lung disease, and other chronic medical problems. While adults have reported increased rates of thrombotic events, studies have shown no increased rate of stroke in children.[68] The mortality data for children in the United States as of June 2021 reported by the American Academy of Pediatrics was 327 while the CDC reported 452 deaths. With more than 4 million pediatric COVID cases, the mortality rate would therefore be calculated to be lower than 0.008%.[69] In addition, studies have reported up to 50% of the reported deaths are patients that died with COVID rather than from COVID.[70]

The Role of Testing

While initially few pediatric cases were reported, this has gradually increased with time. Initially, both the lack of testing materials and the prioritization of adults with underlying medical conditions may have artificially lowered this rate.[71] Almost three quarters of pediatric EDs reported that they were initially limited in their ability to test for COVID-19, with over 65% stating that they only tested if the patient was to be admitted and clinically suspected of having COVID-19.[72] The testing criteria has evolved over time to include all those admitted, requiring medical procedures/sedation, with close contacts, in high-risk living situations (prison, group homes), and clinical suspicion for COVID.

Children have been shown to have similar viral loads in the nasopharynx to adults. Even asymptomatic children can have high viral loads, which can complicate contact tracing and trying to limit disease spread.[73,74] Despite this, in family cases, it is rarely the child who is identified as the source patient. This is encouraging for school openings, as elementary aged children have some of the lowest risk of infections, and are more commonly infected by adults rather than other children.[75]

Who Can Be Discharged?

One of the greatest challenges during this pandemic, especially as it stretched an already taxed medical system, was the question of who could be safely discharged home. To help in this, a severity index was developed to risk-stratify those with COVID-19. Patients were divided into asymptomatic, mild, moderate, severe, and critical categories. They were considered mild if they had symptoms of a fever, upper respiratory illness, abdominal pain, diarrhea, but no abnormal vital signs or physical exam findings. Moderate disease encompassed those with pneumonia, fever, wheezing, but no dyspnea. Severe disease was often appreciated one week into the course of illness with fever, cough, or diarrhea. Patients might have central cyanosis but their oxygen saturation remained above 92%. Critical disease was defined as having respiratory failure, central nervous system, or myocardial involvement, acute renal failure, or shock.

Discharge Instructions

Children with no underlying medical condition that placed them at a higher risk, and were not hypoxic, were considered safe for discharge home. Fortunately, this encompassed the vast majority of patients. They were told to stay at home and self-isolate pending test results. Once they were confirmed to have COVID either clinically or by test result, they are to quarantine at home for 10 days after diagnosis.

When to Admit

The decision of whom to admit can be complicated. While patients with moderate-to-severe disease, cyanosis, hypoxia, or impaired respiratory drive should be admitted, consideration should also be applied to children with mild disease who have risk factors for severe disease.[76] Approximately 5% of pediatric patients may present with hypoxia, but luckily <1% have critical illness.[4] Of those

requiring pediatric intensive care unit (PICU) admission, over 80% had underlying medical conditions that placed them at a higher risk.[77] Those that meet criteria for Multi-inflammatory Syndrome of Children (MIS-C) also warrant admission. MIS-C is a new condition presenting in children under 21 years of age who present with fever, elevated inflammatory markers, categorized as severe, with multiple organ system involvement. They must have no alternative diagnosis and either confirmed or high clinical suspicion for COVID at the time of diagnosis or within the previous 4 weeks.[78] Patients are often found to have an elevated d-dimer, brain natiuretic peptide (BNP), ferritin, and troponin[79] (**Fig. 14.7**).

This is confusing as it can present similarly to Kawasaki disease, but there are a few key differences. Kawasaki often presents in a younger child, while MIS-C patients can present in older children and with intense abdominal pain, cardiac dysfunction, and a decreased platelet count[80–82] (**Table 14.4**).

Treatment Protocols

Fortunately, the majority of children are either asymptomatic or have mild disease. Interestingly, studies have shown that 17% of asymptomatic children had X-ray findings, but current recommendation show no indication for routine radiologic imaging in asymptomatic or children with mild disease. Due to the highly contagious nature of the COVID-19 virus, changes had to be made to not only how care was delivered, but also the type of care provided. EDs developed split-flow models where patients with COVID-like symptoms were placed in specially designated areas to minimize exposure to not only emergency room (ER) staff, but also other patients. Resuscitation teams were scaled back, so that only essential people were in the room. Equipment in these rooms was also analyzed—by limiting what was in the room to the bare essentials (for respiratory and circulatory support) it helped with flow

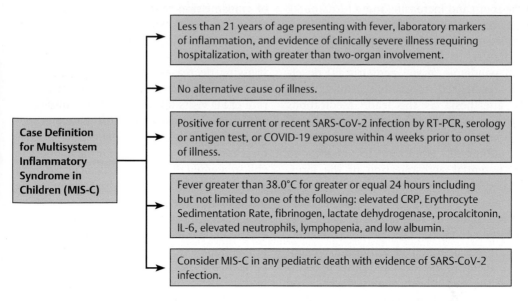

Case Definition for Multisystem Inflammatory Syndrome in Children (MIS-C)

- Less than 21 years of age presenting with fever, laboratory markers of inflammation, and evidence of clinically severe illness requiring hospitalization, with greater than two-organ involvement.

- No alternative cause of illness.

- Positive for current or recent SARS-CoV-2 infection by RT-PCR, serology or antigen test, or COVID-19 exposure within 4 weeks prior to onset of illness.

- Fever greater than 38.0°C for greater or equal 24 hours including but not limited to one of the following: elevated CRP, Erythrocyte Sedimentation Rate, fibrinogen, lactate dehydrogenase, procalcitonin, IL-6, elevated neutrophils, lymphopenia, and low albumin.

- Consider MIS-C in any pediatric death with evidence of SARS-CoV-2 infection.

Fig. 14.7 Case definition for multisystem inflammatory syndrome in children (MIS-C).[80–82]

Table 14.4 MIS-C vs. Kawasaki disease[80–82]

Parameters	MIS-C	Kawasaki Disease
Age	Older children and adolescent, Median age 8–11 years	Infant and young children, 76% of affected children <5 years
Sex ratio	Male/Female 1:1 to 1.2:1	Male/Female 1.5:1 to 1.7: 1
Race and ethnicity	Black and Hispanic descent	Asian descent
Gastrointestinal symptoms	Very Common (53–92%)	Less common (≈20%)
Myocardial dysfunction and shock	Common, 73% elevated BNP, 50% elevated troponin levels, 48% receive vasoactive support	Less common, 5% receive vasoactive support
Organ dysfunction	Multiorgan dysfunction common	Multiorgan dysfunction not common
Inflammatory markers	Highly elevated CRP, ferritin, procalcitonin, and D-dimer, lymphopenia and thrombocytopenia	Elevated CRP, D-dimer and thrombocytosis, usually normal ferritin; thrombocytopenia is rare
Treatment	IVIG, Corticosteroids, IL-1 blocker IL-6 inhibitors	IVIG, Corticosteroids, IL-1 blockers
Outcome	Fatality rate 1.4–1.7%	Fatality rate 0.01 %

MIS-C, muftisystem inflammatory syndrome in children; KD, Kawasaki disease; BNP, B-type natriuretic peptide; CRP, C-reactive protein; IVIG, intravenous immunoglobulin.

in the room and increasing room turnaround. Some departments made special containers wrapped in plastic bags similar to Broslow cart drawers to aid this process.[83] During the initial pandemic, many pediatric ED developed specialized intubation teams, often with anesthesia as the lead.[9] Medications were also adapted to limit exposure to staff and other patients. Most hospitals switched from albuterol nebulizers to inhalers to limit potential aerosolization of the virus. Similarly, epinephrine for severe croup treatment was switched from aerosolized to intramuscular. The role of telemedicine was expanded, which not only permitted continued care but also helped to minimize exposure to medical providers and other patients. Overall, the medical community worked to be able to continue to provide care, but also to try to ensure safety for their staff.

The emergence of MIS-C demonstrated that while most children had mild illness, they could also be critically ill with COVID. Like adults, the majority of care is supportive with respiratory and cardiovascular support. Most patients were treated with IV fluids, aspirin, or IV immunoglobulins, and able to be discharged in under a week. Children that were diagnosed with MIS-C are recommended to follow up with a pediatric cardiologist within 3 weeks.

However, some children required vasopressors (rarely extra corporeal membrane oxygenator (ECMO) for inotropic support. Anticoagulants, including enoxaparin, were recommended due to the concern for thrombosis, and antibiotics should be given only with a significant concern for sepsis. Other treatments included steroids for patients in shock, along with interleukin receptor antagonists.

What We've Learned

While quarantines and lockdowns impacted the spread of normal pediatric illnesses, there was an overall increase in the evaluation of children for febrile and respiratory illnesses. This is supported by increased rates of transmission outside the family in areas where the lockdown was delayed.[84] Pediatric emergency visits during the pandemic decreased significantly, with some reports showing decreases of 70%, and pediatrician visits went down 40% as well.[85] Overall the rate of ED visits for nonemergent causes dramatically decreased.[86] Unfortunately, especially in the height of the pandemic, we saw increased acuity and rates of critical illness in children when they came to the ED.[87] Not only was there a higher odds ratio for admission, but also an increased percentage of negative outcomes, including mental health visits.[88] This may be due to delay in care and delayed presentation, from both parent's inability to perform a thorough physical exam likely limited their effectiveness in identifying some of the critical cases.[85] While telemedicine visits increased, the inability to perform a thorough physical exam likely limited their effectiveness in identifying some of the critical cases. As children overall appear to have a milder course of illness with COVID than adults, this delay in care may have contributed to worse outcomes than COVID itself.

MIS-C was identified in children similar to the "cytokine storm" of severe COVID in adults, causing multiorgan dysfunction and severe inflammation, similar to Kawasaki disease and Toxic Shock syndrome. Unlike adults, this can be delayed, sometimes presenting one month after initial infection. In addition, children are more likely to have a milder course than adults, with less radiographic and laboratory abnormalities. They are less likely to develop ARDS, and fortunately MIS-C appears to be less severe than the adult "cytokine storm.[89]

As their volumes drop, many pediatric departments limited their hours, with decreased staffing. In an effort to help their overwhelmed adult counterparts, they flexed to train staff and providers in treating older patients. Nonclinical personnel received additional training and were tapped as a resource for "surge staffing" when needed.[4] EDs critically reviewed their response to the pandemic, and identified not having proper

PPE, isolation rooms, simulation training, and proper contingency plans as the biggest deficits.

Conclusion

Luckily, children were found to have a lower rate of infection than adults, with less cases of severe and critical illness. This may be in part related to government shutdowns and quarantines that limited their movement outside of the home. Rates of pediatric visits to both primary care and the ED were noted to plummet during the pandemic.[90–94] While this may be related to overall decreased rates of other respiratory viruses and infections during the pandemic, likely fear of contracting the virus in a medical setting contributed to this drop as well.[90–94] Unfortunately, there are some reports of increased acuity and rates of admission for the patients that did present to the ED. This stresses the importance of maintaining medical care during the pandemic, as routine and critical care should not be delayed due to fear.[90–94]

Pregnant Women

The effect of COVID-19 on pregnant women is multifactorial. Many of the normal milestones of pregnancy were either cancelled or altered in a way that few could have imagined. Lockdowns caused baby showers to be cancelled; partners were limited or excluded from routine visits and screening exams. In addition, during the initial pandemic, some institutions did not allow partners to be present during labor. Even now, many hospitals are placing limits on not only who can be in the delivery room, but also how many people are allowed to be present.[95]

Risk Stratification

Pregnant women are at a higher risk from respiratory illnesses and severe pneumonia because of particular physiologic changes that make them more susceptible to hypoxia.[96–101]

As their uterus enlarges, it causes decreased lung volumes. Women are also slightly immunocompromised during pregnancy.[96–101] These factors, in addition to altered hormone levels, can make pregnant women more vulnerable to rapid deterioration, especially with respiratory illnesses, which can put both mother and fetus at an increased risk.[96–101] Of pregnant women with COVID, the vast majority (90%) could be discharged without a need for emergent delivery of the baby. However, of those admitted, early research revealed a 25% case fatality rate. Over three quarters required oxygen, and between 20 and 40% required mechanical ventilation.[96–101] This is significant, as it was found to be over twice the rate of nonpregnant women.[98] They were also found to be at a higher risk for worse complications of COVID during their second and third trimesters.[99] Several factors were identified as an increased risk for severe disease and death, including obesity, diabetes, and age over 40. Laboratory markers of an elevated d-dimer and IL-6 were also associated with an increased risk of severe and critical disease.[98–102] Incidents of severe disease in pregnant women included ARDS, disseminated intravascular coagulation (DIC), and renal failure.[100] Despite all of this, there is no reported increase in either stillbirth or neonatal death rate.[98–102]

The Role of Testing

Due to slight immunocompromised state of pregnancy and the higher complication rate with COVID, it was recommended that all pregnant women be screened before prenatal visits and at the time of delivery. If they were found to be positive, it was recommended that they be isolated from other pregnant patients. In addition, any pregnant woman with COVID-like symptoms should be presumed to be positive until proven otherwise. Likewise, any partner of a patient with confirmed or presumed COVID should be considered to be positive as well.

Who Can Be Discharged?

Pregnant women with mild disease and no high risk factors were found to have a <5% chance of severe disease, so they are safe for discharge. Women with moderate disease and risk factors should be admitted, due to a higher risk of complications (**Fig. 14.8**).

The Modified Early Obstetric Warning Score (MEOWS) was developed in the United Kingdom to improve maternal mortality rates by allowing for easier recognition of women who were critically ill.[102] This used vital signs as an early detector of deterioration, with a specificity of 79% and a sensitivity of 89% for predicting maternal mortality.[102] It is widely used in the United Kingdom and has been shown to decrease mortality, but is not as commonly utilized in the United States. While not yet statistically analyzed for COVID, a modified MEOWS has been used to identify pregnant patients at risk for severe and critical illness[103,104] (**Table 14.5**).

Discharge Instructions

Pregnant women should be counseled to closely follow up with their obstetricians. They are encouraged to maintain their hydration, check for fever at least twice daily, and use a home pulse oximeter to monitor their oxygen level. Prolonged bed rest should be avoided due to the increased risks of thrombotic complications. They should also closely monitor for fetal movement and contractions, and emergently contact their obstetrician for any change as this could indicate fetal compromise. They are advised to follow up with their obstetrician at least every 1 to 2 days. Telehealth has proven to be a valuable asset in this follow-up care, and routine visits and screening ultrasounds should be delayed for at least 2 to 4 weeks after the onset of symptoms to decreased exposure, unless the pregnancy is considered high risk.[105]

When to Admit

Clinicians should consider admitting pregnant patients with mild disease who have more than one comorbidity or those with moderate-to-severe disease.[98] Women who require oxygen, have an elevated respiratory rate, or have signs of clinical respiratory distress should also be admitted. The MEOWS can be used to identify those who need either more emergent obstetric evaluation or admission. Patients with a MEOWS of 0 to 1 are considered normal, and do not require further intervention. A score of 2 to 3 would not require a same-day evaluation; patients should contact their doctor and inform them

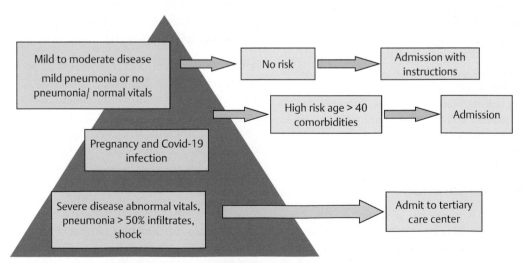

Fig. 14.8 Algorithm for the disposition of pregnant patients with COVID-19. Modified from Boushra et al.[98]

Table 14.5 Modified Early Obstetric Warning Score (MEOWS).[103]

Vital sign	Normal	Light zone	Dark zone
Respiratory rate	11–19/min	20–24/min	≤ 10/min ≥ 25/min
Oxygen saturation, only if respiratory rate triggers	96–100%		≤ 95%
Temperature	36.0–37.4°C	35.1–35.9°C 37.5–37.9°C	≤ 35.0°C ≥ 38.0°C
Maternal heart rate	60–99/min	50–59/min 100–119/min	≤ 49/min ≥ 120/min
Systolic blood pressure	100–139 mm Hg	90–99 mm Hg 140–159 mm Hg	≤ 89 mm Hg ≥ 160 mm Hg
Diastolic blood pressure	50–89 mm Hg	40–49 mm Hg 90–99 mm Hg	≤ 39 mm Hg ≥ 100 mm Hg
AVPU neurological response	A: Alert		V: Voice P: Pain U: Unresponsive

of symptoms. A score of 4 to 5 is considered unstable, and these patients should be evaluated by their physician within 30 minutes. Most concerning is a score above 6, as these patients are critically ill, and should be evaluated within the next 10 minutes.[106] ICU admission should be considered for pregnant women with severe or critical disease, with end-organ failure.[103,105] In addition, those with severe disease should be hospitalized at a facility with both adult and neonatal ICUs.[88,89]

Treatment Protocols

Similar to nonpregnant patients, obstetric clinicians should wear a mask (ideally N-95), and can use COVID testing to help mitigate the mother's risk level.[99–101] Any women who gives birth outside of the hospital should wear a mask, and be presumed to have COVID until proved otherwise. Women with clinical or confirmed COVID should also wear a mask to protect clinical staff. For COVID-positive patients, the neonate can remain with its mother, but she and the child should be kept in isolation. The mother should continue to wear a mask, as there is a risk of cross-infection to the fetus from skin contact

and respiratory droplets.[97–101] In addition, as COVID has been shown to be present in fecal matter, there is at least a theoretical increased risk of transmission to the fetus during vaginal deliveries.[89]

Treatment protocols for pregnant women are relatively similar to nonpregnant women. Dexamethasone has been shown to be safe in pregnancy, and had decreased rates of mortality during the RECOVERY trial. Convalescent plasma trials also included lactating and pregnant women, and showed no adverse effects, but not necessarily any improvement in death rates.[25] While pregnant women were not involved in remdesivir trials for COVID, it was used safely for both the Marberg and Ebola virus.[98] Chloroquine and hydroxychloroquine while given initially during the pandemic are no longer recommended. In addition, they should be used with great caution during pregnancy due to the risk of causing arrhythmias and crossing the maternal–fetal barrier.[98]

Pregnant women with COVID are recommended to receive prophylaxis low-molecular-weight heparin (LMWH) for a minimum of 10 days, and consideration for providing therapeutic doses in critical patient should be given due to the increased risk of thrombosis. While steroids are safe in pregnancy, similar to nonpregnant adults, they should not be given routinely to all patients. They are an adjunct for severe disease, and also to promote lung maturity if preterm delivery is necessary or eminent. Similar to nonpregnant adults, IV fluids should be given cautiously, unless there are signs of cardiovascular compromise. Clinicians should aim to keep pulse oximetry above 95%, and early oxygen use can be of great benefit. For women with severe or critical disease, early intubation is advised if there is concern for worsening respiratory failure.[98-101] However, when intubating pregnant women, clinicians should be aware that they can desaturate more rapidly than nonpregnant patients. In addition, while proning is often recommended with COVID, this can be technically more difficult in pregnancy, especially in advanced stages.[98-101] ECMO is also an option for critical patients with respiratory and cardiovascular failure.

What We've Learned

Similar to pediatrics, there is concern that delay in medical care due to concern for exposure to COVID can lead to worse outcomes. Therefore, it is important that routine prenatal care be stressed and made available even during a pandemic.[107] While it is theoretically possible for a mother to infect the fetus while pregnant, samples taken during cesarean sections have disproven this.[105,107-109] In addition, samples of breast milk have not been shown to contain the virus, so current recommendations do not restrict breast-feeding, though pumping and bottle feeding is encouraged. Studies have shown that infections in early pregnancy were associated with a higher rate of miscarriage.[105,107-109] Cardiomyopathy, along with increased rates of hypertension, has also been described with COVID.[108] Pregnancy was also associated with a 14% rate of severe pneumonia, and if present in the third trimester, correlated with increased neonatal morbidity.[109] Of pregnant women

with COVID, over 50% had a C-section, and almost one-third ended up in the ICU, with ~3% mortality. There was a 14% miscarriage rate and another 14% gave birth <37 weeks gestation. For these neonates, 11.3% required admission to the neonatal ICU, with a 2% perinatal death rate.[89,105,107-109]

Conclusion

Pregnant women are at an increased risk for COVID due to anatomic and physiologic changes during pregnancy that make them more susceptible to respiratory illness. While the number of pregnant women diagnosed with COVID was lower than the general public, they were found to have worse outcomes once admitted. The MEOWS was developed to help risk-stratify pregnant women with COVID, and provides a useful tool on follow-up care and disposition. When diagnosed, they can often be treated similarly to nonpregnant women; however, hydroxychloroquine and routine steroids should not be given. If they require intubation this may be technically more difficult, and they are more likely to quickly desaturate. They do not need to be separated from the neonate after delivery, but should mask to avoid infecting them. Overall, infection in pregnancy was associated with a higher rate of miscarriage, especially if infected early in pregnancy. There was also 14% of preterm delivery, but luckily only a 2% death rate of neonates.

We have learned and will continue to learn a great deal from the worldwide pandemic of what is COVID-19. As vaccination rates are increasing and treatment plans are being developed, there is a small glimmer of hope from our recent statistics that infectious rates are decreasing and severity of illness is dropping in the United States.

References

1. Christine A., Henley SJ, Mattocks, L, et al. Decreases in COVID-19 cases, emergency department visits, hospital admissions, and deaths among older adults following

the introduction of COVID-19 vaccine—United States, September 6, 2020–May 1, 2021. MMWR Morb Mortal Wkly Rep 2021;70:858–864

2. Hartnett KP, Kite-Powell A, DeVies J, et al; National Syndromic Surveillance Program Community of Practice. Impact of the COVID-19 pandemic on emergency department visits—United States, January 1, 2019–May 30, 2020. MMWR Morb Mortal Wkly Rep 2020;69(23):699–704

3. Pandemic Influenza Plan—Update IV. (December 2017) US Department of Health and Human Services Center for Disease Control and Prevention. www.cdc.gov. Accessed July 25, 2021. https://www.cdc.gov

4. Lange SJ, Ritchey MD, Goodman AB, et al. Potential indirect effects of the COVID-19 pandemic on use of emergency departments for acute life-threatening conditions—United States, January–May 2020. MMWR Morb Mortal Wkly Rep 2020;69(25):795–800

5. Degesys NF, Wang RC, Kwan E, Fahimi J, Noble JA, Raven MC. Correlation between N95 extended use and reuse and fit failure in an emergency department. JAMA 2020; 324(1):94–96

6. Lindsley WG, Martin SB Jr, Thewlis RE, et al. Effects of ultraviolet germicidal irradiation (UVGI) on N95 respirator filtration performance and structural integrity. J Occup Environ Hyg 2015;12(8):509–517

7. Nguyen LH, Drew DA, Graham MS, et al; Coronavirus Pandemic Epidemiology Consortium. Risk of COVID-19 among front-line health-care workers and the general community: a prospective cohort study. Lancet Public Health 2020;5(9):e475–e483

8. Fraymovich S, Levine DA, Platt SL. A blueprint for pediatric emergency resource reallocation during the COVID-19 pandemic: an NYC hospital experience. Pediatr Emerg Care 2020;36(9):452–454

9. Levy Y, Frenkel Nir Y, Ironi A, et al. Emergency department triage in the era of COVID-19: the Sheba Medical Center experience. Isr Med Assoc J 2020;22(8):470–475

10. Miller NM, Jones I, Russ S, et al. A model for rapid emergency department expansion for the COVID-19 pandemic. Am J Emerg Med 2020;38(10):2065–2069

11. Al-Sadeq DW, Nasrallah GK. The incidence of the novel coronavirus SARS-CoV-2 among asymptomatic patients: a systematic review. Int J Infect Dis 2020;98:372–380

12. Hanson KE, Caliendo AM, Arias CA, et al. Infectious Diseases Society of America guidelines on the diagnosis of COVID-19: serologic testing. Clin Infect Dis 2020; ciaa1343 10.1093/cid/ciaa1343

13. Dinnes J, Deeks JJ, Berhane S, et al; Cochrane COVID-19 Diagnostic Test Accuracy Group. Rapid, point-of-care antigen and molecular-based tests for diagnosis of SARS-CoV-2 infection. Cochrane Database Syst Rev 2021; 3:CD013705

14. Dinnes J, Deeks JJ, Adriano A, et al; Cochrane COVID-19 Diagnostic Test Accuracy Group. Rapid, point-of-care antigen and molecular-based tests for diagnosis of SARS-CoV-2 infection. Cochrane Database Syst Rev 2020; 8:CD013705

15. Rousan LA, Elobeid E, Karrar M, Khader Y. Chest x-ray findings and temporal lung changes in patients with COVID-19 pneumonia. BMC Pulm Med 2020;20(1):245

16. Bernheim A, Mei X, Huang M, et al. Chest CT findings in Coronavirus disease-19 (COVID-19): Relationship to duration of infection. Radiology 2020;295(3):200463

17. Pivetta E, Goffi A, Tizzani M, et al; Molinette MedUrg Group on Lung Ultrasound. Lung ultrasonography for the diagnosis of SARS-CoV-2 pneumonia in the emergency department. Ann Emerg Med 2021;77(4): 385–394

18. Tobin MJ. Basing respiratory management of COVID-19 on physiological principles. Am J Respir Crit Care Med 2020,201(11): 1319–1320

19. Hernandez-Romieu AC, Adelman MW, Hockstein MA, et al; and the Emory COVID-19 Quality and Clinical Research Collaborative. Timing of intubation and mortality among critically ill Coronavirus disease 2019 patients: a single-center cohort study. Crit Care Med 2020;48(11):e1045–e1053

20. Thompson AE, Ranard BL, Wei Y, Jelic S. Prone positioning in awake, nonintubated patients with COVID-19 hypoxemic respiratory failure. JAMA Intern Med 2020; 180(11):1537–1539

21. Drake TM, Fairfield CJ, Pius R, et al; ISARIC4C Investigators. Non-steroidal anti-inflammatory drug use and outcomes of COVID-19 in the ISARIC Clinical

Characterisation Protocol UK cohort: a matched, prospective cohort study. Lancet Rheumatol 2021;3(7):e498–e506

22. Brown S, Carpenter C, Farmer B, et al. Emergency Department COVID-19 Management Tool. Acep.org. Published May 1, 2021. https://www.acep.org/globalassets/sites/acep/media/covid-19-main/acep-covid-19-ed-management-tool.pdf. Accessed July 25, 2021

23. Steel PAD, Carpenter CR, Fengler B, Cantrill S, Schneider S. Calculated decisions: ACEP ED COVID-19 management tool. Emerg Med Pract 2021;23(Suppl 7):CD1–CD6

24. Populations at Risk. Acep.org. Published July 13, 2021. https://www.acep.org/corona/covid-19-field-guide/risk-stratification/populations-at-risk/. Accessed July 25, 2021

25. Horby P, Lim WS, Emberson JR, et al; RECOVERY Collaborative Group. Dexamethasone in hospitalized patients with Covid-19. N Engl J Med 2021;384(8):693–704

26. Niaid-Rml C. Coronavirus Disease 2019 (COVID-19) Treatment Guidelines. Nih.gov. Published July 8, 2021. https://files.covid19treatmentguidelines.nih.gov/guidelines/covid19treatmentguidelines.pdf. Accessed July 25, 2021

27. Young K. NEJM Journal Watch: Summaries of and commentary on original medical and scientific articles from key medical journals. Jwatch.org. https://www.jwatch.org/fw117729/2021/04/22/nih-updates-covid-19-treatment-guidelines. Accessed July 25, 2021

28. Faust JS. Major NIH-funded trial of convalescent plasma in Covid-19 outpatients stopped early due to futility. Brief19.com. https://brief19.com/2021/02/28/major-nih-funded-trial-of-convalescent-plasma-in-covid-19-outpatients-stopped-early-due-to-futility. Accessed July 25, 2021

29. Gottlieb RL, Nirula A, Chen P, et al. Effect of bamlanivimab as monotherapy or in combination with etesevimab on viral load in patients with mild to moderate COVID-19: a randomized clinical trial. JAMA 2021;325(7):632–644

30. Walker M. FDA shrinks scope of convalescent plasma for COVID-19. MedpageToday. Published February 5, 2021. https://www.medpagetoday.com/infectiousdisease/covid19/91071. Accessed July 25, 2021

31. Terry M. Regeneron's antibody cocktail cuts progression to symptomatic COVID-19. Biospace.com. Published April 12, 2021. https://www.biospace.com/article/regeneron-s-antibody-cocktail-cuts-progression-to-symptomatic-covid-19/. Accessed July 25, 2021

32. The REMAP-CAP, ACTIV-4a, and ATTACC Investigators Therapeutic Anticoagulation with Heparin in Critically Ill Patients with Covid-19. New England Journal of Medicine. 2021;385(9):777-789. doi:10.1056/NEJMoa2103417

33. Paranjpe I, Fuster V, Lala A, et al. Association of treatment dose anticoagulation with in-hospital survival among hospitalized patients with COVID-19. J Am Coll Cardiol 2020;76(1):122–124

34. Chow JH, Khanna AK, Kethireddy S, et al. Aspirin use is associated with decreased mechanical ventilation, intensive care unit admission, and in-hospital mortality in hospitalized patients with Coronavirus disease 2019. Anesth Analg 2021;132(4):930–941

35. Behera P, Patro BK, Singh AK, et al. Role of ivermectin in the prevention of SARS-CoV-2 infection among healthcare workers in India: A matched case-control study. PLOS ONE. 2021;16(2):1-12. doi:10.1371/journal.pone.0247163

36. Arshad S, Kilgore P, Chaudhry ZS, et al; Henry Ford COVID-19 Task Force. Treatment with hydroxychloroquine, azithromycin, and combination in patients hospitalized with COVID-19. Int J Infect Dis 2020;97:396–403

37. RECOVERY Collaborative Group. https://www.recoverytrial.net/results

38. Pan H, Peto R, Henao-Restrepo AM, et al; WHO Solidarity Trial Consortium. Repurposed antiviral drugs for Covid-19: interim WHO solidarity trial results. N Engl J Med 2021;384(6):497–511

39. Tardif J-C, Bouabdallaoui N, L'Allier PL, et al; COLCORONA Investigators. Colchicine for community-treated patients with COVID-19 (COLCORONA): a phase 3, randomised, double-blinded, adaptive, placebo-controlled, multicentre trial. Lancet Respir Med 2021;9(8):924–932

40. Lenze EJ, Mattar C, Zorumski CF, et al. Fluvoxamine vs placebo and clinical deterioration in outpatients with symptomatic

COVID-19: a randomized clinical trial. JAMA 2020;324(22):2292–2300

41. Ramakrishnan S, Nicolau DV Jr, Langford B, et al. Inhaled budesonide in the treatment of early COVID-19 (STOIC): a phase 2, open-label, randomised controlled trial. Lancet Respir Med 2021;9(7):763–772

42. Parasher A. COVID-19: current understanding of its pathophysiology, clinical presentation and treatment. Postgrad Med J 2021;97(1147):312–320

43. CDC. National Syndromic Surveillance Program (NSSP): Emergency Department Visits Percentage of Visits for COVID-19-Like Illness (CLI) or Influenza-like Illness (ILI) September 29, 2019–April 4, 2020. Data as of April 9, 2020. Cdc.gov. Published June 26, 2020. https://www.cdc.gov/corona virus/2019-ncov/covid-data/covidview /04172020/covid-like-illness.html. Accessed July 25, 2021

44. Nogueira PJ, Nobre MA, Nicola PJ, Furtado C, Vaz Carneiro A. Excess mortality estimation during the COVID-19 pandemic: Preliminary data from Portugal. Acta Med Port 2020;33(6):376–383

45. Baldi E, Sechi GM, Mare C, et al; Lombardia CARe Researchers. Out-of-hospital cardiac arrest during the Covid-19 outbreak in Italy. N Engl J Med 2020;383(5):496–498

46. Shekhar AC, Effiong A, Ruskin KJ, Blumen I, Mann NC, Narula J. COVID-19 and the prehospital incidence of acute cardiovascular events (from the nationwide US EMS). Am J Cardiol 2020;134:152–153

47. Mattson CL, Tanz LJ, Quinn K, Kariisa M, Patel P, Davis NL. Trends and geographic patterns in drug and synthetic opioid overdose deaths—United States, 2013–2019. MMWR Morb Mortal Wkly Rep 2021;70(6):202–207

48. Slavova S, Rock P, Bush HM, Quesinberry D, Walsh SL. Signal of increased opioid overdose during COVID-19 from emergency medical services data. Drug Alcohol Depend 2020;214(108176):108176

49. Usul E, Şan I, Bekgöz B. The effect of the COVID-19 pandemic on the anxiety level of emergency medical services professionals. Psychiatr Danub 2020;32(3-4):563–569

50. Cabañas JG, Williams JG, Gallagher JM, Brice JH. COVID-19 pandemic: the role of EMS physicians in a community response effort. Prehosp Emerg Care 2021;25(1):8–15

51. Murphy DL, Barnard LM, Drucker CJ, et al. Occupational exposures and programmatic response to COVID-19 pandemic: an emergency medical services experience. Emerg Med J 2020;37(11):707–713

52. Giwa AL, Desai A, Duca A. Novel 2019 coronavirus SARS-CoV-2 (COVID-19): an updated overview for emergency clinicians. Emerg Med Pract 2020;22(5):1–28

53. American Medical Association. Crisis standards of care: guidance from the AMA Code of Medical Ethics. Ama-assn.org. http:// www.ama-assn.org/delivering-care/ethics/ crisis-standards-care-guidance-ama-code-medical-ethics. Accessed July 25, 2021

54. COVID-19 pandemic patient surge: preparing for crisis care. NYC Health Department. Nyc. gov. https://www1.nyc.gov/assets/doh/ downloads/pdf/imm/covid-19-patient-surge-crisis-care.pdf. Accessed July 25, 2021

55. Patel J. "Department of Health | Emergency Medical Services." The Official Web Site for The State of New Jersey. State.nj.us. http:// www.state.nj.us/health/ems/. Accessed July 25, 2021

56. Department of health for the State of New Jersey. www.nj.gov. https://www.nj.gov/ health/. Accessed July 25, 2021

57. Community Paramedicine Introduction– Rural Health Information Hub. Ruralhealth info.org. http://www.ruralhealthinfo.org/ topics/community-paramedicine. Accessed July 25, 2021

58. Marrazzo F, Spina S, Pepe PE, et al; AREU 118 EMS Network. Rapid reorganization of the Milan metropolitan public safety answering point operations during the initial phase of the COVID-19 outbreak in Italy. J Am Coll Emerg Physicians Open 2020;1(6):1240–1249

59. Spina S, Marrazzo F, Migliari M, Stucchi R, Sforza A, Fumagalli R. The response of Milan's Emergency Medical System to the COVID-19 outbreak in Italy. Lancet 2020;395(10227):e49–e50

60. Al J. Flattening the COVID-19 curve: the unique role of emergency medical services in containing a global pandemic. Isr Med Assoc J. Published online 2020

61. Glatman-Freedman A, Bromberg M, Ram A, et al. A COVID-19 call center for healthcare providers: dealing with rapidly evolving

health policy guidelines. Isr J Health Policy Res 2020;9(1):73

62. Wong CA, Ming D, Maslow G, Gifford EJ. Mitigating the impacts of the COVID-19 pandemic response on at-risk children. Pediatrics 2020;146(1):e20200973

63. Wang C, Zhao P. Critical concerns about 2019 novel coronavirus infection in pediatric population. Mayo Clin Proc 2020;95(6):1295–1296

64. Parri N, Lenge M, Buonsenso D; Coronavirus Infection in Pediatric Emergency Departments (CONFIDENCE) Research Group. Children with Covid-19 in pediatric emergency departments in Italy. N Engl J Med 2020;383(2):187–190

65. Hartford EA, Keilman A, Yoshida H, et al. Pediatric emergency department responses to COVID-19: transitioning from surge preparation to regional support. Disaster Med Public Health Prep 2021;15(1):e22–e28

66. Yonker LM, Shen K, Kinane TB. Lessons unfolding from pediatric cases of COVID-19 disease caused by SARS-CoV-2 infection. Pediatr Pulmonol 2020;55(5):1085–1086

67. Dong Y, Mo X, Hu Y, et al. Epidemiology of COVID-19 among children in China. Pediatrics 2020;145(6):e20200702

68. Pavlakis S, McAbee G, Roach ES. Fear and understanding in the time of COVID-19. Pediatr Neurol 2020;111:37–38

69. Children and COVID-19. State-level data report. Aap.org. https://services.aap.org/en/pages/2019-novel-coronavirus-covid-19-infections/children-and-covid-19-state-level-data-report/. Accessed July 25, 2021

70. Kushner LE, Schroeder AR, Kim J, Mathew R. "For COVID" or "with COVID": classification of SARS-CoV-2 hospitalizations in children. Hosp Pediatr 2021;11(8):e151–e156

71. CDC. Information for pediatric healthcare providers. Cdc.gov. Published July 14, 2021. https://www.cdc.gov/coronavirus/2019-ncov/hcp/pediatric-hcp.html. Accessed July 25, 2021

72. Matera L, Nenna R, Rizzo V, et al. SARS-CoV-2 pandemic impact on pediatric emergency rooms: a multicenter study. Int J Environ Res Public Health 2020;17(23):8753

73. Panahi L, Amiri M, Pouy S. Clinical characteristics of COVID-19 infection in newborn and pediatrics: a systemic review. Arch Acad Emerg Med. 2020;8(1):e50.

74. Tan RMR, Ong GY-K, Chong S-L, Ganapathy S, Tyebally A, Lee KP. Dynamic adaptation to COVID-19 in a Singapore paediatric emergency department. Emerg Med J 2020;37(5):252–254

75. Lee B, Raszka WV Jr. COVID-19 transmission and children: the child is not to blame. Pediatrics 2020;146(2):e2020004879

76. Naseri A, Hosseini M-S. Do not neglect the children: considerations for COVID-19 pandemic. Indian Pediatr 2020;57(6):583–584

77. Jamjoom RS. Coronavirus Disease 2019 (COVID-19) in pediatric emergency. Presentation and disposition. Saudi Med J 2021;42(1):105–109

78. Shulman ST. Pediatric Coronavirus disease-2019-associated multisystem inflammatory syndrome. J Pediatric Infect Dis Soc 2020;9(3):285–286

79. Walker DM, Tolentino VR. COVID-19: the effects on the practice of pediatric emergency medicine. Pediatr Emerg Med Pract 2020;17(Suppl 6-3):1–15

80. Multisystem Inflammatory Syndrome in Children (MIS-C) Associated with Coronavirus Disease. 2019 (COVID-19). Cdc.gov. Published May 15, 2020. https://emergency.cdc.gov/han/2020/han00432.asp. Accessed July 25, 2021

81. Whittaker E, Bamford A, Kenny J, et al; PIMS-TS Study Group and EUCLIDS and PERFORM Consortia. Clinical characteristics of 58 children with a pediatric inflammatory multisystem syndrome temporally associated with SARS-CoV-2. JAMA 2020;324(3):259–269

82. Lee M-S, Liu Y-C, Tsai C-C, Hsu J-H, Wu J-R. Similarities and Differences Between COVID-19-Related Multisystem Inflammatory Syndrome in Children and Kawasaki Disease. Frontiers in Pediatrics. 2021;9:573. doi:10.3389/fped.2021.640118

83. Diaz MCG, Dawson K. Use of simulation to develop a COVID-19 resuscitation process in a pediatric emergency department. Am J Infect Control 2020;48(10):1244–1247

84. Dopfer C, Wetzke M, Zychlinsky Scharff A, et al. COVID-19 related reduction in pediatric

emergency healthcare utilization—a concerning trend. BMC Pediatr 2020;20(1):427

85. Ciacchini B, Tonioli F, Marciano C, et al. Reluctance to seek pediatric care during the COVID-19 pandemic and the risks of delayed diagnosis. Ital J Pediatr 2020;46(1):87

86. Valitutti F, Zenzeri L, Mauro A, et al. Effect of population lockdown on pediatric emergency room demands in the era of COVID-19. Front Pediatr 2020;8:521

87. Angoulvant F, Ouldali N, Yang DD, et al. Coronavirus disease 2019 pandemic: impact caused by school closure and national lockdown on pediatric visits and admissions for viral and nonviral infections—a time series analysis. Clin Infect Dis 2021;72(2):319–322

88. Sheridan DC, Cloutier R, Johnson K, Marshall R. Where have all the emergency paediatric mental health patients gone during COVID-19? Acta Paediatr 2021;110(2):598–599

89. Zimmermann P, Curtis N. COVID-19 in children, pregnancy and neonates: a review of epidemiologic and clinical features. Pediatr Infect Dis J 2020;39(6):469–477

90. Lubrano R, Villani A, Berrettini S, et al. Point of view of the Italians pediatric scientific societies about the pediatric care during the COVID-19 lockdown: what has changed and future prospects for restarting. Ital J Pediatr 2020;46(1):142

91. Vierucci F, Bacci C, Mucaria C, et al. How COVID-19 pandemic changed children and adolescents use of the Emergency Department: the experience of a secondary care pediatric unit in Central Italy. SN Compr Clin Med 2020;2(11):1–11

92. Kruizinga MD, Peeters D, van Veen M, et al. The impact of lockdown on pediatric ED visits and hospital admissions during the COVID19 pandemic: a multicenter analysis and review of the literature. Eur J Pediatr 2021;180(7):2271–2279

93. Luijten MAJ, van Muilekom MM, Teela L, et al. The impact of lockdown during the COVID-19 pandemic on mental and social health of children and adolescents. Qual Life Res 2021; 10.1007/s11136-021-02861-x

94. Sokoloff WC, Krief WI, Giusto KA, et al. Pediatric emergency department utilization during the COVID-19 pandemic in New York City. Am J Emerg Med 2021;45:100–104

95. HEALTH ADVISORY. Multisystem Inflammatory Syndrome in Children (MIS-C) Associated with Coronavirus Disease 2019 (COVID-19). Sanantonio.gov. Published May 14, 2020. https://covid19.sanantonio.gov/files/assets/public/files/healthcare-providers/novel-coronavirus-health-advisory-mis-c.pd. Accessed July 25, 2021

96. Chen H, Guo J, Wang C, et al. Clinical characteristics and intrauterine vertical transmission potential of COVID-19 infection in nine pregnant women: a retrospective review of medical records. Lancet 2020; 395(10226):809–815

97. Diriba K, Awulachew E, Getu E. The effect of coronavirus infection (SARS-CoV-2, MERS-CoV, and SARS-CoV) during pregnancy and the possibility of vertical maternal-fetal transmission: a systematic review and meta-analysis. Eur J Med Res 2020;25(1):39

98. Boushra MN, Koyfman A, Long B. COVID-19 in pregnancy and the puerperium: a review for emergency physicians. Am J Emerg Med 2021;40:193–198

99. Donders F, Lonnée-Hoffmann R, Tsiakalos A, et al; Isidog Covid-Guideline Workgroup. ISIDOG recommendations concerning COVID-19 and pregnancy. Diagnostics (Basel) 2020;10(4):243

100. Rasmussn SA. Coronavirus disease 2019 (COVID-19) and pregnancy: what obstetricians need to know. Am J OB&G Published online 2020.

101. Rezaie S. Impact of anatomic and physiologic changes of pregnancy on respiratory failure and intubation. Rebel EM. Published online December 6, 2020

102. Cook CA. Implementing the modified early obstetric warning score (MEOWS) to detect early signs of clinical deterioration and decrease maternal mortality. J Obstet Gynecol Neonatal Nurs 2014;43:S22

103. Poon LC, Yang H, Dumont S, et al. ISUOG Interim Guidance on coronavirus disease 2019 (COVID-19) during pregnancy and puerperium: information for healthcare professionals: an update. Ultrasound Obstet Gynecol 2020;55(6):848–862

104. Irish maternity early warning system (IMEWS) version 2. Gov.ie. Published February 1, 2019. https://www.gov.ie/en/

collection/517f60-irish-maternity-early-warning-system-imews-version-2/. Accessed July 25, 2021

105. López M, Gonce A, Meler E, et al; on behalf of the COVID Collaborative Group. Coronavirus disease 2019 in pregnancy: a clinical management protocol and considerations for practice. Fetal Diagn Ther 2020;47(7):519–528

106. Lemoine S, Chabernaud J-L, Travers S, Prunet B. COVID-19 in pediatric patients: what the prehospital teams need to know. Arch Pediatr 2020;27(5):281–282

107. Salsi G, Seidenari A, Diglio J, Bellussi F, Pilu G, Bellussi F. Obstetrics and gynecology emergency services during the coronavirus disease 2019 pandemic. Am J Obstet Gynecol MFM 2020;2(4):100214

108. Schwartz DA. The effects of pregnancy on women with COVID-19: maternal and infant outcomes. Clin Infect Dis 2020; 71(16):2042–2044

109. Juan J, Gil MM, Rong Z, Zhang Y, Yang H, Poon LC. Effect of coronavirus disease 2019 (COVID-19) on maternal, perinatal and neonatal outcome: systematic review. Ultrasound Obstet Gynecol 2020;56(1): 15–27

110. Carenzo L, Costantini E, Greco M, et al. Hospital surge capacity in a tertiary emergency referral centre during the COVID-19 outbreak in Italy. Anaesthesia. 2020;75(7): 928-934. doi:https://doi.org/10.1111/anae. 15072

111. Cavalcanti AB, Zampieri FG, Rosa RG, et al. Hydroxychloroquine with or without azithromycin in mild-to-moderate covid-19. N Engl J Med. 2020;383(21):2041-2052

15   COVID-19 and Anesthesia

Wouter Jonker and Anish Patil

Introduction

The role of anesthetists in acute healthcare has expanded significantly in recent decades from being originally a theater-based specialty to one now that has a broader basis in provision of services in out-of-theater locations, e.g., radiology and cardiac suites as well as critical care and transport medicine.[1] In spite of this, the role of the anesthetist is often underrecognized by the public and patients.[2-4] Even within the healthcare environment, the differentiation between the anesthetist and the intensivist is often unclear.[1,5] This is possibly due to the fact that these multiskilled clinicians often work in both these roles. The COVID-19 pandemic demanded many changes in the provision of anesthesia as well as where anesthetist provided their services. In this chapter we hope to provide the reader with insight into the changes on how anesthesia provision has changed during the pandemic as well as illustrate the role of anesthetists in these changes.

Anesthetists were required for safe and effective perioperative care of patients with COVID-19 as well as played significant roles in informing staff (AoA),[6,7] patients (CPOC),[8] and policy makers[9] on how to deal with this pandemic and its aftermath.

Anesthesia nontechnical skills or similar systems[10-12] are now part of many training programs, providing anesthetists with tools and experience in situational awareness, decision-making, teamworking, and leadership abilities to manage the tasks and challenges of the COVID-19 pandemic.

Preoperative

Anesthetists as part of the perioperative team played a central role in the development of local and national escalation plans including updating those as new information became available (AoA).[13-15] Pathways for emergency, urgent, and elective surgery for COVID-19 positive (or unknown) and COVID-19 negative patients, frequently referred to as "red and green" pathways, were established. In many hospitals, states, and even countries nonurgent surgery was postponed during surges.[15] This was to prevent unnecessary exposure of patients to the high-infection-risk hospital environment and to allow redeployment of staff for escalation capacity.

Information and advice provided to patients and relatives during preoperative assessments, often via phone or telemedicine, played a large role in ensuring adherence to preop isolation recommendations, screening guidelines, as well as relieve patient concerns around attending for surgery during the pandemic. This guidance was needed to protect patients from COVID-19-associated mortality, prevent transmission between patients, as well as protect staff so that services could be maintained.

An early meta-analysis revealed that perioperative mortality, complication, and rate of ICU admission among surgical COVD-19 patients were very high. Up to one death for every five COVID-19 patients undergoing surgical procedures were found.[16]

Strategies to decrease perioperative mortality included provision of lower risk anesthetic techniques and alternative management other than surgical procedures.

Intraoperative Management

The anesthetic management of patients during the COVID-19 outbreak had to adapt. Changes to routine practice included among others training in infection control and donning and doffing personal protective equipment (PPE), minimizing staff numbers in theaters, and performing procedures whenever possible under regional techniques.[17] Specific changes to airway management with the aim to decrease aerosol generation were recommended.

Initial recommendations were based on experiences gained during SARS and MERS outbreaks which found an odds ratio between HCWs exposed to and not exposed to AGPs for risk of transmission of SARS-CoV-1 during tracheal intubation, tracheostomy, and suction before intubation to be as high as 6.6, 4.2, and 3.5, respectively.[18]

Throughout the COVID-19 pandemic the message has been that HCWs who perform airway management (e.g., bag-mask ventilation, tracheal intubation and extubation) are at risk of viral infection from contact, droplets, and aerosol spread.[19]

This as well as the limited supply of PPE resulted in clinicians designing and using physical barriers, e.g., plastic sheets or hard plastic intubation boxes in an attempt to provide an additional barrier to infection. Their use was short lived after Emergency Use Authorization by the U.S. FDA was withdrawn after concerns that these devices actually made intubation more difficult and that operating room airflow may be interrupted by these barriers.[20-22]

Subsequent recommendations are continuously updated as more evidence becomes available.[23,24] Recent publications of contrasting evidence about aerosol generation during airway management are generating considerable debate.[25,26] The occupational risk has been found to be lower for those working in UK anesthesia and ICUs[6] compared to other front-line workers.[27-29] There are many potential reasons for this and will require further research. Reasons put forward include availability of PPE, experience in infection control precautions, well-ventilated environments of theaters and ICUs, frequency of droplet and aerosol generation events on wards occurring more commonly than AGPs in operating theaters and ICUs, and the secretions of viable virus that rapidly decreases after 9 to 10 days.[30]

Initial data around protection afforded by vaccinations are encouraging but hasn't yet resulted in significant change in recommendations.

Current advice continues to be based on social distancing, diligent compliance with hand washing, strict adherence to PPE protocols, as well as the use of intubation and extubation checklists.

Specific recommendations for airway management remain in place: insertion of HEPA filters at Y-piece of breathing circuits, optimal preoxygenation before induction with tight seal facemask to reduce risk of hypoxemia, positive pressure bag-mask ventilation after induction to be avoided unless the patient experiences oxygen desaturation, and minimize disconnections of breathing circuits. For optimal intubating conditions, patients should be anesthetized with full muscle relaxation. Videolaryngoscopy is recommended as first-line strategy for airway management. If emergent invasive airway access is indicated, a surgical technique such as scalpel-bougie-tube, rather than an aerosolizing generating procedure, such as transtracheal jet ventilation, is recommended.[23] Additional recommendations for pediatric patients include administering anxiolytic medications, intravenous anesthetic inductions, tracheal intubation using cuffed tracheal tubes, use of inline suction catheters, and modifying workflow to recover patients from anesthesia in the operating room.[19]

Capacity Increase

The exponential growth in COVID-19 positive cases across the world followed by the associated increase in hospital attendances and admissions affected all levels of healthcare from community services, general practices, chronic and acute hospital services, i.e., emergency departments, diagnostic, medical, and surgical services all the way to intensive care.

Breaches of critical care capacity required surge capacity to be developed in nearly all acute hospitals. Areas that could function as escalation critical care areas were identified. Many factors had to be considered including medical gas supplies, ventilation, equipment, and staffing. Expanding the footprint of intensive care outside traditional intensive care units required staff to step up where the services of intensive care clinicians were overstretched. Operating theaters provided additional isolation capacity especially if negative pressure capability were present. These as well as postanesthesia care units were adjusted, equipped, and staffed to function as escalation intensive care spaces. Staff, from within the perioperative environment, were suitably skilled to be redeployed to temporarily increase capacity. The skills of anesthetists in airway management, mechanical ventilation, and sedation as well as training that most likely included rotations through critical care were natural fit to meet the demand. Resources and training for managing COVID-19 patients in these areas were forthcoming.[31,32] Guidance on how anesthesia machines could be utilized as back-up ventilators, when there were insufficient ICU ventilators, was provided by manufacturers (ASAHQ-pdf).

Oxygen supply and demand capability should be carefully considered. The maximum flow per minute via central pipeline supply during periods of peak demand as well as volume capacity of liquid O_2 supply or oxygen cylinder manifolds determined the number of patients that could be cared for as well as what type of ventilation could be offered. This was especially relevant where high-flow nasal cannula oxygen was provided to multiple patients.

Staff Wellbeing

It should not come as a surprise that wellbeing in healthcare workers in general would be adversely affected by a disease outbreak. After all, the health service is the primary frontline in a pandemic. This is coupled with the fact that mental wellbeing in healthcare staff was already being examined prior to the pandemic,[33] and if anything, COVID-19 has served to exacerbate the situation. As anesthetists have played a special role in the pandemic, this has led to specific wellbeing considerations for them.

There has been an increase in workload for a significant chunk of our healthcare staff population. In a 2020 survey, nearly two-thirds of anesthetists were suffering with increased mental burden as a direct result of the additional work pressures of COVID-19 (RCOA).

Another key factor contributing to staff wellbeing is their perceived ability to care for their patients. Almost half of anesthetists felt unconfident in the system's ability to provide a safe surgical service to patients during a future COVID-19 surge (RCOA). If a doctor feels as though they cannot perform their job effectively and safely, it will have obvious implications for their wellbeing.

Finally, the pandemic has especially led to a unique set of challenging circumstances for anesthetists in training, particularly in their novice stage. This specific cohort of new anesthetists relies very heavily on elective surgical lists to gain vital experience and develop their clinical and procedural skills. Cancellation of these lists due to COVID-19 has led to a generation of new trainees who are behind their predecessors in terms of completed case numbers. It has also led to a change in the way clinical skills are being taught to them. For example, it is well known that bag-mask ventilation is one of the most fundamental, lifesaving skills for any anesthetist to have. However, in some countries, videolaryngoscopy has been introduced as a default airway management technique in order to avoid the aerosol-generating nature of bagging. In some centers, dedicated senior airway management teams[34] have been set up to limit staff exposure, many of which exclude junior trainees.[35] This lack of training in airway management skills, especially for a new anesthetist, is destined to cause significant anxiety and stress.

Of course, there are other challenges too, such as the effect on the personal lives of staff. Anesthetists have, however, recognized and responded to these implications for staff wellbeing. The Royal College of Anaesthetists has made key recommendations to the NHS that they remediate staff for flexible time worked, ensure sufficient staff numbers, and place resources in staff wellbeing.[36] The Association of Anaesthetists released multiple wellbeing resources, including a guide and a successful webinar series to help doctors deal with their mental health. It also provides a guide to recognizing the signs and symptoms of a doctor in difficulty. These include traits such as low work rate, frequent absences, and avoidance of the doctor by other colleagues.[37] While steps that directly address mental wellbeing are being taken, other indirect interventions have an impact that may not be immediately obvious. Logistical considerations are a good example of a stressor that may have a bigger impact on our wellbeing than we realize. Many UK health trusts and local authorities have attempted to mitigate this by providing free parking, food, and new rest facilities.[38]

Conclusion

The COVID-19 pandemic presented the biggest challenge to modern healthcare that we are likely to experience in our lifetimes. The extreme pressure and at times collapse of healthcare systems challenged all healthcare workers. These challenges included among many changes to current practice, redeployment to different areas and learning and implementation of new practices. The information tsunami that came upon clinicians in itself added to the burden. Thankfully as the pandemic continues, more and more evidence-based guidelines and recommendation are released. In the provision of anesthesia it seems that the more we learn, the more it seems that best practice aligns with business as usual, just with better PPE.[39]

References

1. Bennett S, Grawe E, Jones C, Josephs SA, Mechlin M, Hurford WE. Role of the anesthesiologist-intensivist outside the ICU: opportunity to add value for the hospital or an unnecessary distraction? Curr Opin Anaesthesiol 2018;31(2):165–171

2. Smith A, Mannion S. Irish patients knowledge and perception of anaesthesia. Ir Med J 2013;106(2):50–52

3. Gottschalk A, Seelen S, Tivey S, Gottschalk A, Rich G. What do patients know about anesthesiologists? Results of a comparative survey in an U.S., Australian, and German university hospital. J Clin Anesth 2013; 25(2):85–91

4. Acosta-Martínez J, Guerrero- Domínguez R, López-Herrera-Rodríguez D, Sánchez-Carrillo F. Rol del anestesiólogo: punto de vista de los pacientes. Rev Colomb Anestesiol 2016;44:121–127

5. Parry-Jones AJ. Anaesthetist or intensivist? Editorial Hosp Med 2004;65(9):516–517, discussion 517–518

6. Anaesthetic management of patients during a COVID-19 outbreak. https://anaesthetists. org/Home/Resources-publications/ Anaesthetic-Management-of-Patients-During-a-COVID-19-Outbreak. Accessed 22 August 2021

7. Kearsley R, Duffy CC. The COVID-19 information pandemic: how have we managed the surge? Anaesthesia 2020;75(8):993–996

8. https://cpoc.org.uk/patients/guidance-adult-patients-having-operation-during-covid-19. Updated Nov 2020. CPOC-FAQ for patients having an operation during the pandemic. pdf. Accessed 22 August 2021

9. Ferguson K, Johnston PW. Law, litigation and learning: a legacy from COVID-19. Anaesthesia 2020;75(11):1428–1431

10. Flin R, Patey R, Glavin R, Maran N. Anaesthetists' non-technical skills. Br J Anaesth 2010;105(1):38–44
11. Doumouras AG, Hamidi M, Lung K, et al. Non-technical skills of surgeons and anaesthetists in simulated operating theatre crises. Br J Surg 2017;104(8):1028–1036
12. Gaba DM. Crisis resource management and teamwork training in anaesthesia. Br J Anaesth 2010;105(1):3–6
13. Guidance on the management of scheduled services for adults in acute hospitals during the COVID-19 era. https://www.hse.ie/eng/about/who/acute-hospitals-division/covid-19-guidance/guidance-on-the-management-of-scheduled-services-for-adults-in-acute-hospitals-during-the-covid-19-era.pdf. Accessed 22 August 2021
14. COVID-19 and Elective Surgery. https://www.asahq.org/in-the-spotlight/coronavirus-covid-19-information/elective-surgery. Accessed 22 August 2021
15. Moletta L, Pierobon ES, Capovilla G, et al. International guidelines and recommendations for surgery during Covid-19 pandemic: A Systematic Review. Int J Surg 2020;79:180–188
16. Abate SM, Mantefardo B, Basu B. Postoperative mortality among surgical patients with COVID-19: a systematic review and meta-analysis. Patient Saf Surg 2020;14:37
17. Uppal V, Sondekoppam RV, Landau R, El-Boghdadly K, Narouze S, Kalagara HKP. Neuraxial anaesthesia and peripheral nerve blocks during the COVID-19 pandemic: a literature review and practice recommendations. Anaesthesia 2020;75(10):1350–1363
18. Tran K, Cimon K, Severn M, Pessoa-Silva CL, Conly J. Aerosol generating procedures and risk of transmission of acute respiratory infections to healthcare workers: a systematic review. PLoS One 2012;7(4):e35797
19. Matava CT, Kovatsis PG, Lee JK, et al; PeDI-Collaborative. Pediatric airway management in COVID-19 patients: consensus guidelines from the Society for Pediatric Anesthesia's Pediatric Difficult Intubation Collaborative and the Canadian Pediatric Anesthesia Society. Anesth Analg 2020;131(1):61–73
20. Baker PA, von Ungern-Sternberg BS, Engelhardt T. Desperate times breed desperate measures: About valiance or foolhardiness. Paediatr Anaesth 2020;30(6):634–635
21. Brown H, Preston D, Bhoja R. Thinking outside the box: a low-cost and pragmatic alternative to aerosol boxes for endotracheal intubation of COVID-19 patients. Anesthesiology 2020;133(3):683–684
22. Tighe NTG, McClain CD, Vlassakova BG, et al. Aerosol barriers in pediatric anesthesiology: Clinical data supports FDA caution. Paediatr Anaesth 2021;31(4):461–464
23. Foley Lorraine J, Urdaneta Felipe, Berkow Lauren, et al. Difficult airway management in adult COVID-19 patients: statement by the Society of Airway Management. Anesthesia Analgesia March 12, 2021. 10.1213/ANE.0000000000005554
24. Matava CT, Peyton J, von Ungern-Sternberg BS. Pediatric airway management in times of COVID-19: a review of the evidence and controversies. Curr Anesthesiol Rep 2021;1–5
25. Brown J, Gregson FKA, Shrimpton A, et al. A quantitative evaluation of aerosol generation during tracheal intubation and extubation. Anaesthesia 2021;76(2):174–181
26. Dhillon RS, Rowin WA, Humphries RS, et al; Clinical Aerosolisation Study Group. Aerosolisation during tracheal intubation and extubation in an operating theatre setting. Anaesthesia 2021;76(2):182–188
27. Houlihan CF, Vora N, Byrne T, et al; Crick COVID-19 Consortium; SAFER Investigators. Pandemic peak SARS-CoV-2 infection and seroconversion rates in London frontline health-care workers. Lancet 2020;396(10246):e6–e7
28. Shields A, Faustini SE, Perez-Toledo M, et al. SARS-CoV-2 seroprevalence and asymptomatic viral carriage in healthcare workers: a cross-sectional study. Thorax 2020;75(12):1089–1094
29. Eyre DW, Lumley SF, O'Donnell D, et al; Oxford University Hospitals Staff Testing Group. Differential occupational risks to healthcare workers from SARS-CoV-2 observed during a prospective observational study. eLife 2020;9:e60675

30. Cook TM, Lennane S. Occupational COVID-19 risk for anaesthesia and intensive care staff: low-risk specialties in a high-risk setting. Anaesthesia 2021;76(3):295–300

31. European Society of Intensive Care Medicine Academy courses. https://academy.esicm.org/blocks/activityvisualization/layout_browseall.php?tab=covidESICM. Accessed 22 August 2021

32. Information, guidance and resources supporting the understanding and management of Coronavirus (COVID-19). https://icmanaesthesiacovid-19.org/. Accessed 22 August 2021

33. Looseley A, Wainwright E, Cook TM, et al; SWeAT Study Investigator Group. Stress, burnout, depression and work satisfaction among UK anaesthetic trainees; a quantitative analysis of the satisfaction and wellbeing in anaesthetic training study. Anaesthesia 2019;74(10):1231–1239

34. https://www.asahq.org/in-the-spotlight/coronavirus-covid-19-information/ purposing-anesthesia-machines-for-ventilators. Accessed 22 August 2021

35. Sneyd JR, Mathoulin SE, O'Sullivan EP, et al. Impact of the COVID-19 pandemic on anaesthesia trainees and their training. Br J Anaesth 2020;125(4):450–455

36. Royal College of Anaesthetists. View from the frontline of anaesthesia during COVID-19. https://rcoa.ac.uk/policy-communications/policy-public-affairs/views-frontline-anaesthesia-during-covid-19-pandemic-July2020

37. Association of Anaesthetists. 2021. https://anaesthetists.org/Portals/0/PDFs/Guidelines%20PDFs/Vital_Signs_in_Anaesthesia2020.pdf?ver=2020-03-31-170128-410. Accessed 28 August 2021

38. WFSAQH. 2021. https://resources.wfsahq.org/wp-content/uploads/atow-444-00.pdf. Accessed 28 August 2021

39. McGrath BA, Brenner MJ, Warrillow SJ. Tracheostomy for COVID-19: business as usual? Br J Anaesth 2020;125(6):867–871

16 Tracheostomy during COVID-19 Pandemic

Christopher de Souza, Anish Patil, Srinivasan Ramnathan, Kiran Shekade, Prakash Jiandani, and Rosemarie de Souza

Introduction

Tracheostomy has been termed an aerosol-generating procedure in the COVID-19 pandemic. As a result, concerns have been raised regarding the safe performance of the tracheostomy procedure. During the first wave in 2020 there were some who advised deferral of the procedure as it was thought that healthcare workers (HCWs) would be exposed and therefore likely contract the viral infection.

It was thought that by deferring the procedure the patient would enter a phase where they would be less infectious and so posed less of a danger of transmitting the disease to those who were performing the procedure.

Some authors have pointed out that such a course is from the perspective of the healthcare deliverers. How did such decisions affect patients on whom such procedures were to be conducted? These were pertinent and relevant questions which needed to be answered.

Tracheostomy in COVID-19 Situations

Many papers have been published subsequently on this subject. Many questions have been answered. However, the long-term effects of these decisions will only be answered by careful follow-up of these survivors.

Early experience with SARS CoV-2 in China showed that HCWs involved in the tracheostomy were at greater risk (odds ratio 4.15) than those who were not. This led to guidelines of donning a fully enhanced personnel protection equipment (PPE). This included protective surgical gown, N95 mask, helmet/face shields, gloves, and boots.

At the beginning of the COVID-19 pandemic, many treating physicians were pessimistic about tracheostomy and whether it would make any difference to the course of the disease. Since they held such an opinion, they considered deferral as a means to protect the HCWs who would have been involved in the performance of the tracheostomy.

They also postulated that during proning the tracheostomy tube would likely get obstructed.

Early on in the pandemic in 2020, there was a rush to place patients on invasive mechanical ventilation (IMV).[1] After some time it became apparent that most patients could be managed with noninvasive oxygenation (NIMV) and the numbers requiring IMV dropped significantly. This in turn caused the numbers requiring tracheostomy to also decline.

Some reports point out that the N95 mask was the single most important piece of equipment needed when performing the tracheostomy procedure.

The N95 masks are effective at filtering 99.5% of particles >0.75 µm which travels within aerosol particles which are >1 µm. Thus, the N95 mask protects the wearer from the virus.

Timing

Some studies have clearly shown that early tracheostomy leads to better outcomes in terms of survivorship as well as being weaned off IMV.[2]

Conversely delayed tracheostomy was associated with poorer survivorship and lengthy and costly delay in weaning off the ventilator.

Early tracheostomy was labeled as tracheostomy performed by day 10 of being placed on IMV.

Timing of tracheostomy was significantly associated with the length of stay,[3] 40 days for early tracheostomy (tracheostomy done within 10 d of being intubated) versus 49 days for late/deferred tracheostomy. Competing risks models with death as the competing risk demonstrated that late tracheostomy was 16% less likely to get off the ventilator.

Early tracheostomy led to early discharge from hospital.[4] Enhanced PPEs for the operating surgeons was associated with low rates of transmission.[5] More importantly, early tracheostomy was associated with diminished risk of mortality.

Many papers[4,6,7] concede that there was no way of accurately determining the degree of infectivity and the viral load. It was thought that since the viral loads were thought to reduce substantially by day 8 the viral particles would also be less. So performance of tracheostomy by day 10 was thought not to pose as serious a possibility of disease transmission as previously thought.[8,9]

However, all personnel involved in the procedure had as a protocol to don a full and complete PPE when performing the tracheostomy.[10,11]

Recent data clearly demonstrates[12] that even after upper respiratory tract samples become negative, lower respiratory tract samples can remain positive for up to 39 days. The correlation between positive results by quantitative PCR viral testing and infectivity is currently being investigated.[13]

Data also demonstrates that patients with the severe form of the disease present with a much higher viral load that decreases slowly.[14]

Another factor that should influence decision making is the presence of comorbidities. Patients with no comorbidities do much better than those with health issues.

Many studies during the second wave demonstrated that very few HCWs developed COVID-19 following tracheostomy.[15–17]

These studies focused on the following factors[18]: (1) safety for surgeons, (2) appropriate timing of tracheostomy, (3) whether outcomes were pulmonary or influenced by tracheostomy.

Recommended protocols for tracheostomy in COVID-19 are currently as follows[19–21]:

- Mandatory adequate PPE for the operating personnel. This includes surgical gown, N95 mask, helmet/face shield, cap, gloves, boots/appropriate footwear.
- Site to perform tracheostomy. Most prefer to do it by the bedside. Transporting the patient to the operating room runs the risk of dissemination of disease.
- Precautions to reduce time of exposure to infected elements. Speed of performing tracheostomy is important especially once the trachea is about to be opened. At that time the ventilator should be placed on standby. Once the trachea is opened the tracheostomy tube should be inserted correctly and swiftly.
- To avoid complications, delays, and confusion, a well-established tracheostomy team should be in place. Everyone in the team is expected to know their role and exactly how the procedure is to be conducted safely and efficiently.
- Open versus percutaneous tracheostomy is the team's choice and they should be familiar with both.

Our Protocol

Tracheostomy to be conducted at the earliest when it is apparent that the patient will need prolonged IMV support.

We have an established team of personnel familiar with open and percutaneous tracheostomies. At times we conducted hybrid procedures especially if the patient was obese. An incision was taken in the neck until the trachea was distinctly visible and palpable.

All tracheostomies were conducted by the bedside.

We favored the percutaneous tracheostomy procedure because it was quick and safe and as time went by expertise and confidence of performing it reliably, safely, and efficiently grew exponentially.

We record our technique which is simple, efficient, and safe and is replicable. These guidelines can help even inexperienced surgeons to conduct a safe tracheostomy procedure using the percutaneous technique.

Procedure with Percutaneous Tracheostomy

- Patient positioning: The neck should be extended and the area prepped.

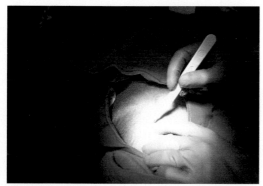

Fig. 16.1 Short horizontal incision over the trachea.

- The endotracheal tube withdrawn to 17 cm to the incisor teeth.
- Infiltration with anesthetic solution.
- Two-centimeter horizontal incision (**Fig. 16.1**).
- Injection into the trachea: The syringe should have its plunger withdrawn and if bubbles are seen it indicates that the trachea has been entered correctly (**Fig. 16.2**). If not, then the endotracheal tube needs to be withdrawn further. Resistance can be felt when injecting into the trachea if the endotracheal tube has not been withdrawn enough. Withdrawing the ET will help the surgeon to correctly identify the trachea.
- The syringe is withdrawn and the J-wire is inserted through the needle. The surgeon will be able to feel the wire enter the trachea.
- The red spigot is threaded through the J-wire and the trachea is dilated (**Figs. 16.3–16.5**).
- This is removed and the bigger white dilator is then threaded into the J-wire and the tracheal opening is further dilated (**Figs. 16.6** and **16.7**).
- The ventilator is now put on standby in order to prevent aerosolization of infected fluids.
- Insertion of the dilator is a very important step as it provides an opening large enough for the tracheostomy

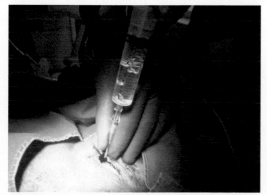

Fig. 16.2 Injecting into the trachea. Aspiration reveals bubbles, confirming that the trachea is entered.

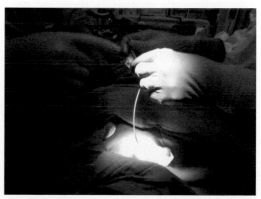

Fig. 16.3 The first red dilator is threaded through the guidewire.

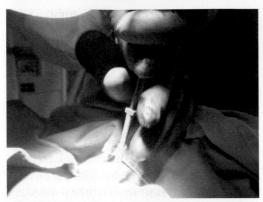

Fig. 16.4 The short red dilator is then pushed through the skin and into the trachea.

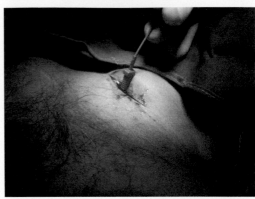

Fig. 16.5 The red dilator is inserted into the trachea.

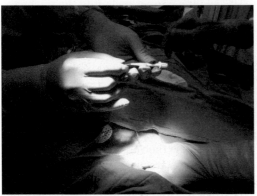

Fig. 16.6 The white and larger dilator is then threaded into the J-wire.

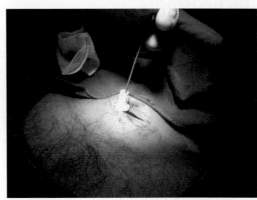

Fig. 16.7 The white dilator is then used to dilate the tracheal opening further.

tube to be inserted. The tracheal dilator should be inserted into the trachea and then the jaws of the forceps opened sufficiently enough to allow the passage of the tracheostomy tube to allow it to enter smoothly. The trachea is dilated horizontally as well as vertically (**Figs. 16.8** and **16.9**).

• The dilator is removed, and the tracheostomy is then threaded and inserted. Once inserted into the trachea, the cuff is inflated and secured (**Fig. 16.10**).

The ventilator is then connected to the tracheostomy tube. All parameters are checked to determine correct placement of the tracheostomy tube.

Conclusion

Early tracheostomy is in general advocated for patients requiring IMV support. The benefits of early intervention include shortened hospital stay, early weaning off ventilator support, and decreased mortality. Once HCWs have donned recommended PPEs, risk of transmission of disease is negligible. Percutaneous tracheostomy in our hands has been quick, devoid of complications when performing tracheostomies on COVID-19-affected patients. An established and experienced team should perform tracheostomy on COVID-19 patients. They should be familiar with both open and percutaneous methods. They should be able to perform this by the bedside.

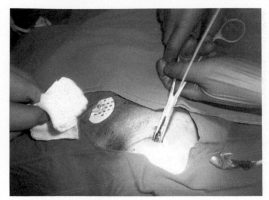

Fig. 16.8 The metal dilator is also threaded through the guidewire and then dilates the tracheal opening first in the vertical plane.

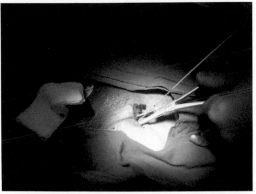

Fig. 16.9 The metal dilator then dilates the opening in the horizontal plane. This should be enlarged enough to allow passage of the tracheostomy tube.

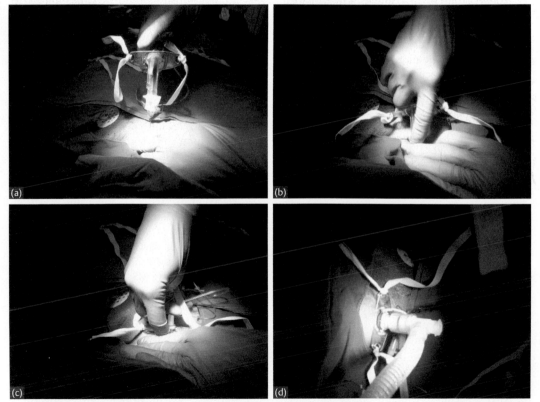

Fig. 16.10 (**a**) Tracheostomy tube after being threaded through the guidewire is inserted into the trachea. At all times the guidewire should be in place. (**b**) The tracheostomy tube is advanced through the J-wire. (**c**) The tracheostomy tube is now correctly placed in the trachea and can be safely connected to the ventilator. (**d**) The tracheostomy tube is inserted into the trachea.

References

1. Chao TN, Harbison SP, Braslow BM, et al. Outcomes after tracheostomy in Covid 19 patients. Ann Surg 2020;272(3):e181–e186
2. Cazzador D, Franchella S, Navalesi P. Tracheostomy during Covid 19 pandemic: in search of lost timing. JAMA Otolaryngol Head Neck Surg 2020;146(10):981–982
3. Bertroche JT, Pipkorn P, Zolkind P, Buchman CA, Zevallos JP. Negative pressure aerosol cover for COVID 19 tracheostomy. JAMA Otolaryngol Head Neck Surg 2020;146(7): 672–674
4. Rosano A, Martinelli E, Fusina F, et al. Early percutaneous tracheostomy in corona virus disease 2019. Associated with removal of tracheostomy tube at ICU discharge. A cohort study of 121 patients. Crit Care Med 2020;4752: 10.1097/cm
5. Tay JK, Khoo ML, Loh WS. Surgical considerations for tracheostomy during the covid 19 pandemic. Lessons learned from the severe acute respiratory syndrome outbreak. Published online March 31. JAMA Otolaryngol Head Neck Surg 2020; 10.1001/jamaoto2020.0764
6. Goldman RA, Swendseid B, Cognetti DM. Comment on tracheotomy in Covid-19 patients: why delay or avoid? Letters to the editor. Otolaryngol Head Neck Surg 2021;164(3):684
7. McGrath BA, Brenner MJ, Warrillow SJ, et al. Tracheostomy in the COVID-19 era: global and multidisciplinary guidance. Lancet Respir Med 2020;8(7):717–725
8. Kwak PE, Connors JR, Benedict PA, et al. Early outcomes from early tracheostomy for patients with covid 19. JAMA Otolaryngol Head Neck Surg 2021;147(3):239–244
9. Kwak PE, Persky MJ, Angel L, Rafeq S, Amin MR. Tracheostomy in Covid 19 patients Why delay or avoid? Letters to the editor. Otolaryngol Head Neck Surg 2021;164(3): 683–684
10. Givi B, Schiff BA, Chinn SB, et al. Safety recommendations for evaluation and surgery of the head and neck during the covid 19 pandemic. JAMA Otolaryngol Head Neck Surg 2020;146(6):579–584
11. Heyd CP, Desiato VM, Nguyen SA, et al. Tracheostomy protocols during COVID-19 pandemic. Head Neck 2020;42(6): 1297–1302
12. Avilés-Jurado FX, Prieto-Alhambra D, González-Sánchez N, et al. Timing, complications and safety of tracheotomy in critically ill patients with Covid 19. JAMA Otolaryngol Head Neck Surg 2020;147(1):1–8
13. Aviles Jurado FX, Vilaseca I. Letter to the editor. JAMA Otolaryngol Head Neck Surg April 22, 2021
14. Andriolo BN, Andriolo RB, Saconato H, Atallah AN, Valente O. Early versus late tracheostomy for critically ill patients. Cochrane Database Syst Rev 2015;1:CD007271
15. Chiesa-Estomba CM, Lechien JR, Calvo-Henríquez C, et al. Systematic review of international guidelines for tracheostomy in COVID-19 patients. Oral Oncol 2020;108: 104844
16. Staibano P, Levin M, McHugh T, Gupta M, Sommer DD. Association of tracheostomy with outcomes in patients with Covid-19 and SARS-COV2 transmission among health care professional. A systematic review and meta-analysis. JAMA Otolaryngol Head Neck Surg 2021;147(7):646–655
17. Thal AG, Schiff BA, Ahmed Y, et al. Tracheotomy in a high volume center during the COVID 19 pandemic. Evaluating the surgeon's risk. Otolaryngol Head Neck Surg 2021;164(3):522–527
18. Fiacchini G, Tricò D, Ribechini A, et al. Evaluation of the incidence and potential mechanisms of tracheal complications in patients with covid 19. JAMA Otolaryngol Head Neck Surg 2021;147(1):70–76
19. Schultz MJ, Teng MS, Brenner MJ. Timing of tracheostomy for patients with Covid 19 in the ICU-setting precedent in unprecedented times. JAMA Otolaryngol Head Neck Surg 2020;146(10):887–888
20. Sommer DD, Engels PT, Weitzel EK, et al. Recommendations from the CSO-HNS taskforce on performance of tracheotomy during the COVID-19 pandemic. J Otolaryngol Head Neck Surg 2020;49(1):23
21. Takhar A, Walker A, Tricklebank S, et al. Recommendation of a practical guideline for safe tracheostomy during the COVID-19 pandemic. Eur Arch Otorhinolaryngol 2020; 277(8):2173–2184

17

Donning and Doffing

Christine Filippone

Introduction

Emerging pathogens are defined as novel etiological agents that have been recently introduced in a population. The most recent emerging novel virus is severe acute respiratory syndrome coronavirus 2 (SARS-CoV-2), which created a global pandemic. SARS-CoV, a member of the coronaviridae family, is known to infect the horseshoe bat and in late 2019 "jumped" into a human host, thus resulting in a worldwide pandemic. In the human population, SARS-CoV causes a respiratory disease called coronavirus disease 19 (COVID-19). Many viruses such as influenza viruses and SARS-CoV-2 affect the respiratory tract and are transmitted by respiratory secretions and aerosol droplets. Effective measures for preventing their transmission in a health care setting include following infection prevention practices. As the virus evolves in the human population, so do the science, diagnostic measures, treatment modalities, and prevention strategies. Sharing updated information regarding the various aspects of the disease caused by the virus will help in managing and controlling emerging viral infections better.[1]

A multipronged approach is needed in decreasing the transmission of SARS-CoV-2. This approach in health care includes universal masking, social distancing, use of personal protective equipment (PPE), implementation of isolation precautions, hand hygiene, and vaccination. This chapter will focus on the use of infection prevention measures to prevent the transmission of infection to patients and health care providers (HCPs).

General Infection and Prevention Practice in an Acute Care Setting

General Infection Prevention Practices

During the SARS-CoV-2 pandemic, the Centers for Disease Control and Prevention (CDC) recommends using standard precautions with additional infection prevention and control practices in the care of all patients. Some additional practices include screening for symptoms of COVID-19, adherence to source control of respiratory secretions with the use of a mask, and social distancing.[2]

Entrances of the Facility

Screening of persons entering the facility is an important strategy to identify persons with symptomatic disease. Persons need to be screened by asking for the presence of the following symptoms: fever, cough, shortness of breath (SOB), chills, myalgia, headache, congestion, ageusia, and anosmia. Persons entering the building should also be queried if they have been diagnosed with COVID-19 in the past 10 days or exposed to a person with COVID-19 in the past 14 days. Persons who respond positively to any of the questions should be restricted from access and referred for evaluation.[3]

Hospital-Wide Locations

Signage regarding infection prevention practices, facemask, screening, hand hygiene, respiratory etiquette, and social distancing should be visible at the entrances and strategic locations such as waiting areas, dining areas, and elevators. Limiting the number of persons in elevators should be posted to ensure proper distancing.

Social distancing is a vital strategy to prevent the transmission of COVID-19. Reminders such as markings should be placed on the floor, indicating 6-feet separation when anticipated waiting for lines. Seating in waiting areas should spatially be separated by 6 feet. Strategically place alcohol-based hand sanitizers (ABHRs) with 60 to 95% alcohol throughout the building. In attempts to decrease transmission of COVID-19, visitors and unnecessary personnel should be restricted or limited during high prevalence of transmission.[3]

General Guidelines for the Use of Masks

Studies reveal that asymptomatic patients can transmit the infection to others due to the presence of high viral loads in the upper respiratory tract.[4–6] Therefore, masks are essential in the strategy for the source control of respiratory secretions from persons who are speaking, sneezing, or coughing. Well-fitting facemasks are required to be worn by all persons older than 2 years within the health care facility and by all HCPs.

To limit the potential for contamination, the HCP should consider wearing the same mask and eye protection throughout their work shift. If the HCP needs to remove the mask or eye protection, perform hand hygiene before and after removing PPE.

Breakroom Areas

The potential for exposure to SARS-CoV-2 can also occur from other employees as well as patients. Maintaining social distancing as well as source control of respiratory secretion during meal and break time is essential. Signage with the appropriate number of persons should be posted inside the breakroom

and meeting rooms. The use of plastic barriers is an additional measure to decrease potential exposure to respiratory secretions during mealtime. High-efficiency particulate air (HEPA) filters in breakrooms and eating locations are an added measure in decreasing the transmission of infection.

Routine Care for Patients Not Diagnosed with SARS-CoV-2

Facemasks covering the patient's nose and mouth should be worn at all times to manage source control of respiratory secretions. During mealtime, the facemask may be removed and replaced as soon as possible. Patients may remove their mask when alone in their rooms but the mask should be donned as soon as other persons are in the room or upon leaving the room.

As part of the daily and ongoing assessment of the patient, the HCP should include screening for symptoms of COVID-19 and monitor temperature and oxygen saturation. Transmission-based precautions (TBPs) should be implemented for any unexplained fever or symptoms of COVID-19. HCPs should wear an N95 respirator or a well-fitting facemask with a nosepiece. When donning the facemask, the HCP must conform the nosepiece to the face in a smooth fashion and secure the mask tight to the face and ensure that there are no gaps on either side of the mask. Eye protection from respiratory secretions should be worn during all patient encounters.

Patients with Suspected/Confirmed SARS-CoV-2 Infection

Patient Placement and Isolation Precautions

Those persons who have been in close contact with someone who has COVID-19 need to be quarantined for 14 days from the last exposure. Persons who have mild-to-moderate illness and are stable may be quarantined at home in a private room. Persons who have tested positive for COVID-19 in the previous 3 months do not need to quarantine.[7]

Hospitalization is required for COVID-19-positive persons who are acutely ill or are decompensating. Patients with suspected or confirmed COVID-19 should be admitted in a private room with a bathroom; the door should be closed, and the patient should be placed on transmission-based isolation precautions. Patients may be grouped together in a semiprivate room if they have lab-confirmed COVID-19 infection and no other infectious disease or respiratory pathogen is identified. Designating patient care units for confirmed or suspected SARS-CoV-2 patients with assigned staff is a strategy to limit HCPs' exposures and conserve PPE.[2]

Patients should wear their masks at all times, except when eating or drinking. Maintain a barrier between patients by using a privacy curtain or plastic barrier. Patients should be kept alone if they cannot keep their facemask on or are symptomatic despite negative SARS-CoV-2 tests. Ideally, aerosol-generating procedures (AGPs) should take place in a negative pressure room.[2] Aerosol-generating procedures are considered; "open suctioning of airways, sputum induction, cardiopulmonary resuscitation, endotracheal intubation and extubations, bronchoscopy, manual ventilation and non-invasive ventilation" such as bilevel positive airway pressure (BiPAP) and continuous positive airway pressure (CPAP). Other procedures that may create aerosolization are nebulizer administration and high-flow oxygen delivery.[8]

Transmission-Based Precautions

TBPs are based upon the routes transmission of a suspected or confirmed pathogen to another person. The transmission of a pathogen depends on many factors such as the infectiousness of the pathogen, the type of care the HCP is providing, the proximity of the HCP and the patient, use of PPE, and compliance with hand hygiene.

The SARS-CoV-2 virus is approximately 0.1 μm in diameter. Respiratory droplets produced by speaking, coughing, and sneezing are divided into two sizes; large droplets (>5 μm in diameter) and small droplets ($\leq$5 μm in diameter). Large respiratory droplets fall to the ground rapidly, are transmitted over short distances, and settle onto surfaces and contaminate the environment or patient room. Patients with infectious diseases that produce large droplets are placed on droplet precautions. Small respiratory droplets can remain suspended in the air for a significant period of time as droplet nuclei. These droplet nuclei can be inhaled. Aerosolized particles (<5 μm in diameter) may be generated from infected patients, especially during AGPs. Therefore, the implementation of airborne isolation precautions is recommended. N95 masks are manufactured to remove more than 95% of all particles that are at least 0.3 μm in diameter. Measurements of particle filtration of N95 masks reveal they are efficacious in filtering approximately 99.8% of particles with a diameter of approximately 0.1 μm.[9]

HCPs can contaminate themselves by touching contaminated surfaces with their hands and subsequently touching their mucous membranes (eyes, nose, and mouth) during doffing PPE or if hand hygiene is not performed when indicated. SARS-CoV-2 pathogen has been recovered from surfaces several weeks after contact.[10] The remaining stability of the infectious virions on surfaces varies depending on the type of surface, the temperature, and the humidity of the environment. Note that the stability of the virus on plastic is greater than that on copper or steel.[11] Due to the potential for the environment to become contaminated, contact precautions are also recommended.

Negative Pressure Rooms and Airborne Isolation Precautions

Airborne isolation refers to the isolation of patients infected with organisms spread by airborne droplet nuclei less than 5 μm in diameter. Negative pressure rooms are required to be designed using the single-pass approach bringing clean air from a clean area to the contaminated area. Several factors impact the actual negative pressure level, such as the differences in the supply air volume and the exhaust air volume, airflow paths, and airflow openings as well as room size. To maintain negative pressure in a room, the exhaust air volume needs to be 10% larger than the supply air volume. Six to twelve air changes per hour are needed to ensure the room is under negative pressure, so airflow direction is from the adjacent outside space such as the hallway into the room.[12] The air in the negative pressure room is preferably exhausted to the outside 25 feet away from intake areas but may be recirculated, provided that the return air is filtered through a HEPA filter.[13]

Negative pressure rooms should be prioritized for a suspected or confirmed COVID-19 patients receiving AGPs. A complete list of AGPs has not been determined for two primary reasons: limited data from studies supporting which procedures would generate infectious aerosols and difficulty in determining if transmissions during AGPs are due to the aerosolization of infectious particles. In general, coughing, sneezing, talking, and breathing can create aerosolization of respiratory particles, but some procedures may create uncontrolled respiratory secretions and place HCPs at an increased risk of exposure to respiratory pathogens. These procedures include open suctioning, sputum induction, cardiopulmonary resuscitation, intubation and extubation, supplemental oxygenation using BiPAP or CPAP, bronchoscopy, and manual ventilation. There are limited studies to confirm if aerosolized particles from medications administered through a nebulizer or high-flow oxygen delivery are infectious.[14,15]

General Care

All persons entering a patient's room with suspected or confirmed COVID-19 are to practice TBPs, perform hand hygiene, and wear the appropriate PPE. Persons at the most significant risk of infection are those who have prolonged, unprotected close contact, defined as within 6 feet for 15 minutes or longer, with a confirmed SARS-CoV-2-infected symptomatic or asymptomatic person. This risk can be reduced by practicing social distancing, performing hand hygiene, and wearing appropriate PPE.[8]

To decrease the exposure of employees to suspected or confirmed cases of SAR-CoV-2, bundling of care should be implemented when feasible. Reallocating duties such as surface cleaning of the patient room or dietary tray distribution to a few personnel also helps decrease HCPs' exposure. Dedicated equipment should be used for a suspected or confirmed SARS-CoV-2 patients. If dedicated equipment is not available, all equipment needs to be cleaned and disinfected according to the manufacturer's recommendations. When delivering care to a patient, limit exposure to the environment as much as possible and limit the traffic into the patient's room.

Use routine care for linens and dietary items; no additional precautions are needed. Waste generated from a patient should be contained in strong bags and entirely closed before disposal. Tissues or other respiratory care items used by the patient to manage source control of sneezes or coughs should be immediately disposed of in the trash, followed immediately by hand hygiene.

Measures should be implemented to limit the movement of the patient throughout the facility. Transporting or transferring patients outside of their room should be limited to medically necessary procedures. If the patient needs to be transported to another department, the HCP in the receiving department should be notified in advance to prevent any delays and to facilitate immediate entrance into the exam room, expedited exam, and a quick turnaround to bring the patient back to his room. During transport, the patient should have a facemask and a clean sheet covering the stretcher or wheelchair. The transport vehicle needs to be cleaned after use.[3]

There is insufficient evidence to determine if the following additional measures impact the risk of transmission, but some HCPs may implement the following:

- Donning headwear.
- Removing clothing and immediately washing items worn at work.
- Showering upon entering the home environment.
- Dedicating shoes specific for work.

Cleaning and Disinfection

Environmental surfaces can become contaminated with infectious organisms. The virus can be detected on surfaces such as bedrails and floors for a prolonged period of time. The survival time of the virus depends on several factors, including the initial virus concentration, type and smoothness of the surface, temperature, and relative humidity.[16,17] The transmission of pathogens usually occurs due to contamination of the hands of the HCP from the patient or their environment. The HCP can then contaminate other patients, employees, equipment, or themselves unless strict adherence to donning and doffing, isolation precautions, and hand hygiene are performed.

Cleaning and disinfection and hand hygiene are integral components of reducing the incidence of all health care–acquired infections. Cleaning may be a one-step or two-step process depending upon the product's Environmental Protection Agency (EPA) registration. A multistep process requires the surface to be first cleaned and then disinfected. Inactivation of the SARS-CoV-2 virus could be achieved within 1 minute using common disinfectants, such as 70% ethanol or 0.1% sodium hypochlorite.[18] The EPA List

N is a compilation of all agents with activity against SAR-CoV-2.[19]

Cleaning is an essential first step because it lowers the number of organisms and bioburden from surfaces, but it does not kill the organisms. Cleaning is done with soap or detergent and water with the physical act of removing the organisms from surfaces or decreasing the bioburden on the surface. Disinfecting is the second step and is carried out using chemicals to eliminate or kill germs on surfaces or objects. This process does not necessarily clean dirty surfaces or remove germs, but killing germs on a surface after cleaning can further lower the risk of spreading infection. All surfaces must be thoroughly cleaned before disinfection can occur.[8,20,21]

The Use of Adjunct Technology for Disinfection

The use of electrostatic sprayers or foggers and ultraviolet germicidal irradiation for the disinfection of patient rooms and surfaces is considered adjunct technology for terminal cleaning of the environment. This process is only performed when the room is vacant and cleaned, curtains are removed, and linens and other moveable equipment are not present in the room. Special training and competency of personnel utilizing the adjunct technology are needed.[22]

The Severity of Illness Criteria

The severity of illness from COVID-19 can range from mild to critical. Patients with mild illness present with various symptoms, including fever, cough, sore throat, malaise, headache, muscle pain with or without SOB, dyspnea, or abnormal chest imaging. Patients with moderate illness due to COVID-19 present with a clinical picture or imaging evidence of lower respiratory disease and oxygen saturation (SpO_2) of 94% or more on room air at sea level. Patients with severe illness due to COVID-19 present with a respiratory rate of more than 30 breaths per minute, SpO_2 of less than 94% on room air at sea level, or a decrease from baseline of more than 3% in patients who have chronic hypoxia, a ratio of arterial partial pressure of oxygen to fraction of inspired oxygen (PaO_2/F_IO2) of less than 300 mg Hg, or infiltrates in greater than 50% of the lungs.[23] In a large case study conducted in China, 81% of persons were classified as experiencing mild disease, 15% were classified as severe, and 5% were critically ill.[24]

Duration and Discontinuation of Isolation for Patients with COVID

The duration of natural immunity to this virus continues to be under investigation. In patients recovering from mild-to-moderate COVID-19 infection, a replication-competent virus has not been recovered after 10 days from symptom onset.[25] Patients recovering from severe COVID-19 infection may shed replication-competent virus after up to 20 days. Severely immunosuppressed patients may shed replication-competent virus beyond 20 days.[25] The presence of SARS-CoV-2 RNA may be recovered from upper respiratory tract specimens up to 12 weeks after symptom onset.[25]

Reinfection of SARS-CoV-2 is possible, and the impact of the variant strains on reinfection requires further studies.[2,25] One study identified an 84% lower risk of reinfection in patients with a previous history of COVID-19.[26] Patients who have recovered from COVID-19 infection and remain asymptomatic and have a positive SARS-CoV-2 polymerase chain reaction (PCR) test 90 days after the initial infection represent persistent shedding of the virus. If patients become symptomatic during the 90 days following an initial infection with COVID-19 and an evaluation does not identify the etiology of the symptoms, retesting and evaluating for reinfection with SARS-CoV-2 should be done in consultation with an infectious disease expert.[25]

The test-based strategy for the discontinuation of TBPs is not routinely recommended due to the prolonged detection of the virus in the upper respiratory tract. Around 88 to 95% of patients infected with COVID-19 do not have replication-competent virus after 10 to 15 days of symptoms onset. Some patients who have recovered from COVID-19 may continue to have SARS-CoV-2 RNA detected in their upper respiratory specimens for as long as 12 weeks after symptom onset. Evidence of prolonged detection of the virus as long as 143 days after an initial positive test is noted in immunocompromised patients.[25] The virus recovered from these patients does not have replication-competent virus.[25]

A test-based strategy may be helpful in severely immunocompromised patients, and there is concern that the patient is still infectious for more than 20 days. Severely immunocompromised is defined by the CDC as patients "on chemotherapy for cancer, being within one year of receiving a hematopoietic stem cell or organ transplant, untreated human immunodeficiency virus (HIV) infection with a CD4 T lymphocyte count of < 200, combined primary immunodeficiency disorder and receipt of prednisone > 20 mg/day for more than 14 days."[23]

The CDC has outlined criteria utilizing the test-based strategy and a symptom-based strategy for the discontinuation of TBPs. A test-based strategy for the discontinuation of TBPs for patients with COVID-19 has challenges due to the prolonged presence of the virus in the upper respiratory tract. Therefore, the use of the symptom-based strategy may provide a more conservative approach for discontinuing TBPs. As results of studies and new information are acquired, practice will change based upon recent evidence. Symptomatic patients may discontinue isolation if there are resolution of fever without fever-reducing medication, improved respiratory symptoms, and negative SARS-CoV-2 PCR test results from at least two consecutive respiratory specimens collected more than 24 hours apart. Asymptomatic patients may discontinue isolation if they have negative SARS-CoV-2 PCR test results from at least two consecutive respiratory specimens collected more than 24 hours apart.[23]

The symptom-based strategy to discontinue TBPs for patients with COVID-19 considers the severity of illness and includes the days since symptoms onset, the presence of a fever, and the clinical improvement of the patient's symptoms. Mild illness is defined as persons who have various symptoms, including fever, cough, sore throat, malaise, headache, and muscle pain without SOB, dyspnea, or abnormal chest imaging. Moderate illness is defined as persons who have clinical or imaging evidence of lower respiratory disease. Severe illness is seen in persons with a respiratory rate of more than 30 breaths per minute, SpO_2 of less than 94% on room air at sea level, or a decrease from baseline of more than 3% in persons with chronic hypoxemia, a ratio of arterial partial pressure of oxygen to fraction of inspired oxygen (PaO_2/F_IO_2) of less than 300 mm Hg, or infiltrates in greater than 50% of the lungs. Persons with respiratory failure, septic shock, and multisystem failure are considered critically ill.[23]

TBPs can be discontinued 10 days after symptoms onset in asymptomatic persons with COVID-19 who present with a mild-to-moderate illness provided there is a resolution of fever for at least 24 hours, without fever-reducing medication and in the presence of improving clinical symptoms. For persons with COVID-19 who present with a severe critical illness, TBPs can be discontinued 20 days after symptom onset. Severely immunosuppressed persons may continue to have replication-competent virus for more than 20 days and require testing and further evaluation.[25]

Discontinuation of Empiric Transmission-Based Precautions for Patients with Suspected COVID

The decision to discontinue TBPs for suspected COVID-19 can be made based on one negative SARS-CoV-2 PCR test result from a respiratory specimen. If the person remains suspect for COVID-19 infection, maintain TBPs and secure a second SARS-CoV-2 PCR test. The provider's clinical judgment and suspicion of COVID-19 infection should determine whether to continue to discontinue empiric TBPs.[23]

HCPs who enter the room of a suspected or confirmed SARS-CoV-2 patient should adhere to TBPs and use an N95 mask or equivalent or higher-level respirator, gown, gloves, and eye protection. Hand hygiene remains the cornerstone of infection prevention and should be performed before and after all patient contact and contact with potentially contaminated surfaces, before donning, and after doffing PPE. Hand hygiene may be performed by using ABHRs containing at least 60% alcohol or using soap and water for at least 20 seconds.

Personal Protective Equipment for the Care of Suspected or Confirmed COVID-19 Patient

PPE is worn to minimize exposure to blood and body fluid. PPE includes gloves, gowns, masks or respirators, and eye protection. Employers need to provide PPE following Occupational Safety and Health Administration (OSHA) PPE Standards (29 CFR 1910). All PPE should be readily available and consist of a safe design, and should be maintained in a clean manner. Employers are required to provide training that includes when to use PPE, what PPE is necessary, how to properly don and doff PPE as well as dispose of or properly disinfect and maintain PPE, and the limitations of PPE.[27]

Hand hygiene is to be performed before donning and after doffing gloves. Nonsterile gloves are used upon entry into the patient room and need to be changed if they become torn or heavily contaminated. Limit contact with contaminated surfaces when in the patient's room. Remove gloves before leaving the patient room and perform hand hygiene. A clean gown should be worn upon entry into a patient room and discarded after use. The gown should be fluid-resistant and provide coverage of the front and the entire length of the arm. An N95 respirator (equivalent or higher-level respirator) or facemask (if a respirator is unavailable) is needed before entering the patient's room. Other respirators include powered air-purifying respirators (PAPRs), controlled air-purifying respirator (CAPR), or elastomeric respirators. When performing AGPs, use N95 respirators or respirators that provide a higher level of protection.[8]

AGPs include open suctioning, sputum induction, cardiopulmonary resuscitation, intubation and extubation, supplemental oxygenation using BiPAP or CPAP, bronchoscopy, and manual ventilation. There are limited studies to confirm if aerosolized particles from medications administered through a nebulizer or high flow oxygen delivery are infectious.[8,14]

Remove disposable masks or respirators after leaving the patient's room unless practicing extended use or reuse. Use care when removing PAPRs and CAPRs to prevent contamination and clean according to the manufacturer's recommendations. Perform hand hygiene after touching the mask or respirator.

When selecting eye protection, consider the ability of the device to protect against bodily fluids (respiratory secretions), ensure that the device fits appropriately, covering the front and sides of the face, and is comfortable, and ascertain that the vision is not restricted or distorted, the device does not interfere with any other PPE (such as the facemask or respirator), and the device is cleanable. Eye protection may include goggles or a face shield. HCPs' eyeglasses are not sufficient to protect against bodily fluids. Eye protection needs to be applied before entering the patient's room and remove after leaving the patient's room unless practicing extended use. Use care when removing eye protection to prevent contamination, and clean according to the manufacturer's recommendations. Perform hand hygiene after touching the eye protection.[27,28]

Reusable PPE must be adequately cleaned, including the proper contact time for the disinfecting agent. The PPE is to be stored in a clean, breathable bag or container (not a plastic bag) and labeled with the HCP name.[27]

Donning and Doffing Personal Protective Equipment When Caring for Patients with Suspected or Confirmed COVID-19

More than one donning and doffing method may be acceptable. It is crucial that the HCP receives comprehensive training and demonstrates competency in the use of PPE.[29] The training should include the concept of what aspect of the PPE is "contaminated" and what aspect is "clean," and how to prevent contamination of PPE, including not touching PPE once donned and limiting the contact of surfaces within the patient's environment. The curriculum should also include the type of PPE needed, when the HCP needs to don the PPE, how to don and doff the PPE, the limitations and proper care of the PPE, and the disposal of PPE.[27]

Doffing potentially contaminated PPE needs to be performed in a mindful, deliberate manner to prevent self-contamination. The fit test is required for the N95 mask worn by the HCP and PPE donned before entering the patient's room. Do not touch or adjust the mask or eye protection in an effort to prevent contamination of PPE. Hand hygiene is to be performed before donning, after doffing gloves, as contamination can occur during the doffing process.

Donning

- Identify and secure the necessary PPE to don.
- Perform hand hygiene.
- Put on the isolation gown. Thoroughly cover the torso from neck to knees, arms to the end of wrists, and wrap around the back. Tie all the ties on the gown.
- Put on NIOSH-approved N95 mask. A fit test needs to be performed for the specific mask being used. If the mask has a nosepiece, it should be fitted to

the nose with both hands and should not be bent or tented. Gently apply firm pressure along the upper portion of the mask to fit close to the face. Do not pinch the nosepiece. The mask should be extended under the chin. Both your mouth and nose should be protected. Fit check mask by performing a seal check by blowing air out with your hands cupped over the mask and ensuring no air leakage is felt.
- Some HCPs don a facemask over the N95 mask to prevent further contamination.
- Put on a face shield or goggles. Select the proper eye protection to ensure good visualization but it should not interfere with the fit of the mask.
- Don gloves to extend to cover wrists.

Doffing

- Remove gloves and gown in one motion by gently pulling the gown from the chest area and breaking the ties only touching outside of gown only with gloved hands. While removing the gown, roll the gown inside out into a bundle. As you are removing the gown, peel off the gloves simultaneously, only touching the inside of the gloves and gown with your bare hands. Dispose of in regular trash.
- Exit the patient's room.
- Perform hand hygiene.
- Remove eye protection. Remember that the outside of the eye protection is contaminated: do not touch the outside of the eye protection. Carefully remove eye protection by grabbing the straps or stem of googles pulling away from the head and face. Do not touch the front of the face shield or goggles.
- Remove the masks. Remember the front of the mask is contaminated: do not touch the front of the mask.
  - Facemask: Carefully untie or unhook from the ears, pull away from the

face without touching the front of the mask.
  - N95 mask: Remove the bottom strap by touching only the strap and bring it carefully over the head. Grasp the top strap and bring it carefully over the head, and then pull the N95 mask away from the face without touching the front of the mask.
- Perform hand hygiene.[29]

If reusing eye protection:
- Don gloves and clean the outside of the face shield or goggles with an approved agent and place them in a clean, breathable bag (not a plastic bag) labeled with the HCP's name.
- Perform hand hygiene.[28]

References

1. Parvez MK, Parveen S. Evolution and emergence of pathogenic viruses: past, present, and future. Intervirology 2017;60(1–2):1–7
2. Centers for Disease Control and Prevention. Interim infection prevention and control recommendations or patients with suspected or confirmed coronavirus disease 2019 (COVID-19) in healthcare settings. Available at: https://www.esrdnetwork.org/sites/default/files/Infection%20and%20Prevention%20-%20CDC.pd. Accessed April 18, 2021
3. Centers for Disease Control and Prevention. Interim infection prevention and control recommendations for healthcare personnel during the coronavirus disease 2019 (COVID-19) pandemic. Available at: https://www.cdc.gov/coronavirus/2019-ncov/hcp/infection-control-recommendations.html#print. Accessed March 15, 2021
4. Ferretti L, Wymant C, Kendall M, et al. Quantifying SARS-CoV-2 transmission suggests epidemic control with digital contact tracing. Science 2020;368(6491):eabb6936
5. Tan J, Shousheng L, Zhuang L, et al. Transmission and clinical characteristics of asymptomatic patients with SARS-CoV-2 infection [online]. Future Virol 2020. doi:10.2217/fvl-2020-0087
6. World Health Organization. Transmission of SARS-CoV-2: implications for infection

prevention precautions. Available at: https://www.who.int/news-room/commentaries/detail/transmission-of-sars-cov-2-implications-for-infection-prevention-precautions. Accessed March 17, 2020

7. Centers for Disease Control and Prevention. When to quarantine: stay home if you might have been exposed to COVID-19. Available at: https://www.cdc.gov/coronavirus/2019-ncov/if-you-are-sick/quarantine.html#print. Accessed March 15, 2021

8. Centers for Disease Control and Prevention. Clinical questions about COVID-19: questions and answers. Revised March 4, 2021. Available at: https://www.cdc.gov/coronavirus/2019-ncov/hcp/faq.html. Accessed March 15, 2021

9. Rengasamy S, Shaffer R, Williams B, Smit S. A comparison of facemask and respirator filtration test methods. J Occup Environ Hyg 2017;14(2):92–103

10. Moriarty LF, Plucinski MM, Marston BJ, et al; CDC Cruise Ship Response Team; California Department of Public Health COVID-19 Team; Solano County COVID-19 Team. Public health responses to COVID-19 outbreaks on cruise ships - worldwide, February-March 2020. MMWR Morb Mortal Wkly Rep 2020;69(12):347–352

11. Bar-On YM, Flamholz A, Phillips R, Milo R. SARS-CoV-2 (COVID-19) by the numbers. eLife 2020;9:e57309

12. Jinkyun C, Kyunghun W, Byungseon SK. Improved ventilation system for removal of airborne contamination in airborne infectious isolation rooms. Available at: https://www.ashrae.org/technical-resources/ashrae-journal/featured-articles/improved-ventilation-system-for-removal-of-airborne-contamination-in-airborne-infectious-isolation-rooms. Accessed March 15, 2021

13. Rosenbaum RA, Benyo JS, O'Connor RE, et al. Use of a portable forced air system to convert existing hospital space into a mass casualty isolation area. Ann Emerg Med 2004;44(6):628–634

14. Tran K, Cimon K, Severn M, Pessoa-Silva CL, Conly J. Aerosol generating procedures and risk of transmission of acute respiratory infections to healthcare workers: a systematic review. PLoS One 2012;7(4):e35797

15. World Health Organization. Modes of transmission of virus causing COVID-19: implications for IPC precaution recommendations. Available at: https://www.who.int/news-room/commentaries/detail/modes-of-transmission-of-virus-causing-covid-19-implications-for-ipc-precaution-recommendations. Accessed March 17, 2021

16. National Institutes of Health. Study suggests new coronavirus may remain on surfaces for days. Available at: https://www.nih.gov/news-events/nih-research-matters/study-suggests-new-coronavirus-may-remain-surfaces-days#:~:text=Scientists%20found%20that%20SARS%2D,to%20protect%20against%20infection. Accessed April 15, 2021

17. van Doremalen N, Bushmaker T, Morris DH, et al. Aerosol and surface stability of HCoV-19 (SARS-CoV-2) compared to SARS-CoV-1. medRxiv 2020 (e-pub ahead of print). doi:10.1056/NEJMc2004973

18. Centers for Disease Control and Prevention. Best practices for environmental cleaning in healthcare facilities: in resource-limited settings. Available at: https://www.cdc.gov/hai/pdfs/resource-limited/environmental-cleaning-RLS-H.pdf. Accessed March 15, 2021

19. United States Environmental Protection Agency. About List N: disinfectants for coronavirus (COVID-19). Available at: https://www.epa.gov/coronavirus/about-list-n-disinfectants-coronavirus-covid-19-0. Accessed March 15, 2021

20. Centers for Disease Control and Prevention. Cleaning & disinfecting environmental surfaces. Available at: https://www.cdc.gov/oralhealth/infectioncontrol/faqs/cleaning-disinfecting-environmental-surfaces.html. Accessed April 15, 2021

21. Centers for Disease Control and Prevention. Environmental cleaning procedures. Available at: https://www.cdc.gov/hai/prevent/resource-limited/cleaning-procedures.html. Accessed April 15, 2021

22. Centers for Disease Control and Prevention. Safety precautions when using electrostatic sprayers, foggers, misters, or vaporizers for surface disinfection during the COVID-19 pandemic. Available at: https://www.cdc.gov/coronavirus/2019-ncov/php/

eh-practitioners/sprayers.html#print. Accessed April 15, 2021

23. Centers for Disease Control and Prevention. Discontinuation of transmission-based precautions and disposition of patients with SARS-CoV-2 infection in healthcare settings. Available at: https://www.cdc.gov/coronavirus/2019-ncov/hcp/disposition-hospitalized-patients.html. Accessed March 15, 2021

24. Wu Z, McGoogan, JM. Characteristics of and important lessons from the coronavirus disease 2019 (COVID-19) outbreak in China: summary of a report of 72, 314 cases from the Chinese Center for Disease Control and Prevention. JAMA 2020;323(13):1239-1242

25. Centers for Disease Control and Prevention. Ending isolation and precautions for people with COVID-19: interim guidance. Available at: https://www.cdc.gov/coronavirus/2019-ncov/hcp/duration-isolation.html#print. Accessed March 15, 2021

26. Hall VJ, Foulkes S, Charlett A, et al; SIREN Study Group. SARS-CoV-2 infection rates of antibody-positive compared with antibody-negative health-care workers in England: a large, multicentre, prospective cohort study (SIREN). Lancet 2021;397(10283):1459–1469

27. Occupational Safety and Health Administration. Personal protective equipment. Available at: https://www.osha.gov/sites/default/files/publications/osha3151.pdf. Accessed March 15, 2021

28. Centers for Disease Control and Prevention. Using personal protective equipment (PPE). Available at: https://www.cdc.gov/coronavirus/2019-ncov/hcp/using-ppe.html. Accessed March 15, 2020

29. Centers for Disease Control and Prevention. Use of personal protective equipment (PPE) when caring for patients with confirmed or suspected COVID-19. Available at: https://www.cdc.gov/coronavirus/2019-ncov/hcp/preparedness-resources.html. Accessed March 15, 2021

18   Outpatient Management

Jose Iglesias, Amit Setya, and Paul Marik

Introduction

During the early days of the pandemic there was no known early effective treatment for outpatients with COVID-19. Initial treatment was symptomatic care with antipyretics, analgesics, antitussives, bronchodilators, and antibiotics.[1-3] Patients were advised to go to the emergency room if they could not breathe or they noticed their "lips to turn blue."[1,4] This approach led to patients present late in their disease during the pulmonary phase of the disease.[3,5] During the pulmonary phase of the disease a large proportion of patients require oxygen and many deteriorate requiring intensive care admission thus overwhelming hospital resources.[3,5-7] Antiviral therapy with Remdesivir is less effective during this phase which is characterized by severe inflammation and thrombosis.[3,6,8] With the exception of monoclonal antibody therapy for high-risk patients, in the majority of western developed countries such as the United States, United Kingdom, France, and Germany, public health authorities (national institutes of health (NIH), national health service (NHS), food and drug administration (FDA)) offer no effective outpatient management protocols.[1,9-14] In terms of outpatient therapies, there remains a paucity of large randomized, double-blinded placebo-controlled trial. Studies evaluating potential candidate agents for outpatient therapy have included investigator-led studies, observational, small placebo-controlled trials, and open label studies. This approach has been criticized by evidence-based medicine (EBM) purists as being small, underpowered, and containing significant bias.[2,3,6,12,14] Meta-analysis performed by different groups have yielded conflicting reports. Although application of the principles of EBM is the gold standard approach to care, this may not be feasible or appropriate during a pandemic.[3,6] It is the opinion of the authors that the reliance on large trials by "the Ivory Tower" evidence-based purists has led to some degree of therapeutic nihilism.

Many clinicians caring for patients afflicted with COVID-19 have based their treatment decisions based on what we have learned about the virology, the clinical phases, and the pathophysiology of disease to devise early treatment protocols.[3,6,8] COVID-19 disease progression can be characterized by an asymptomatic viremic phase, a symptomatic viremic phase, an early inflammatory pulmonary phase, and a late pulmonary phase.[3,6,8,15] As the disease progresses viral-induced injury decreases, and a hyperinflammatory coagulopathic state ensues. Using this approach, timing of treatment has been based on knowledge of the phases of disease employing antivirals, immunomodulatory, anti-inflammatory, and antithrombotic agents.[6,8,15] Proponents of early outpatient multifaceted treatment such as McCullough, Zelenko, Marik, the Front line critical care consortium (FLCCC), and others have devised early multifaceted protocols that have the potential to decrease the severity and burden of disease.[3,6,15-17] The current therapeutic arsenal for outpatient therapy includes nutraceuticals, repurposed agents that have shown potential as antiviral and anti-inflammatory agents. This chapter will review the principles of early treatment based on the phases of the disease. It is important to note that this chapter covering early outpatient treatment includes nutraceuticals, repurposed medications, and agents that have demonstrated basic science evidence of potential benefit or low-level evidence of benefit. Many of these protocols have not undergone the thorough, evidence-based scrutiny in large, randomized placebo-controlled trials which in the current crisis is difficult to perform. In contrast to western developed nations, many countries' health authorities have developed outpatient protocols.

We briefly discuss potential agents and timing of therapy in outpatients. For a more detailed discussion on therapeutic agents, we refer you to Chapter 12.

Paradigm of Early Treatment: The Phases of Disease and Treatment

Infection with SARS-CoV-2 results in COVID-19 disease, which generally progresses through at least three distinct phases during the clinical course of disease, and therapy should be directed with this understanding.[6,8,15,18] The early viremic phase progresses from an asymptomatic to a symptomatic phase and is associated with rapid viral replication followed by activation of the innate and adaptive immunity (approximately day 1–7).[8,15,18] An appropriate immune response results in viral clearance and resolution of symptoms.[15,18] However, in a proportion of patients even as viral load decreases, dead viral particles, viral proteins, and pseudovirions generate a dysregulated immune response, and an exaggerated increase in proinflammatory macrophages and cytokines (**Fig. 18.1**). The net result is an organizing pneumonia and in some patients progressive hypoxemia respiratory failure and the cytokine storm.[8,18,19]

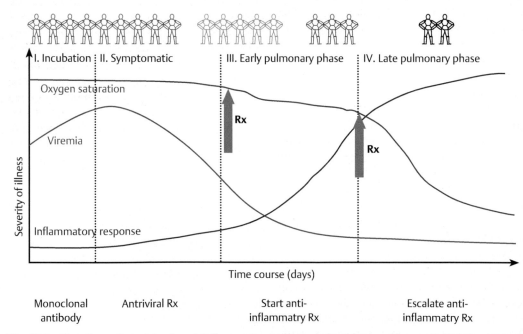

Fig. 18.1 Timeline of viral load and inflammatory response. In this paradigm antiviral therapy and administration of monoclonal therapy in high-risk patients, effectiveness is greatest during viremic phase of disease. Used with permission from PE Marik.

Risk Stratification and Early Therapy

In approximately 80% of patients SARS-CoV-2 infection is either asymptomatic or self-limited.[3,5,20,21] However, in the remaining 20% of individuals disease progress is severe, with a high risk of morbidity and mortality.[1] Therefore, patients likely to derive the greatest benefit of early treatment are those with comorbidities, age 60 or greater, those with underlying comorbidities regardless of age, and moderately ill patients regardless of age-displaying dyspnea.

Home Monitoring

Patients diagnosed with COVID-19 should be instructed on frequent home pulse-oximetry monitoring. Patient monitoring can be performed using telehealth.[22-24] Although the field of home pulse oximetry is complex and is beyond the scope of this chapter, suffice to say that inexpensive nonmedical use pulse oximeters have been compared to those approved for medical use and have demonstrated reasonable accuracy in arterial oxygen saturations between 90 and 99%.[22-24] Smart phone pulse oximeters have been found to lack accuracy for home monitoring and the use of these devices is discouraged. Hospital or urgent care evaluation is advised when saturation falls below 94. At this level early identification helps those patients who are at high risk for clinical decompensation and require in-person evaluation.[22-24] Initially it was thought that pulse oximetry in individuals of brown or black color would be inaccurate; however, this is usually when oxygen saturations fall below 80% which is way below the threshold that would raise alarm in the outpatient management of COVID-19.[22-24] Measurement should be taken using the index finger. There should be no nail polish on the persons nail. After allowing approximately 1 minute to allow for a clear pulse signal recording, proceed with obtaining readings. Only readings associated with a strong pulse signal should be recorded. Measurement should be observed over 1 minute and the average reading should be recorded. Reading should be obtained indoors with individual at rest; however, if patients' clinical course dictates readings can be measured with walking or increased activity.[22-24]

It is pertinent to note that in western developed nations patients are usually hospitalized when oxygen therapy is required; it is not unfeasible to utilize all noninvasive oxygenation methods in the outpatient settings in areas where hospital resources are limited or overburdened.

Phases of Disease and Treatment

Viremic Phase

Monoclonal Antibody Therapy

Monoclonal neutralizing antibodies directed against SARS-CoV-2 have been implemented in clinical trials and have obtained emergency use agreement (EUA) for the treatment of high-risk patients with COVID-19.[9,11,25,26] Combination monoclonal antibody therapy seems to be more effective than monotherapy.[27] A Cochrane review of monoclonal therapy revealed that outpatient therapy with bamlanivimab/etesevimab compared to placebo decreased hospitalization by day 29.[28] Casirivimab/imdevimab compared to placebo was found to reduce hospital admissions or death.[10,11] We recommend early implementation of these agents in patients who are at high risk for hospitalization, worsening disease, or death.

Oral Antiviral Agents

Hydroxychloroquine (HCQ) and Chloroquine (CQ)

Chloroquine and hydroxychloroquine due to in vitro antiviral effects and immunomodulatory effects were one of the first medications repurposed for the management of COVID-19.[29,30] Both agents are zinc ionophores facilitating zinc uptake into the intracellular compartment where zinc can exert antiviral activity.[31,32] In Wuhan, China, initial reports by Gao demonstrated that CQ improved the clinical course of COVID-19 pneumonia and shortened duration of disease; however, this study to date has not released datasets.[33]

Hydroxychloroquine given along with zinc and azithromycin initially demonstrated clinical benefits in terms of symptom resolution, decreased hospitalization, and mortality in multiple retrospective and large observational studies.[34-39] However, prospective randomized controlled trials and Cochrane group meta-analysis demonstrated no clinical benefit.[30,40-43] Observational and retrospective data on early outpatient therapy employing HCQ have demonstrated improved clinical symptoms and decrease hospitalization rates.[34-39] There have been very little prospective randomized trials employing HCQ. Many of these trials have been stopped prematurely for futility and unknown reasons.[40,41,44] Schwartz et al, in a randomized double-blind study that did not reach enrollment goals and terminated early, enrolled patients with up to 12 days of symptoms, demonstrated no clinical benefit in the HCQ group.[41] The Together trial was a randomized trial comparing HCQ, lopinavir/ritonavir against placebo. This trial found no difference in resolution. The trial was terminated early due to futility and it is unclear if this trial is representative of early therapy.[40] Skipper et al performed a randomized double-blind trial evaluating HCQ versus placebo and demonstrated no clinical benefit of HCQ.[44] It is pertinent to note that the placebo employed in this trial did not use inert substance and there was PCR confirmed cases in only 58% of patients.[44] Thus there remains controversy regarding HCQ; regardless it is still incorporated in some outpatient early protocols. If HCQ or CQ is used in protocols for outpatient therapy, it is prudent to monitor for QTc interval prolongation and drug–drug interactions.

Interferon

Type 1 interferons (IFNs) are a group of cytokines which are one of the bodies' innate immune response defenses against viral infection.[45,46] They possess antiviral properties and are known to inhibit viral proteases.[47,48] In patients with advancing age, comorbidities, and a subset of patients at high risk for progression, there may be a blunted IFN response to SARS-CoV-2 infection. In addition SARS-CoV-2 proteins particularly open reading frame (ORF) 3b, ORF 6, and nucleocapsid are known to inhibit expression of IFNs.[46] From a pathophysiological standpoint, Mosaddeghi et al demonstrated that individuals with an initial decreased expression of IFN during the early stages of infection had a higher risk of mortality.[46,49] The investigators proposed early therapy with IFN.[46] Thus, there has been a significant interest in employing IFN therapy in patients with infection. In a meta-analysis, Nakhlband and colleagues demonstrated that the administration of subcutaneous IFN-β1 in conjunction with antiviral therapy improved hospital length of stay and mortality in hospitalized patients with COVID-19.[47] In a randomized, outpatient, placebo-controlled trial comparing IFN-λ1 versus placebo, Feld et al demonstrated an accelerated viral clearance particularly in those with high viral loads.[50] Idelsis et al in a randomized controlled trial of intramuscular injection of IFN-α2b and IFN-γ demonstrated improved viral clearance and improved symptoms in patients with COVID-19.[51] In a large retrospective study with over 1,400 patients, inhalational therapy with 5 million units bid of IFN-α2b therapy observed that early treatment within 0 to 2 days of symptom onset resulted in decreased need for mechanical ventilation and mortality.[52] In those patients where treatment was initiated 3 to 5 days later from symptom onset, clinical outcomes were noted to be poor.[52]

Favipiravir

Favipiravir (FAV) is an orally administered antiviral agent that has demonstrated a broad-spectrum in vitro and in vivo antiviral activity against many negative-stranded RNA viruses.[53] Similar to Remdesivir it is an inhibitor of RNA polymerase.[53] In hospitalized patients there has been encouraging results in improved rates of recovery, viral shedding, and trend in decreasing rates of the need for mechanical ventilation.[53-55] The ability of oral administration makes FAV an attractive agent for early outpatient protocols. Based on the interim results of a Russian phase II/III demonstrating improved viral clearance and resolution of symptoms in patients with moderate COVID-19, the agent has been approved for outpatient and inpatient use by Russian health authorities.[56] FAV is also approved for the treatment of COVID-19 by Indian health authorities.[57] It is important to note that the dosages employed for COVID-19 1,600 to 2,000 mg bid day 1 followed by 600 to 800 mg bid for up to 14 days may result in side effects such as hyperuricemia elevated transaminases and significant gastrointestinal side effect.[58,59] Furthermore, FAV is teratogenic, and appropriate contraceptive measures should be employed.[58] There are some pertinent drug–drug interactions such as sulfonylurea toxicity-associated hypoglycemia.[59]

Antibiotics

Azithromycin (AZA) and Doxycycline (DOXY)
Although AZA and DOXY have demonstrated antiviral properties and have been employed in outpatient treatment protocols,[60] it is the opinion of the authors that there is no benefit in adding these patients to outpatient protocols unless there is a suspicion of an underlying secondary infection.

Nitazoxanide
Nitazoxanide (NTZ), an oral antiprotozoal agent, has demonstrated in-vitro and in-vivo antiviral activity and has been employed in small clinical trials against a variety of viruses.[61,62] In a small, double-blind randomized placebo-controlled trial involving 50 hospitalized patients, NTZ 600 mg bid started within 3 days of symptoms and 36 hours of admission, investigators demonstrated a significant reduction in hospital length of stay, greater resolution to SARS-CoV-2 PCR negativity, and a reduction in inflammatory

markers.[63] In a randomized clinical trial employing 500 mg of NTZ, treatment with NTZ resulted in a greater reduction of viral load compared with placebo. The study demonstrated no difference in clinical outcomes.[64] Cadegiani et al in a prospective observational trial, the Pre-Andro trial, observed that early treatment with azithromycin combined with either HCQ, ivermectin, or NTZ was associated with a marked reduction in viral shedding, hospitalizations, respiratory compromise, need for mechanical ventilation, and the development of post-COVID complications.[65] Historically, the agent has demonstrated reasonable safety and tolerability profile.

Ivermectin
Interest in ivermectin (IVM), an antiparasitic agent, with known in-vitro and in-vivo antiviral activity as a potential therapeutic agent against SARS-Cov-2 began when Caly et al demonstrated marked in-vitro anti-SARS-CoV-2 activity.[66] In addition IVM possesses anti-inflammatory and immune-modulating properties mainly acting in the NFK-β pathway of inflammation.[67-69] Since the initial antiviral in-vitro discovery by Caly et al, there have been numerous clinical studies performed, and for reasons unknown, there has been a significant amount of controversies.[70-72] There has been conflicting evidence regarding IVM and improved clinical outcomes. However, in at least two meta-analysis which included over 28 randomized controlled trials, 78% improvement was noted in important clinical outcomes.[70-72] A website analysis of 63 studies on the use of IVM for COVID-19 treatment found that early treatment was associated with a 61% improvement in lowering hospitalizations, a 66% improvement in clinical recovery, a 68% improvement in viral clearance, and a 37% decrease in mortality.[73] In contrast, the Cochrane database and the study by Roman et al, which evaluated fewer studies, found no statistically significant differences in important clinical outcomes or mortality.[74] Currently, there are several clinical trials in progress.

Symptomatic Phase

Fluvoxamine

Fluvoxamine (FLUV), although not an antiviral agent per se, exerts antiviral effects by inhibiting endolysosomal viral trafficking. Studies have demonstrated that early therapy with FLUV may prevent clinical deterioration in COVID-19 patients.[75,76] Lenz et al in a double-blind placebo-controlled trial involving outpatients demonstrated that 100 mg of FLUV given three times a day prevented clinical deterioration and lower hospitalization rates when compared to placebo.[77] Similarly, Boulware et al in a prospective trial observed lower need for hospitalization in patients receiving early treatment with FLUV.[78] FLUV has many pleiotropic effects that make it an important agent in the early outpatient management of COVID-19.[75,79] These include antiviral effects via inhibition of lysosomal trafficking, functionally inhibiting sphingomyelinase preventing viral entry, anti-inflammatory effects, inhibition of mast cell degranulation and antithrombotic effects by inhibiting platelet aggregation. Together these effects suggest that FLUV may be effective in all stages of the disease and have the potential to mitigate the cytokine storm.[75,77]

Budesonide

In an open-label randomized controlled phase 2 early treatment trial comparing inhaled budesonide 400 µg two puffs two times a day to usual care started within 7 days of onset of mild treatment demonstrated that early treatment with inhaled budesonide decreased duration of symptoms, need for urgent care visits, and need for hospitalization.[80] The study was terminated early due to superiority of budesonide treatment. The Principal trial, a much larger study that enrolled patients age 65 or greater with symptoms for 14 days or less and at high risk for adverse outcomes, randomized 692 patients to inhaled budesonide 800 µg two times a day for 14 days versus 968 patients to usual care.[81] Patients randomized to budesonide treatment demonstrated a statistically significant difference in improved time to recovery.[81,82] There was a trend toward decreased hospitalizations and mortality in the treatment group; however, this did not meet Bayesian analysis superiority threshold.[81] Thus, budesonide is an ideal candidate for use in outpatient COVID-19 treatment protocols, although an inhaled corticosteroid can be utilized in the symptomatic and pulmonary phases of the disease.[81,82]

Antithrombotic Agents

Aspirin

The pathophysiologic hallmark of COVID-19 disease is its inflammatory, thrombotic, and coagulopathic nature. Aspirin possesses both anti-inflammatory and antithrombotic properties. There is observational evidence that aspirin has the potential to improve clinical outcomes.[83] In two large propensity matched retrospective analysis, the investigators observed that use of aspirin pre-COVID-19 diagnosis was associated with a marked decrease in mortality.[84,85] Chow et al observe that aspirin use within 7 days of diagnosis and 24 hours of admission was associated with a decreased risk of need for mechanical ventilation, ICU admission, and hospital mortality.[84] To date, there are no prospective trials involving aspirin use in outpatients. The authors feel that if there is no contraindication in the initiation of aspirin, it should be included as an agent in early outpatient treatment protocols. In patients already on aspirin pre-COVID-19 diagnosis, aspirin should not be discontinued unless there is a clear-cut indication for discontinuation.

Heparin

Heparin, an anticoagulation and antithrombotic prophylaxis, has proven to improve clinical outcomes in hospitalized patients.[86-90] However, although most likely it has not been employed as outpatient therapy in western developed nations, it is not inconceivable for its incorporation in outpatient protocols in areas with scarce hospital resources.

Antiandrogen Therapy

Epidemiological data has demonstrated that male sex is a risk factor for adverse outcomes, and interest in antiandrogen treatment as a therapeutic agent has been explored. Early trials with differing agents such as dutasteride, spironolactone, and proxalutamide have demonstrated promise as repurposed agents that can be employed in decreasing hospitalization, decreasing inflammatory markers, and improving radiographic abnormalities.[91-94] In an observational study of an electronic health record database involving over 6 million individuals, a sample of 3,057 COVID-19 patients receiving androgen deprivation therapy appeared to have less severity of disease.[95] An outpatient double-blind placebo-controlled trial demonstrated that proxalutamide decrease hospitalization in COVID-19 patients compared to standard of care.[96] Thus, androgen deprivation is a potential agent that can be employed in a multimodal outpatient management protocol in COVID-19.

Statins/Fenofibrate

Although used clinically to lower low density lipoprotein (LDL) cholesterol, statins possess antithrombotic, anti-inflammatory, and immunomodulatory properties.[97-99] In silico molecular docking has demonstrated that statins bind effectively to SARS-CoV-2 major protease and have potential antiviral properties.[97] In addition by decreasing cell membrane cholesterol they may inhibit viral cellular penetration. An in vitro experiment demonstrated simvastatin was able to inhibit SARS-CoV-2 nucleocapsid protein-induced endothelial cell activation and monocyte adhesion to activated endothelium.[98,100] Several observational studies have demonstrated that statin use within 30 days of hospital admission for COVID-19 decreased mortality.[99,101-103] A propensity matched retrospective study during the height of the pandemic in China involving over 13,000 patients of which 1,219 received statins, investigators observed that statin use was significantly associated with a markedly lower risk of death.[103]

In vitro data has demonstrated that fenofibrate stimulates ACE2 dimerization and inhibits receptor-binding domain (RBD) and ACE2 binding, exerting an antiviral effect.[104,105] Fenofibrate increased the glycosphingolipid sulfatide which inhibits viral entry through the cell membrane.[105]

Nutraceuticals

Many nutraceuticals possess adaptogenic, antioxidant, anti-inflammatory, and immunomodulating properties that make them ideal agent to employ in early outpatient therapeutic regimens.[106] Nutraceuticals of interest include vitamin D, ascorbic acid, bioflavonoids, and small molecules such as melatonin and quercetin.[106] Extensive review of these agents is beyond the scope of this chapter; however, we will discuss the major agents employed.

Vitamin D

Observational studies have demonstrated that individuals who live in northern latitudes where vitamin D deficiency is prevalent have worse clinical outcomes when they develop SARS-CoV-2 infection and COVID-19 disease.[107-110] Prior to the pandemic, there was evidence mounting that low vitamin D levels in critically ill persons was associated with a higher risk of developing acute respiratory distress syndrome (ARDS).[111] Low vitamin D levels are highly correlated with increased risk of SARS-CoV-2 infection and adverse outcomes.[109,110,112,113] Vitamin D has many pleiotropic effects involving the immune system, including modulating expression of antiviral defensins which inhibit viral entry and replication, immunomodulatory effects on professional antigen-presenting cells, and anti-inflammatory effects reducing levels of proinflammatory cytokines.[107,109,113-115] In addition, vitamin D via its action on inducing the anti-inflammatory, antiproliferative, antifibrotic, antiapoptotic and vasodilatory ACE2/Ang 1-7/MasR arm of the renin angiotensin system (RAS) downregulating the vasoconstrictive arm of pulmonary renin angiotensin system.[107,109,113,115] Vitamin D deficiency may result in an increase in the activation of the vasoconstrictive, proliferative, proinflammatory, profibrotic arm of pulmonary angiotensin system mediated by Ang 2.[107,109,113,115] Thus vitamin D may prevent or ameliorate the severe lung injury which occurs in patients with severe COVID-19. In a meta-analysis involving over 10,000 patients, supplementation with vitamin D decreased the risk of respiratory infections. Many observational studies have demonstrated that low vitamin D level in patients with COVID-19 is associated with poor clinical outcomes.[109,110,112,113] In a small clinical study high-dose vitamin D supplementation for 7 days resulted in significant conversions of SARS-CoV-2 RT-PCR to negative status, thus suggesting that vitamin D supplementation resulted in decreased viral clearance.[116] Castillo et al in a small randomized trial involving hospitalized patients demonstrated that administration of 25-OH vitamin D (calcifediol) administered for 3 to 7 days when added to a regimen of HCQ and azithromycin significantly reduced severity of disease and need for ICU admission when compared to HCQ and azithromycin treatment alone.[117] Lakkireddy et al performed an open-label randomized trial involving mild to moderately ill hospitalized patients with COVID-19 and demonstrated that administration of high-dose vitamin D for up to 10 days reduced inflammatory markers.[118]

Thus, due to its relatively short-term nontoxic effects, immune-modulating properties, and anti-inflammatory and antiviral effects, vitamin D is ideal for potentially preventing infection and severity of disease and should be incorporated in early and prophylactic treatment protocols against COVID-19.

Quercetin

Flavonoids such as quercetin possess immunomodulatory, anti-inflammatory, and antioxidant properties. In addition, there is mounting in vitro evidence that quercetin possesses the ability to inhibit polymerases, proteases, and many other enzymes necessary for viral replication.[119–124] In addition, studies have demonstrated that quercetin can bind to viral capsid proteins, thus potentially preventing viral assembly.[122,124–126] A recent open-label randomized controlled trial of nonhospitalized patients demonstrated that quercetin added to standard care led to a reduction in the length of hospital stay need for increased noninvasive oxygen delivery and ICU admission.[127] In a small open-label randomized controlled trial involving 42 consecutive patients with COVID-19, Quercetin Phytosome added to standard care revealed a significant amelioration of symptoms, decreased inflammatory markers, and increased viral clearance in the treatment group compared to standard care.[119] In the clinical trials to date quercetin demonstrates very low toxicity, intolerance, and appears safe to use. Coadministration with ascorbic acid seems to potentiate the antiviral, anti-inflammatory effects of both agents.[120] Due to ease of use and safety profile, quercetin is an ideal agent for early outpatient treatment protocols.

Ascorbic Acid

There is both in vitro and in vivo evidence that ascorbic acid (AA) possesses antiviral, anti-inflammatory, antioxidant, and immune-modulating properties.[128–131] Humans lack the enzymatic machinery to synthesize AA and require supplementation to have adequate levels. Hypovitaminosis of AA is common in critical illness.[130] Several studies in patients with pneumonia and sepsis demonstrate that AA levels are depleted.[130,132,133] In addition, AA acts synergistically with and is able to recycle quercitin.[120] AA is necessary cofactor in the synthesis of catecholamines, enhances the synthesis of IFN production, limits proinflammatory cytokine end organ injury, and inhibits the activation of the NLRP3 inflammasome.[132,134–141] COVID-19 infection leads to intracellular disruption via its viroporin proteins activating immune-signaling inflammasome NLRP3.[142,143] Activation of NLRP inflammasome plays a critical role in the increased production of inflammatory cytokines resulting in the cytokine storm.[142] Experimental evidence supports that AA inhibits the activation of NLRP by scavenging mitochondrial reactive oxygen species (ROS).[142,143] Two large meta-analyses involving critically ill patients demonstrated that intravenous vitamin C administration showed no adverse reactions, reduced the need for fluids and vasopressor support, and reduced intubation time.[144,145] In summary, due to the pleiotropic effects of AA on important physiologic functions, its properties as powerful antioxidant/ROS scavenger, and previous successful clinical use as a pharmacologic agent in the treatment of hyperinflammatory conditions, AA should be considered in the outpatient management of COVID-19.

Melatonin

Melatonin possesses pleiotropic actions including antiviral, free radical scavenging, anti-inflammatory, and immune-modulating properties.[76,146–148] Furthermore, melatonin via a melatonergic-mitochondrial pathway can alter effector immune cell phenotype from a proinflammatory to an anti-inflammatory-quiescent phenotype, thus possibly attenuating the cytokine storm.[149–151] There is significant in vitro and in vivo evidence that melatonin possesses the ability to prevent end organ injury caused by lethal viral infections.[146,147,152–157] In particular in an in vitro model of Ebola-induced endothelial injury, melatonin attenuated endothelial injury. Melatonin prevented multiorgan injury in several animal models of sepsis and in two small clinical trials administration of melatonin to neonates with sepsis melatonin improved clinical outcomes and prevented lipoperoxidation, a marker of oxidant injury.[147,154,157–160] A recent study utilizing a large network database maintained by the Cleveland Clinic investigators observed that after adjusting for confounding variables, melatonin use was associated with a significant decrease in the development of SARS-CoV-2 infection in individuals using melatonin.[161] Melatonin possesses an excellent safety profile and self-limited adverse symptoms related to intolerance. Although the exact efficacious dose for COVID-19 has not been determined, the agent is ideal for early treatment protocols.

Zinc

Zinc is an essential cofactor in proper immune cell function and low zinc levels has been associated with poor clinical outcomes in patients with COVID-19 disease.[162] Inflammatory states such as infection have been known to cause depletion of Zinc.[163–165] In addition, zinc depletion and deficiency increase the severity of inflammatory states.[163–165] Zinc has antioxidant and anti-inflammatory properties via a feedback loop involving NFK-β, thereby decreasing proinflammatory cytokine expression.[166] Zinc may possess antiviral properties. Zinc administered in addition with a zinc ionophore such as HCQ was implemented as a therapeutic strategy in the early days of the pandemic.[32,163,167] In a retrospective analysis of zinc as an add-on therapy to HCQ and azithromycin, Carlucci et al. observed that zinc was associated with improved clinical outcomes in hospitalized patients with COVID-19.[39] Short-term therapy with zinc is associated with little toxicity and appears to have a good margin of safety.

Conclusion

In western developed nations, public health bodies have offered very little recommendations regarding early outpatient treatment of COVID-19. Agents that have been employed in early treatment by clinicians are relatively inexpensive and available. The majority of these agents under the clinician's supervision have reasonable margins of safety. Although most of the agents employed in outpatient management have not undergone large randomized controlled trials, it is the authors' opinion that the bedside clinician employing his knowledge of pathophysiology of COVID-19 and the preclinical and clinical data available can overcome the therapeutic nihilism that exists today in the early treatment of this disease.

References

1. https://www.covid19treatmentguidelines.nih.gov/management/clinical-management/nonhospitalized-adults–therapeutic-management/

2. Payne JD, Sims K, Peacock C, Welch T, Berggren RE. Evidence-based approach to early outpatient treatment of SARS-CoV-2 (COVID-19) infection. Proc Bayl Univ Med Cent 2021;34(4):464–468

3. McCullough PA, Kelly RJ, Ruocco G, et al. Pathophysiological basis and rationale for early outpatient treatment of SARS-CoV-2 (COVID-19) infection. Am J Med 2021;134(1):16–22

4. https://health.usnews.com/conditions/articles/when-are-coronavirus-symptoms-bad-enough-to-warrant-going-to-the-hospital

5. Moghadas SM, Shoukat A, Fitzpatrick MC, et al. Projecting hospital utilization during the COVID-19 outbreaks in the United States. Proc Natl Acad Sci U S A 2020;117(16):9122–9126

6. McCullough PA, Alexander PE, Armstrong R, et al. Multifaceted highly targeted sequential multidrug treatment of early ambulatory high-risk SARS-CoV-2 infection (COVID-19). Rev Cardiovasc Med 2020;21(4):517–530

7. McCullough PA, Vijay K. SARS-CoV-2 infection and the COVID-19 pandemic: a call to action for therapy and interventions to resolve the crisis of hospitalization, death, and handle the aftermath. Rev Cardiovasc Med 2021;22(1):9–10

8. Griffin DO, Brennan-Rieder D, Ngo B, et al. The importance of understanding the stages of COVID-19 in treatment and trials. AIDS Rev 2021;23(1):40–47

9. Dougan M, Nirula A, Azizad M, et al; BLAZE-1 Investigators. Bamlanivimab plus Etesevimab in mild or moderate COVID-19. N Engl J Med 2021;0(0): null. doi:10.1056/NEJMoa2102685

10. Group RC, Horby PW, Mafham M, et al. Casirivimab and imdevimab in patients admitted to hospital with COVID-19 (RECOVERY): a randomised, controlled, open-label, platform trial. *medRxiv*. Published online 2021. doi:10.1101/2021.06.15.21258542

11. Weinreich DM, Sivapalasingam S, Norton T, et al; Trial Investigators. REGN-COV2, a neutralizing antibody cocktail, in outpatients with Covid-19. N Engl J Med 2021;384(3):238–251

12. https://files.covid19treatmentguidelines.nih.gov/guidelines/covid19treatmentguidelines.pdf

13. https://www.england.nhs.uk/coronavirus/secondary-care/management-confirmed-coronavirus-covid-19/clinical-medical-management/

14. https://www.idsociety.org/covid-19-real-time-learning-network/therapeutics-and-interventions/immunomodulators/#antisarscov2

15. https://covid19criticalcare.com/wp-content/uploads/2020/12/FLCCC-Protocols-%E2%80%93-A-Guide-to-the-Management-of-COVID-19.pdf

16. Derwand R, Scholz M, Zelenko V. COVID-19 outpatients: early risk-stratified treatment with zinc plus low-dose hydroxychloroquine and azithromycin: a retrospective case series study. Int J Antimicrob Agents 2020;56(6):106214

17. Turkia M. The history of methylprednisolone, ascorbic acid, thiamine, and heparin protocol and I-MASK+ ivermectin protocol for COVID-19. Cureus 2020;12(12):e12403

18. Marik PE, Varon J, Kory P. Treatment of COVID-19 is critically phase specific. Crit Care Shock 2020;23(5):201–203

19. Kory P, Kanne JP. SARS-CoV-2 organising pneumonia: "Has there been a widespread failure to identify and treat this prevalent condition in COVID-19?". BMJ Open Respir Res 2020;7(1):e000724

20. Zheng Z, Peng F, Xu B, et al. Risk factors of critical & mortal COVID-19 cases: a systematic literature review and meta-analysis. J Infect 2020;81(2):e16–e25

21. Yang F, Shi S, Zhu J, Shi J, Dai K, Chen X. Clinical characteristics and outcomes of cancer patients with COVID-19. J Med Virol 2020;92(10):2067–2073

22. Greenhalgh T, Knight M, Inda-Kim M, Fulop NJ, Leach J, Vindrola-Padros C. Remote management of covid-19 using home pulse oximetry and virtual ward support. BMJ 2021;372:n677

23. Hudson AJ, Benjamin J, Jardeleza T, et al. Clinical interpretation of peripheral pulse oximeters labeled "Not for Medical Use." Ann Fam Med 2018;16(6):552–554

24. Luks AM, Swenson ER. Pulse oximetry for monitoring patients with COVID-19 at home: potential pitfalls and practical guidance. Ann Am Thorac Soc 2020;17(9):1040–1046

25. Siemieniuk RA, Bartoszko JJ, Díaz Martinez JP, et al. Antibody and cellular therapies for treatment of covid-19: a living systematic review and network meta-analysis. BMJ 2021;374(2231):n2231

26. An EUA for bamlanivimab and etesevimab for COVID-19. Med Lett Drugs Ther 2021; 63(1621):49–50

27. Deb P, Molla MMA, Saif-Ur-Rahman KM. An update to monoclonal antibody as therapeutic option against COVID-19. Biosaf Health 2021;3(2):87–91

28. Kreuzberger N, Hirsch C, Chai KL, et al. SARS-CoV-2-neutralising monoclonal antibodies for treatment of COVID-19. Cochrane Database Syst Rev 2021;9(9):CD013825

29. Pan H, Peto R, Henao-Restrepo A-M, et al; WHO Solidarity Trial Consortium. Repurposed antiviral drugs for Covid-19: interim WHO solidarity trial results. N Engl J Med 2021;384(6):497–511

30. Johnston C, Brown ER, Stewart J, et al; COVID-19 Early Treatment Study Team. Hydroxychloroquine with or without azithromycin for treatment of early SARS-CoV-2 infection among high-risk outpatient adults: a randomized clinical trial. EClinicalMedicine 2021;33:100773

31. Shittu MO, Afolami OI. Improving the efficacy of chloroquine and hydroxychloroquine against SARS-CoV-2 may require zinc additives a better synergy for future COVID-19 clinical trials. Infez Med 2020;28(2):192–197

32. Derwand R, Scholz M. Does zinc supplementation enhance the clinical efficacy of chloroquine/hydroxychloroquine to win today's battle against COVID-19? Med Hypotheses 2020;142:109815

33. Gao J, Tian Z, Yang X. Breakthrough: chloroquine phosphate has shown apparent efficacy in treatment of COVID-19 associated pneumonia in clinical studies. Biosci Trends 2020;14(1):72–73

34. Arshad S, Kilgore P, Chaudhry ZS, et al; Henry Ford COVID-19 Task Force. Treatment with hydroxychloroquine, azithromycin, and combination in patients hospitalized with COVID-19. Int J Infect Dis 2020;97:396–403

35. Gautret P, Lagier J-C, Parola P, et al. Hydroxychloroquine and azithromycin as a treatment of COVID-19: results of an open-label non-randomized clinical trial. Int J Antimicrob Agents 2020;56(1):105949

36. Lei Z-N, Wu Z-X, Dong S, et al. Chloroquine and hydroxychloroquine in the treatment of malaria and repurposing in treating COVID-19. Pharmacol Ther 2020;216:107672

37. Million M, Lagier J-C, Gautret P, et al. Early treatment of COVID-19 patients with hydroxychloroquine and azithromycin: a retrospective analysis of 1061 cases in Marseille, France. Travel Med Infect Dis 2020;35:101738

38. Paccoud O, Tubach F, Baptiste A, et al. Compassionate use of hydroxychloroquine in clinical practice for patients with mild to severe Covid-19 in a French university hospital. Clin Infect Dis 2020;ciaa791

39. Carlucci PM, Ahuja T, Petrilli C, Rajagopalan H, Jones S, Rahimian J. Zinc sulfate in combination with a zinc ionophore may improve outcomes in hospitalized COVID-19 patients. J Med Microbiol 2020;69(10): 1228–1234

40. Reis G, Moreira Silva EADS, Medeiros Silva DC, et al; TOGETHER Investigators. Effect of early treatment with hydroxychloroquine or lopinavir and ritonavir on risk of hospitalization among patients with COVID-19: the TOGETHER randomized clinical trial. JAMA Netw Open 2021;4(4): e216468–e216468

41. Schwartz I, Boesen ME, Cerchiaro G, et al; ALBERTA HOPE COVID-19 Collaborators. Assessing the efficacy and safety of hydroxychloroquine as outpatient treatment of COVID-19: a randomized controlled trial. CMAJ Open 2021;9(2):E693–E702

42. Singh B, Ryan H, Kredo T, Chaplin M, Fletcher T. Chloroquine or hydroxychloroquine for prevention and treatment of COVID-19. Cochrane Database Syst Rev 2021;2(2): CD013587

43. Elavarasi A, Prasad M, Seth T, et al. Chloroquine and hydroxychloroquine for the treatment of COVID-19: a systematic review and meta-analysis. J Gen Intern Med 2020;35(11):3308–3314

44. Skipper CP, Pastick KA, Engen NW, et al. Hydroxychloroquine in nonhospitalized

adults with early COVID-19: a randomized trial. Ann Intern Med 2020;173(8):623–631

45. Acharya D, Liu G, Gack MU. Dysregulation of type I interferon responses in COVID-19. Nat Rev Immunol 2020;20(7):397–398

46. Palermo E, Di Carlo D, Sgarbanti M, Hiscott J. Type I interferons in COVID-19 pathogenesis. Biology (Basel) 2021;10(9):829

47. Nakhlband A, Fakhari A, Azizi H. Interferon-beta offers promising avenues to COVID-19 treatment: a systematic review and meta-analysis of clinical trial studies. Naunyn Schmiedebergs Arch Pharmacol 2021;3 94(5):829–838

48. Jagannathan P, Andrews JR, Bonilla H, et al. Peginterferon Lambda-1a for treatment of outpatients with uncomplicated COVID-19: a randomized placebo-controlled trial. Nat Commun 2021;12(1):1967

49. Mosaddeghi P, Shahabinezhad F, Dehghani Z, et al. Therapeutic approaches for COVID-19 based on the interferon-mediated immune responses. Curr Signal Transduct Ther 2021; 16:1

50. Feld JJ, Kandel C, Biondi MJ, et al. Peginterferon lambda for the treatment of outpatients with COVID-19: a phase 2, placebo-controlled randomised trial. Lancet Respir Med 2021;9(5):498–510

51. Idelsis E-M, Jesus P-E, Duncan Roberts Y, et al. Effect and safety of combination of interferon alpha-2b and gamma or interferon alpha-2b for negativization of SARS-CoV-2 viral RNA: preliminary results of a randomized controlled clinical trial. 2020. doi:10.1101/2020.07.29.20164251

52. Yu J, Lu X, Tong L, et al. Interferon-α-2b aerosol inhalation is associated with improved clinical outcomes in patients with coronavirus disease-2019. Br J Clin Pharmacol 2021; n/a(n/a): doi:https://doi.org/10.1111/bcp.14898

53. Ghasemnejad-Berenji M, Pashapour S. Favipiravir and COVID-19: a simplified summary. Drug Res (Stuttg) 2021;71(3): 166–170

54. Cai Q, Yang M, Liu D, et al. Experimental treatment with favipiravir for COVID-19: an open-label control study. Engineering (Beijing) 2020;6(10):1192–1198

55. Dabbous HM, Abd-Elsalam S, El-Sayed MH, et al. Efficacy of favipiravir in COVID-19 treatment: a multi-center randomized study. Arch Virol 2021;166(3):949–954

56. Ivashchenko AA, Dmitriev KA, Vostokova NV, et al. AVIFAVIR for treatment of patients with moderate coronavirus disease 2019 (COVID-19): interim results of a phase II/III multicenter randomized clinical trial. Clin Infect Dis 2021;73(3):531–534

57. Pulla P. Covid-19: India's slow moving treatment guidelines are misleading and harming patients. BMJ 2021;372:n278

58. Łagocka R, Dziedziejko V, Kłos P, Pawlik A. Favipiravir in therapy of viral infections. J Clin Med 2021;10(2):E273

59. Agrawal U, Raju R, Udwadia ZF. Favipiravir: a new and emerging antiviral option in COVID-19. Med J Armed Forces India 2020; 76(4):370–376

60. Ohe M, Furuya K, Goudarzi H. Multidrug treatment for COVID-19. Drug Discov Ther 2021;15(1):39–41

61. Pepperrell T, Pilkington V, Owen A, Wang J, Hill AM. Review of safety and minimum pricing of nitazoxanide for potential treatment of COVID-19. J Virus Erad 2020; 6(2):52–60

62. Silva M, Espejo AL, Pereyra M, et al. Efficacy of nitazoxanide in reducing the viral load in COVID-19 patients. Randomized, placebo-controlled, single-blinded, parallel group, pilot study. *medRxiv*. Published online 2021. doi:10.1101/2021.03.03.21252509

63. Blum VF, Cimerman S, Hunter JR, et al. Nitazoxanide superiority to placebo to treat moderate COVID-19: a Pilot prove of concept randomized double-blind clinical trial. EClinicalMedicine 2021;37:100981

64. Rocco PRM, Silva PL, Cruz FF, et al; SARITA-2 investigators. Early use of nitazoxanide in mild COVID-19 disease: randomised, placebo-controlled trial. Eur Respir J 2021; 58(1):2003725

65. Cadegiani FA, Goren A, Wambier CG, McCoy J. Early COVID-19 therapy with azithromycin plus nitazoxanide, ivermectin or hydroxychloroquine in outpatient settings significantly improved COVID-19 outcomes compared to known outcomes in untreated patients. New Microbes New Infect 2021; 43:100915

66. Caly L, Druce JD, Catton MG, Jans DA, Wagstaff KM. The FDA-approved drug ivermectin inhibits the replication of SARS-CoV-2 in vitro. Antiviral Res 2020;178:104787

67. Hernández-Vásquez A, Vargas-Fernández R, Azañedo D. Considerations on the article

"Antiviral and anti-Inflammatory properties of ivermectin and its potential use in COVID-19". Arch Bronconeumol (Engl Ed) 2020;56(12):832

68. Formiga FR, Leblanc R, de Souza Rebouças J, Farias LP, de Oliveira RN, Pena L. Ivermectin: an award-winning drug with expected antiviral activity against COVID-19. J Control Release 2021;329:758–761

69. Portmann-Baracco A, Bryce-Alberti M, Accinelli RA. Antiviral and anti-inflammatory properties of ivermectin and its potential use in COVID-19. Arch Bronconeumol (Engl Ed) 2020;56(12):831

70. Bryant A, Lawrie TA, Dowswell T, et al. Ivermectin for prevention and treatment of COVID-19 infection: a systematic review, meta-analysis, and trial sequential analysis to inform clinical guidelines. Am J Ther 2021;28(4):e434–e460

71. Kory P, Meduri GU, Varon J, Iglesias J, Marik PE. Review of the emerging evidence demonstrating the efficacy of ivermectin in the prophylaxis and treatment of COVID-19. Am J Ther 2021;28(3):e299–e318

72. Padhy BM, Mohanty RR, Das S, Meher BR. Therapeutic potential of ivermectin as add on treatment in COVID 19: a systematic review and meta-analysis. J Pharm Pharm Sci 2020; 23:462–469

73. https://ivmmeta.com/#tp

74. Roman YM, Burela PA, Pasupuleti V, Piscoya A, Vidal JE, Hernandez AV. Ivermectin for the treatment of COVID-19: a systematic review and meta-analysis of randomized controlled trials. Clin Infect Dis 2021;ciab591

75. Sukhatme VP, Reiersen AM, Vayttaden SJ, Sukhatme VV. Fluvoxamine: a review of its mechanism of action and its role in COVID-19. Front Pharmacol 2021;12:652688

76. Anderson GM. Fluvoxamine, melatonin and COVID-19. Psychopharmacology (Berl) 2021;238(2):611

77. Lenze EJ, Mattar C, Zorumski CF, et al. Fluvoxamine vs placebo and clinical deterioration in outpatients with symptomatic COVID-19: a randomized clinical trial. JAMA 2020;324(22):2292–2300

78. Seftel D, Boulware DR. Prospective cohort of fluvoxamine for early treatment of coronavirus disease 19. Open Forum Infect Dis 2021;8(2):b050

79. Hashimoto K. Repurposing of CNS drugs to treat COVID-19 infection: targeting the sigma-1 receptor. Eur Arch Psychiatry Clin Neurosci 2021;271(2):249–258

80. Ramakrishnan S, Nicolau DV Jr, Langford B, et al. Inhaled budesonide in the treatment of early COVID-19 (STOIC): a phase 2, open-label, randomised controlled trial. Lancet Respir Med 2021;9(7):763–772

81. Group PC, Yu L-M, Bafadhel M, et al. Inhaled budesonide for COVID-19 in people at higher risk of adverse outcomes in the community: interim analyses from the PRINCIPLE trial. *medRxiv*. Published online 2021. doi:10.1101/2021.04.10.21254672

82. Yu L-M, Bafadhel M, Dorward J, et al; PRINCIPLE Trial Collaborative Group. Inhaled budesonide for COVID-19 in people at high risk of complications in the community in the UK (PRINCIPLE): a randomised, controlled, open-label, adaptive platform trial. Lancet 2021;398(10303):843–855

83. Liang H, Ding X, Li H, Li L, Sun T. Association between prior aspirin use and acute respiratory distress syndrome incidence in at-risk patients: a systematic review and meta-analysis. Front Pharmacol 2020;11:738

84. Chow JH, Khanna AK, Kethireddy S, et al. Aspirin use is associated with decreased mechanical ventilation, intensive care unit admission, and in-hospital mortality in hospitalized patients with coronavirus disease 2019. Anesth Analg 2021;132(4):930–941

85. Osborne TF, Veigulis ZP, Arreola DM, Mahajan SM, Röösli E, Curtin CM. Association of mortality and aspirin prescription for COVID-19 patients at the Veterans Health Administration. PLoS One 2021;16(2):e0246825

86. Talasaz AH, Sadeghipour P, Kakavand H, et al. Antithrombotic therapy in COVID-19: systematic summary of ongoing or completed randomized trials. *medRxiv*. Published online 2021. doi:10.1101/2021.01.04.21249227

87. Miesbach W, Makris M. COVID-19: coagulopathy, risk of thrombosis, and the rationale for anticoagulation. Clin Appl Thromb Hemost 2020;26:1076029620938149

88. Levi M, Thachil J, Iba T, Levy JH. Coagulation abnormalities and thrombosis in patients with COVID-19. Lancet Haematol 2020;7(6): e438–e440

89. Zarychanski R. Therapeutic anticoagulation in critically ill patients with Covid-19—preliminary report. *medRxiv*. Published online 2021. doi:10.1101/2021.03.10.21252749

90. Cuker A, Tseng EK, Nieuwlaat R, et al. American Society of Hematology 2021 guidelines on the use of anticoagulation for thromboprophylaxis in patients with COVID-19. Blood Adv 2021;5(3):872–888

91. Cadegiani FA. Repurposing existing drugs for COVID-19: an endocrinology perspective. BMC Endocr Disord 2020;20(1):149

92. Cadegiani FA, McCoy J, Gustavo Wambier C, Goren A. Early antiandrogen therapy with dutasteride reduces viral shedding, inflammatory responses, and time-to-remission in males with COVID-19: a randomized, double-blind, placebo-controlled interventional trial (EAT-DUTA AndroCoV Trial - Biochemical). Cureus 2021;13(2):e13047

93. Cadegiani FA, McCoy J, Gustavo Wambier C, et al. Proxalutamide significantly accelerates viral clearance and reduces time to clinical remission in patients with mild to moderate COVID-19: results from a randomized, double-blinded, placebo-controlled trial. Cureus 2021;13(2):e13492

94. Goren A, Wambier CG, Herrera S, et al. Anti-androgens may protect against severe COVID-19 outcomes: results from a prospective cohort study of 77 hospitalized men. J Eur Acad Dermatol Venereol 2021;35(1):e13–e15

95. Lee KM, Heberer K, Gao A, et al. A population-level analysis of the protective effects of androgen deprivation therapy against COVID-19 disease incidence and severity. *medRxiv*. Published online 2021. doi:10.1101/2021.05.10.21255146

96. McCoy J, Goren A, Cadegiani FA, et al. Proxalutamide reduces the rate of hospitalization for COVID-19 male outpatients: a randomized double-blinded placebo-controlled trial. Front Med (Lausanne) 2021;8:668698

97. Reiner Ž, Hatamipour M, Banach M, et al. Statins and the COVID-19 main protease: *in silico* evidence on direct interaction. Arch Med Sci 2020;16(3):490–496

98. Lee KCH, Sewa DW, Phua GC. Potential role of statins in COVID-19. Int J Infect Dis 2020;96:615–617

99. Russo V, Silverio A, Scudiero F, et al. Preadmission statin therapy and clinical outcome in hospitalized patients with COVID-19: an Italian Multicenter Observational Study. J Cardiovasc Pharmacol 2021;78(1):e94–e100

100. Casari I, Manfredi M, Metharom P, Falasca M. Dissecting lipid metabolism alterations in SARS-CoV-2. Prog Lipid Res 2021;82:101092

101. Cariou B, Goronflot T, Rimbert A, et al; CORONADO investigators. Routine use of statins and increased COVID-19 related mortality in inpatients with type 2 diabetes: Results from the CORONADO study. Diabetes Metab 2021;47(2):101202

102. Marić I, Oskotsky T, Kosti I, et al. Decreased mortality rate among COVID-19 patients prescribed statins: data from Electronic Health Records in the US. Front Med (Lausanne) 2021;8:639804

103. Zhang X-J, Qin J-J, Cheng X, et al. In-hospital use of statins is associated with a reduced risk of mortality among individuals with COVID-19. Cell Metab 2020;32(2):176–187.e4

104. Davies SP, Mycroft-West CJ, Pagani I, et al. The hyperlipidaemic drug fenofibrate significantly reduces infection by SARS-CoV-2 in cell culture models. Front Pharmacol 2021;12:660490

105. Buschard K. Fenofibrate increases the amount of sulfatide which seems beneficial against Covid-19. Med Hypotheses 2020;143:110127

106. Subedi L, Tchen S, Gaire BP, Hu B, Hu K. Adjunctive nutraceutical therapies for COVID-19. Int J Mol Sci 2021;22(4):1963

107. Bilezikian JP, Bikle D, Hewison M, et al. Mechanisms in endocrinology: vitamin D and COVID-19. Eur J Endocrinol 2020;183(5):R133–R147

108. Carpagnano GE, Di Lecce V, Quaranta VN, et al. Vitamin D deficiency as a predictor of poor prognosis in patients with acute respiratory failure due to COVID-19. J Endocrinol Invest 2021;44(4):765–771

109. Getachew B, Tizabi Y. Vitamin D and COVID-19: role of ACE2, age, gender, and ethnicity. J Med Virol 2021;93(9):5285–5294

110. Liu N, Sun J, Wang X, Zhang T, Zhao M, Li H. Low vitamin D status is associated with

coronavirus disease 2019 outcomes: a systematic review and meta-analysis. Int J Infect Dis 2021;104:58–64

111. Dancer RCA, Parekh D, Lax S, et al. Vitamin D deficiency contributes directly to the acute respiratory distress syndrome (ARDS). Thorax 2015;70(7):617–624

112. Crafa A, Cannarella R, Condorelli RA, et al. Influence of 25-hydroxy-cholecalciferol levels on SARS-CoV-2 infection and COVID-19 severity: A systematic review and meta-analysis. EClinicalMedicine 2021;37:100967

113. Kumar R, Rathi H, Haq A, Wimalawansa SJ, Sharma A. Putative roles of vitamin D in modulating immune response and immunopathology associated with COVID-19. Virus Res 2021;292:198235

114. Shi YY, Liu TJ, Fu JH, et al. Vitamin D/VDR signaling attenuates lipopolysaccharide-induced acute lung injury by maintaining the integrity of the pulmonary epithelial barrier. Mol Med Rep 2016;13(2):1186–1194

115. Kong J, Zhu X, Shi Y, et al. VDR attenuates acute lung injury by blocking Ang-2-Tie-2 pathway and renin-angiotensin system. Mol Endocrinol 2013;27(12):2116–2125

116. Rastogi A, Bhansali A, Khare N, et al. Short term, high-dose vitamin D supplementation for COVID-19 disease: a randomised, placebo-controlled, study (SHADE study). Postgrad Med J 2020; postgradmedj-2020-139065 10.1136/postgradmedj-2020-139065

117. Entrenas Castillo M, Entrenas Costa LM, Vaquero Barrios JM, et al. Effect of calcifediol treatment and best available therapy versus best available therapy on intensive care unit admission and mortality among patients hospitalized for COVID-19: A pilot randomized clinical study. J Steroid Biochem Mol Biol 2020;203:105751

118. Lakkireddy M, Gadiga SG, Malathi RD, et al. Impact of daily high dose oral vitamin D therapy on the inflammatory markers in patients with COVID 19 disease. Sci Rep 2021;11(1):10641

119. Di Pierro F, Iqtadar S, Khan A, et al. Potential clinical benefits of quercetin in the early stage of COVID-19: results of a second, pilot, randomized, controlled and open-label clinical trial. Int J Gen Med 2021;14:2807–2816

120. Colunga Biancatelli RML, Berrill M, Catravas JD, Marik PE. Quercetin and vitamin C: an experimental, synergistic therapy for the prevention and treatment of SARS-CoV-2 related disease (COVID-19). Front Immunol 2020;11:1451

121. Mrityunjaya M, Pavithra V, Neelam R, Janhavi P, Halami PM, Ravindra PV. Immune-boosting, antioxidant and anti-inflammatory food supplements targeting pathogenesis of COVID-19. Front Immunol 2020;11:570122

122. Agrawal P, Agrawal C, Blunden G. Quercetin: antiviral significance and possible COVID-19 integrative considerations. Nat Prod Commun 2020;15

123. Saeedi-Boroujeni A, Mahmoudian-Sani M-R. Anti-inflammatory potential of Quercetin in COVID-19 treatment. J Inflamm (Lond) 2021;18(1):3

124. Saakre M, Mathew D, Ravisankar V. Perspectives on plant flavonoid quercetin-based drugs for novel SARS-CoV-2. Beni Suef Univ J Basic Appl Sci 2021;10(1):21

125. Derosa G, Maffioli P, D'Angelo A, Di Pierro F. A role for quercetin in coronavirus disease 2019 (COVID-19). Phytother Res 2021; 35(3):1230–1236

126. Mathioudakis MM, Rodríguez-Moreno L, Sempere RN, Aranda MA, Livieratos I. Multifaceted capsid proteins: multiple interactions suggest multiple roles for Pepino mosaic virus capsid protein. Mol Plant Microbe Interact 2014;27(12):1356–1369

127. Di Pierro F, Derosa G, Maffioli P, et al. Possible therapeutic effects of adjuvant quercetin supplementation against early-stage COVID-19 infection: a prospective, randomized, controlled, and open-label study. Int J Gen Med 2021;14:2359–2366

128. Mohammed BM, Fisher BJ, Kraskauskas D, et al. Vitamin C: a novel regulator of neutrophil extracellular trap formation. Nutrients 2013;5(8):3131–3151

129. Wilson JX. Mechanism of action of vitamin C in sepsis: ascorbate modulates redox signaling in endothelium. Biofactors 2009; 35(1):5–13

130. Marik PE. Vitamin C for the treatment of sepsis: the scientific rationale. Pharmacol Ther 2018;189:63–70

131. Moskowitz A, Andersen LW, Huang DT, et al. Ascorbic acid, corticosteroids, and thiamine

in sepsis: a review of the biologic rationale and the present state of clinical evaluation. Crit Care 2018;22(1):283

132. Abobaker A, Alzwi A, Alraied AHA. Overview of the possible role of vitamin C in management of COVID-19. Pharmacol Rep 2020;72(6):1517–1528

133. Carr AC, Spencer E, Dixon L, Chambers ST. Patients with community acquired pneumonia exhibit depleted vitamin C status and elevated oxidative stress. Nutrients 2020;12(5):E1318

134. May JM, Qu Z-C, Nazarewicz R, Dikalov S. Ascorbic acid efficiently enhances neuronal synthesis of norepinephrine from dopamine. Brain Res Bull 2013;90:35–42

135. Kim Y, Kim H, Bae S, et al. Vitamin C is an essential factor on the anti-viral immune responses through the production of interferon-α/β at the initial stage of influenza a virus (H3N2) infection. Immune Netw 2013;13(2):70–74

136. Pizzicannella J, Fonticoli L, Guarnieri S, et al. Antioxidant ascorbic acid modulates NLRP3 inflammasome in LPS-G treated oral stem cells through NFκB/caspase-1/IL-1β pathway. Antioxidants 2021;10(5):797

137. Ascorbic Acid and Catecholamines. Ascorbic acid and catecholamines. Nutr Rev 1976; 34(6):181–182

138. Carr AC, Shaw GM, Fowler AA, Natarajan R. Ascorbate-dependent vasopressor synthesis: a rationale for vitamin C administration in severe sepsis and septic shock? Crit Care 2015;19:418

139. Cai Y, Li Y-F, Tang L-P, et al. A new mechanism of vitamin C effects on A/FM/1/47(H1N1) virus-induced pneumonia in restraint-stressed mice. BioMed Res Int 2015;2015: 675149

140. Fowler AA III, Truwit JD, Hite RD, et al. Effect of vitamin C infusion on organ failure and biomarkers of inflammation and vascular injury in patients with sepsis and severe acute respiratory failure: the CITRIS-ALI randomized clinical trial. JAMA 2019; 322(13):1261–1270

141. Marik PE, Hooper MH. Adjuvant vitamin C in critically ill patients undergoing renal replacement therapy: What's the right dose? Crit Care 2018;22(1):320

142. Sang X, Wang H, Chen Y, et al. Vitamin C inhibits the activation of the NLRP3 inflammasome by scavenging mitochondrial ROS. In: 2016

143. Shah A. Novel coronavirus-induced NLRP3 inflammasome activation: a potential drug target in the treatment of COVID-19. Front Immunol 2020;11:1021

144. Zhang M, Jativa DF. Vitamin C supplementation in the critically ill: a systematic review and meta-analysis. SAGE Open Med 2018;6:2050312118807615

145. Hemilä H, Chalker E. Vitamin C may reduce the duration of mechanical ventilation in critically ill patients: a meta-regression analysis. J Intensive Care 2020;8:15

146. Colunga Biancatelli RML, Berrill M, Mohammed YH, Marik PE. Melatonin for the treatment of sepsis: the scientific rationale. J Thorac Dis 2020;12(Suppl 1):S54–S65

147. Carrillo-Vico A, Lardone PJ, Naji L, et al. Beneficial pleiotropic actions of melatonin in an experimental model of septic shock in mice: regulation of pro-/anti-inflammatory cytokine network, protection against oxidative damage and anti-apoptotic effects. J Pineal Res 2005;39(4):400–408

148. Bahrampour Juybari K, Pourhanifeh MH, Hosseinzadeh A, Hemati K, Mehrzadi S. Melatonin potentials against viral infections including COVID-19: Current evidence and new findings. Virus Res 2020;287:198108

149. Reiter RJ, Sharma R, Ma Q, Dominquez-Rodriguez A, Marik PE, Abreu-Gonzalez P. Melatonin inhibits COVID-19-induced cytokine storm by reversing aerobic glycolysis in immune cells: a mechanistic analysis. Med Drug Discov 2020;6:100044

150. Boga JA, Coto-Montes A, Rosales-Corral SA, Tan D-X, Reiter RJ. Beneficial actions of melatonin in the management of viral infections: a new use for this "molecular handyman"? Rev Med Virol 2012;22(5): 323–338

151. Anderson G, Carbone A, Mazzoccoli G. Aryl hydrocarbon receptor role in co-ordinating SARS-CoV-2 entry and symptomatology: linking cytotoxicity changes in COVID-19 and cancers; modulation by racial discrimination stress. Biology (Basel) 2020;9(9):E249

152. Cross KM, Landis DM, Sehgal L, Payne JD. Melatonin for the early treatment of COVID-19: a narrative review of current evidence and possible efficacy. Endocr Pract 2021;27(8):850–855

153. Junaid A, Tang H, van Reeuwijk A, et al. Ebola hemorrhagic shock syndrome-on-a-chip. iScience 2020;23(1):100765

154. Ji M-H, Xia D-G, Zhu L-Y, et al. Short- and long-term protective effects of melatonin in a mouse model of sepsis-associated encephalopathy. Inflammation 2018;41(2):515–529

155. Nunes O da S, Pereira R de S. Regression of herpes viral infection symptoms using melatonin and SB-73: comparison with Acyclovir. J Pineal Res 2008;44(4):373–378

156. Silvestri M, Rossi GA. Melatonin: its possible role in the management of viral infections—a brief review. Ital J Pediatr 2013;39(1):61

157. Srinivasan V, Mohamed M, Kato H. Melatonin in bacterial and viral infections with focus on sepsis: a review. Recent Pat Endocr Metab Immune Drug Discov 2012;6(1):30–39

158. El Frargy M, El-Sharkawy HM, Attia GF. Use of melatonin as an adjuvant therapy in neonatal sepsis. J Neonatal Perinatal Med 2015;8(3):227–232

159. El-Gendy FM, El-Hawy MA, Hassan MG. Beneficial effect of melatonin in the treatment of neonatal sepsis. J Matern Fetal Neonatal Med 2018;31(17):2299–2303

160. Lowes DA, Webster NR, Murphy MP, Galley HF. Antioxidants that protect mitochondria reduce interleukin-6 and oxidative stress, improve mitochondrial function, and reduce biochemical markers of organ dysfunction in a rat model of acute sepsis. Br J Anaesth 2013;110(3):472–480

161. Zhou Y, Hou Y, Shen J, et al. A network medicine approach to investigation and population-based validation of disease manifestations and drug repurposing for COVID-19. PLoS Biol 2020;18(11):e3000970

162. Joachimiak MP. Zinc against COVID-19? Symptom surveillance and deficiency risk groups. PLoS Negl Trop Dis 2021;15(1):e0008895

163. Gammoh NZ, Rink L. Zinc in infection and inflammation. Nutrients 2017;9(6):E624

164. Ibs K-H, Rink L. Zinc-altered immune function. J Nutr 2003; 133(5, Suppl 1):1452S–1456S

165. Olechnowicz J, Tinkov A, Skalny A, Suliburska J. Zinc status is associated with inflammation, oxidative stress, lipid, and glucose metabolism. J Physiol Sci 2018;68(1):19–31

166. Jarosz M, Olbert M, Wyszogrodzka G, Młyniec K, Librowski T. Antioxidant and anti-inflammatory effects of zinc. Zinc-dependent NF-κB signaling. Inflammopharmacology 2017;25(1):11–24

167. te Velthuis AJW, van den Worm SHE, Sims AC, Baric RS, Snijder EJ, van Hemert MJ. Zn(2+) inhibits coronavirus and arterivirus RNA polymerase activity in vitro and zinc ionophores block the replication of these viruses in cell culture. PLoS Pathog 2010;6(11):e1001176

19 Telemedicine and the COVID-19 Pandemic

Mika Turkia

Introduction

In comparison to "in-person" medicine, telemedicine, i.e., "remote" or "over a distance" medicine, has another set of advantages and limitations. For example, in a teleconsultation with a patient on a sailboat, diagnostic systems and most medications are unavailable. The clinician has less information to rely on, and in the end has to rely more on intuition and innovation. However, in a telemedicine setting involving a general practitioner at an outpatient clinic remotely consulting an expert such as a pulmonologist, *tele* adds to the usual set of options. Another example of telemedicine could be a constant automated remote monitoring of a patient, with the observing clinician also working remotely at home. Other examples could include a clinician-guided group psychotherapy session over videoconferencing, or robots delivering medications on an isolation ward.

Living participants of a telemedicine setting may be patients, clinicians, family members, or other parties such as officials. A family member or a social worker may participate remotely in an in-person clinical visit. Automated participants may include software agents such as smartphone programs/apps connected to remote monitoring systems, artificial intelligence systems based on machine learning, or traditional expert systems based on descriptive logic programming. They may also include physical robots, which need no protection from aerosols, can be built self-disinfecting, and can work without breaks or rest.[1]

Amid pandemic-related societal closures and social distancing requirements, telemedicine has offered an opportunity to address the ongoing health care needs of patients.

Telemedicine has been applied to the whole treatment process or parts of it, such as an initial diagnosis or a follow-up.

In these days, technological prerequisites for telemedicine are often easy to fulfill. Even low-end smartphones provide the necessary capabilities for videoconferencing. External diagnostic devices providing heart rate or oxygen level monitoring may be utilized through wireless connections provided by the phones. Many "smart" watches and rings have these features built in. There are also experiments with microscopic lenses to be overlaid on smartphone camera lenses to diagnose parasites in blood samples, for example.[2]

Depending on locally available mobile data plans, videoconferencing and remote data monitoring may have an affordable fixed cost or may be relatively expensive. These costs may be offset by reduced need for traveling, for example. A clinician only working remotely may save on office costs. Possibilities depend also on features of existing electronic medical record and prescribing systems.

The return on investment on telemedicine may be larger in developing countries due to less equal access to health care between rural areas and cities.[3] However, also in Western countries, specialists are often concentrated in the cities. Telemedicine may thus equalize access to health care. Fields of medicine depending on touch may be unfeasible or at a disadvantage, although counterexamples such as telesurgery exist. By reducing person-to-person contact, robot-assisted surgery or telesurgery reduces risk of infections for both patients and medical professionals. Telesurgery could provide high-quality surgery in rural areas, battlefields, refugee camps, boats, etc.[4] It allows collaboration among surgeons residing at different locations, reduces need to travel, and may allow more efficient use of surgeons' time, helping to overcome the shortage of surgeons. Operator's physiological tremor can be cancelled, improving accuracy and reducing damage to adjacent healthy tissues, thereby quickening recovery. With new innovations, methods applied in telesurgery could possibly be extended to other fields of medicine, for example, by building general-purpose remote-controlled robots that could utilize ultrasound and other diagnostic devices.

Although it has different set of advantages and disadvantages in comparison to conventional settings, on average the efficacy of telemedicine may not differ much from conventional clinical work. For example, a systematic review of eight randomized controlled trials and three cluster randomized trials about telemedicine in pediatrics revealed that telemedicine was comparable and occasionally more beneficial, compared to in-person visits, with regard to outcomes related to symptom management, quality of life, satisfaction, medication adherence, visit completion rates, and disease progression.[5] Interventions were based on videoconferencing, smartphone-based solutions, and telephone counseling.

Telemedicine during the Pandemic

In the United States, telehealth-provided Medicare primary care visits increased dramatically, from 0.1% in February 2020 to 43.5% in April 2020.[6] This was due to a significant relaxation of telehealth-related regulations during the public health emergency. Telehealth use increased dramatically also among specialists. The highest uptake of telehealth primary care visits occurred in cities, whereas the uptake was somewhat smaller in rural areas with lower incidences of COVID-19. It is estimated that an increased demand in telehealth visits will remain also in the postpandemic era. In a survey of 300 practitioners, the percentage of telehealth visits was 9% before pandemic, 51% amid the first wave, and was expected to remain at 21% postpandemic. With regard to access of care, in one local survey of telemedicine visits in the United States, black and Asian minorities used less telemedicine services than whites, and women used more services than men, indicating that some patient groups may have been less likely to use the services.[7]

The Smart Field Hospital of Wuhan

In March 2020, a field hospital for 20,000 patients was built in Wuhan, with the aim of relieving exhausted health care workers.[8] Patients wore smart bracelets and rings that constantly monitored their vital signs. Autonomous robots screened patients' temperatures, delivered food, drinks, medicines, information, and entertainment to patients. They also disinfected surfaces with UV-C light and cleaned the floors. Due to successful containment of the epidemic, the experiment was short-lived.

In June 2020, a Chinese research group proposed dual-arm robot for isolation wards, capable of remote auscultation and operation of bedside medical instrument touchscreens, equipped with ultrasound stethoscope and UV disinfection device.[9]

A Handheld Remote Physical Examination Platform in COVID-19

In April 2020, the University of Virginia organized a multidisciplinary response team for handling COVID-19 outbreaks in patients of a local postacute and long-term care facility.[10] Using off-the-shelf FDA-approved equipment, the team built a handheld platform that allowed remote physical examination. It integrated videoconferencing with a stethoscope, an otoscope, an oral camera, and wireless vital sign monitoring.

Patients' clinical statuses and vital sign data were reviewed daily in videoconferencing meetings of the facility teams and the university clinical, administrative, and technological experts. Predefined changes in oxygen saturation, respiratory or heart rate, blood pressure, temperature, mental status, or gastrointestinal distress triggered a consultation with university pulmonologist or geriatrician, leading to transfer to a hospital if needed.

Initially, 85% of the patients at the facility tested positive for COVID-19. Median age was 85 years and all had multiple chronic health conditions. Over a month, 27% received telemedicine consultation and 38% required hospitalization, and mortality rate was 12.5%. Other comparable facility outbreaks reported a hospitalization rate of 54% and a mortality rate of 34%. The authors attributed the difference to rapid identification of patients requiring escalation of care, provision of care plans for monitoring and treatment of patients remaining at the facility, confirmation and optimization of goals of care, and coordinated care efforts between the facility and hospital. After the initial experience, the approach has been replicated to other facilities.

Teleconsultation in COVID-19

As an example of COVID-19-related teleconsultation, between March 1 and April 30, 2020, the French medical maritime teleconsultation organization Tele-Medical Assistance Service (TMAS) consulted 51 suspected COVID-19 patients of 15 nationalities in passenger ships, ferries, ocean liners, merchant ships, fishing vessels, and pleasure crafts.[11] In total, 88% presented with fever, 76% with cough, 15% with respiratory distress, 13% with headaches, 2% with diarrhea, 2% with loss of smell, and 2% with loss of taste. A total of 47% were prescribed paracetamol, 10% antibiotics, and 2% antitussive agents. However, 45% were not given a prescription by TMAS but approximately half of them were also attended to by a physician on board.

On closure, 2% were rerouted, 13% evacuated, 20% disembarked, and 65% received treatment on board. The evacuated tested COVID-19 positive in 92% of cases. In addition to the 51 patients, 10 more patients were classified as epidemic-related cases (30% of these were contacts of suspected COVID-19 patients, 10% suffering from isolation, and 60% had a shortage of previously prescribed medication). On average, treatment of one case involved four calls (standard deviation = 4; min = 1; max = 13).

After the National Institutes of Health (NIH) guideline change in early 2021 taking a neutral stance toward ivermectin but the continuing reluctance of most clinicians to prescribe it, several clinicians in the United States begun providing ivermectin prescriptions by teleconsultation.[12]

Tele-Intensive Care Units

In one example in the United States, an existing virtual telecritical care (TCC) system, which involved providing care to critically ill patients through synchronous, two-way audiovisual communication, was expanded with four goals.[13] The first goal was to augment room capacity by equipping non–intensive care unit (non-ICU) rooms with mobile telehealth carts, to expand the pool of available teleintensivists (e.g., allow retired or self-quarantined clinicians to work from home), and to allow nonintensivists to provide bedside critical care with the help of remote guidance by intensivists. The second goal was to minimize exposure of workers to patients by allowing communication without direct exposure, and simultaneously verify that personal protective equipment was used properly. The third goal was to improve bedside team management by enabling instant communication with non-ICU specialists, allow virtual team-based rounding with remote members, and serve as a central point of coordination and communication for evolving clinical algorithms. The fourth goal was to optimize ICU bed utilization by creating a real-time capacity surveillance of confirmed and suspected cases, and centralizing ICU triage decisions. Global supply-chain shortages affected by the pandemic affected purchases of necessary equipment for the TCC system expansion. Use of extension tubing to move ventilators and intravenous pumps to outside the patient's room impaired the ability for TCC intensivists to assess the patient and intervene. Use of personal protective equipment (PPE) by staff impaired bedside audiovisual communications. Language barriers further limited communications. There was a potential for conflicting medical decision making between bedside and virtual providers, and potential of service disruption related to technological issues. Regardless, TCC infrastructure allowed flexible up- and downregulation of capacity. The study also described the components and costs of the carts and home workstations.

A rapid guideline provided recommendations on the organizational management of ICUs during the pandemic.[14] The guideline suggested, among other items, use of mathematical modeling to support surge capacity planning. They also recommended using available communication technology to enable family members to communicate with patients and staff, and engaging family members in rounds and patient care discussions. In addition, the guideline suggested engaging chaplains/spiritual care, social workers, ethics consultants, and patients advocates to provide support to patients and their families. The guideline also advised against using the sequential organ failure assessment (SOFA) score for triaging COVID-19 patients, due to its low performance in predicting outcomes.

In 2012, a centralized tele-ICU service center was established in India, later providing services to 50 hospitals in the United States.[15] During the COVID-19 pandemic, tele-ICU was proposed for alleviating gross shortages of intensivists in India (India had approximately 70,000 ICU beds, and the largest society of critical care medicine in India had approximately 12,000 members, in contrast to a population of approximately

1,350,000,000). However, regulatory guidelines mostly addressed outpatient telemedicine, not inpatient telemedicine including tele-ICU. Also, there was a lack of training and funding. In addition, in India, intensivists provide consultation but are not fully empowered to direct care, creating ambiguities that may be exacerbated in a remote setting.

Patient–Family Communications

Telemedicine was also utilized for tablet-based communications between isolated patients and their family members in cases where patients did not own mobile phones.[16] Tablets were restricted to disallow use of other apps. Privacy regulations required ensuring patient privacy by selecting apps in which only accounts on an allowed contact list could call the patient. Non-HIPAA-compliant apps without centralized administration capabilities added administrative overhead. User-friendliness and familiarity with the chosen app was important in order to reduce the need for support.

Telemedicine in Other Diseases during COVID-19

As an example, in March–May 2020, a buprenorphine clinic in New York assessed feasibility of telemedicine-based opioid treatment with buprenorphine–naloxone in 78 patients with 252 visits.[17] At 8 weeks, 54% of patients remained in care, 27% were referred to community treatment program, and 19% were lost to follow-up. It was concluded that unobserved home induction on buprenorphine–naloxone was safe and feasible.

Medical Conferences by Telemedicine

Organizing medical conferences as videoconferences enables organizing them also during lockdowns and amid air travel restrictions.

The costs of organizing a teleconference may be significantly lower than an in-person conference, with participants also saving on travel and accommodation costs. Thus, people who could not have attended an ordinary conference due to limitations on time or funding may be able to participate, enhancing spread of knowledge of current research. As an example, the Interdisciplinary Conference on Psychedelic Research traditionally organized in Amsterdam, the Netherlands, was moved fully online in September 2020.[18]

Similarly, meetings of national or local medical associations may suddenly be easily available to people in other cities or countries. As an example, the Swedish Network for Psychedelic Science begun organizing member-only weekly webinars with invited international guest speakers that also included videoconferencing interaction between members before and after the invited presentations.[19]

With regard to medical education, specific training for telemedicine has been considered important in order to learn its application across specialties as well as its limitations.[20] Proposed contents of the training include history of telemedicine, discussions on applications, ethics, safety, etiquette and patient considerations, faculty-supervised telehealth encounters, and hands-on diagnostic or therapeutic procedures using telehealth equipment.

Telemedicine and Emotions

Trust and Connection in Teleconsulting

Building and maintaining trust and connection may be more challenging over videoconferencing than in person. Psychiatric patients, for example, may abruptly disconnect if stressed. Clinicians relying a lot on body language reading may find some setups limited. Clinicians with a good skill of interpreting emotional and somatic cues in voice and facial expressions have an advantage. Clinicians with long experience typically have more of the "pattern-recognition" skill needed for intuitive diagnosis. In addition, the skill of utilizing tones of voice to direct emotional states of patients may be of increased importance.

Respectively, clinicians with little experience may find teleconsultation overly demanding. A survey of internal medicine residents in New York revealed residents feeling less confident in managing chronic diseases through telemedicine visits than in-person.[21] Introduction of telemedicine aimed at preventing undertraining of residents and maintaining patient care during lockups.

The ways of projecting a calming presence for an anxious patient may differ. A study comparing a 12-week online program ($n = 37$) and 6-day in-person group ($n = 37$) focused on the development of interpersonal skills (with various methods including mindfulness, breathwork, meditation, and active listening) with pre-, post-, and 1-year follow-up noted that anxiety reduced in the in-person group but not the online group.[22] The pretest anxiety and depression symptoms were much higher in the in-person group, however. Depression was reduced in both groups, although the effect was larger in the in-person group. In both groups, 29% improvement in relation satisfaction was found. The effects were maintained in the follow-up. The authors noted that online programs may not mirror therapeutic efficacy of in-person treatment in every dimension but may play a role regardless.

Teleconsultation may require learning new "trauma-conscious" skills to overcome the limitations. Various breathwork[23] and somatic experiencing[24,25] techniques and vagus nerve[26,27] exercises may be applicable also over videoconferencing (e.g., the basic exercise by Rosenberg[28]). In addition, internal family systems therapy has commonly been applied over teleconsultation.[29]

Technological and Organizational Considerations

Data Security and Regulations

Health care is heavily regulated and telehealth solutions are affected in various ways. In the United States, the HIPAA Privacy Rule places compliance demands on solutions. Other countries may set their own rules, resulting in country- or area-specific solutions.

Only proprietary solutions adhering to local regulations may be available. In the European Union, purchasing a solution may require adhering to rules concerning public contracts. These processes take months or years, blocking response in crises. Countries with little regulation may thus rapidly implement functional ad hoc teleconsultation solutions, whereas countries with extensive regulations may fail to introduce them. In a crisis situation, inflexible regulations may even be unethical, resulting in avoidable deaths.

Therefore, HIPAA rules were relaxed during the pandemic in the United States to allow HIPAA-covered health care providers to provide telehealth services to patients using commonly used apps, even if the application does not fully comply with HIPAA rules.[30] Of the many options, free and open-source Signal Private Messenger is the most recommendable for messaging, voice calls, and one-to-one video calls, balancing first-class security and usability.[31]

For large-scale communication systems, a good option may be the free, open-source solution Matrix (in conjunction with Element. io or other compatible apps), which is in use by the government of France, the German states of Schleswig-Holstein and Hamburg, and Bundeswehr (armed forces) of Germany.[32] The system is, however, also suitable for small groups and can be implemented to use one's own servers or virtual private servers.

Such solutions do not, however, provide integration to existing health care systems. Comprehensive open-source telehealth solutions are rare and their adoption typically require in-house software development expertise.

Custom Software Project Management

Telemedicine may involve custom software development. In these cases, it is advisable to be very clear on the relevance and focus of the system. The aim of telemedicine should not be to foster software consultants. Is the system really necessary and relevant? Does it consistently improve the work conditions, or does some area suffer? What are the maintenance costs? Considering costs, does it provide lifetime net benefit or loss? Does it require less or more of clinicians' time? Does it reform processes to utilize what technology can provide or just copy existing manual processes verbatim? Does it introduce bureaucracy and slowdowns?

An especially difficult area are technological choices. Aiming at "securing the future" by adopting the most conventional current "industry practices" often leads to slow development, high costs for changes, and eventually stagnation. Functional and logic programming languages usually provide smaller (in terms of lines of code), more readable, and maintainable systems.[33,34] A proprietary database Datomic offers records retention by design, preserving all previous states of the data and enabling full review of all changes.[35] Such advanced solutions may provide significant benefits in comparison to mainstream methods.

Minimalism, i.e., providing everything that is needed but not more, is a good philosophy in software development. Also, one should take into account the differing incentives of external consults versus in-house experts and clinicians: fundamentally, an extensive system that is expensive to maintain is in the short-term interests of external consults, whereas it is not in the interests of the patients or the clinicians because of the financial resource drain from clinical work to software maintenance.

Artificial intelligence systems present their own tradeoffs. Deep learning approaches learning from massive datasets typically provide a "black box" system, the internal logic of which cannot be made explicit.[36] This leads to inability to evaluate the system's decisions. Traditional rule-based expert systems require manual descriptions of the rules by which the decisions are made. Decisions of these systems are thus verifiable but derivation of relevant rules from clinical experience or datasets is a complex task.[37]

Conclusion

The aim of telemedicine may be seen as two-fold: first, to augment information, treatment options, or safety in a given situation, with the aim to improve treatment results; and second, to increase cost-effectiveness and demands on medical professionals while maintaining the quality of treatment results. Given these limitations, telemedicine may take many different forms allowed by technological solutions.

During the COVID-19 pandemic, telemedicine has been applied to—in addition to ensuring patient care in general during lock-ups, for example, building a roboticized hospital—a handheld device for remote physical examination of elderly patients of a postacute and long-term care facility, medical maritime teleconsultation, preventing undertraining of medical residents, and perhaps, most importantly, providing tele-ICU services.

Broader application of telemedicine may provide flexibility and increase possibilities for unsupervised patient self-care of routine issues, reducing dependence on and costs of the health care system. The released resources may then be utilized for solving previously ignored or unresolved issues.

References

1. Seidita V, Lanza F, Pipitone A, Chella A. Robots as intelligent assistants to face COVID-19 pandemic. Brief Bioinform 2021; 22(2):823–831
2. Agbana TE, Diehl JC, van Pul F, et al. Imaging & identification of malaria parasites using cellphone microscope with a ball lens. PLoS One 2018;13(10):e0205020
3. Combi C, Pozzani G, Pozzi G. Telemedicine for developing countries. a survey and some design issues. Appl Clin Inform 2016;7(4): 1025–1050
4. Choi PJ, Oskouian RJ, Tubbs RS. Telesurgery: past, present, and future. Cureus 2018;10(5): e2716
5. Shah AC, Badawy SM. Telemedicine in pediatrics: systematic review of randomized controlled trials. JMIR Pediatr Parent 2021; 4(1):e22696
6. U.S. Department of Health & Human Services. HHS issues new report highlighting dramatic trends in Medicare beneficiary telehealth utilization amid COVID-19. 2020. Available at: https://www.hhs.gov/about/news/2020/07/28/hhs-issues-new-report-highlighting-dramatic-trends-in-medicare-beneficiary-telehealth-utilization-amid-covid-19.html
7. Lott A, Campbell KA, Hutzler L, Lajam CM. Telemedicine utilization at an academic medical center during COVID-19 pandemic: are some patients being left behind? Telemed J E Health 2021 (e-pub ahead of print). doi:10.1089/tmj.2020.0561
8. CNBC. What America can learn from China's use of robots and telemedicine to combat the coronavirus. 2020. Available at: https://www.cnbc.com/2020/03/18/how-china-is-using-robots-and-telemedicine-to-combat-the-coronavirus.html
9. Yang G, Lv H, Zhang Z, et al. Keep healthcare workers safe: application of teleoperated robot in isolation ward for COVID-19 prevention and control. Chin J Mech Eng 2020; 33(1):47
10. Harris DA, Archbald-Pannone L, Kaur J, et al. Rapid telehealth-centered response to COVID-19 outbreaks in postacute and long-term care facilities. Telemed J E Health 2021;27(1):102–106
11. Dehours E, Balen F, Saccavini A, Roux P, Houze-Cerfon CH. COVID-19 and French medical maritime teleconsultation. Telemed J E Health 2021;27(4):397–401

12. FrontLineCOVID-19CriticalCareAlliance.How to get ivermectin. 2021. Available at: https://web.archive.org/web/20210316104352/https://covid19criticalcare.com/i-mask-prophylaxis-treatment-protocol/how-to-get-ivermectin/

13. Singh J, Green MB, Lindblom S, Reif MS, Thakkar NP, Papali A. Telecritical care clinical and operational strategies in response to COVID-19. Telemed J E Health 2021; 27(3):261–268

14. Aziz S, Arabi YM, Alhazzani W, et al. Managing ICU surge during the COVID-19 crisis: rapid guidelines. Intensive Care Med 2020;46(7):1303–1325

15. Ramakrishnan N, Tirupakuzhi Vijayaraghavan BK, Venkataraman R. Breaking barriers to reach farther: a call for urgent action on tele-ICU services. Indian J Crit Care Med 2020;24(6):393–397

16. Fang J, Liu YT, Lee EY, Yadav K. Telehealth solutions for in-hospital communication with patients under isolation during COVID-19. West J Emerg Med 2020;21(4):801–806

17. Tofighi B, McNeely J, Walzer D, et al. A telemedicine buprenorphine clinic to serve New York City: initial evaluation of the NYC Public Hospital System's initiative to expand treatment access during the COVID-19 pandemic. J Addict Med. Published online February 5, 2021. doi:10.1097/ADM.0000000000000809

18. Stichting OPEN. Interdisciplinary conference on psychedelic research 2020. 2020. Available at: https://icpr2020.net/

19. The Swedish Network for Psychedelic Science. Available at: https://www.psykedeliskvetenskap.org/about

20. Jumreornvong O, Yang E, Race J, Appel J. Telemedicine and medical education in the age of COVID-19. Acad Med 2020;95(12): 1838–1843

21. Chiu CY, Sarwal A, Jawed M, Chemarthi VS, Shabarek N. Telemedicine experience of NYC Internal Medicine residents during COVID-19 pandemic. PLoS One 2021;16(2):e0246762

22. Church D, Clond M. Is online treatment as effective as in-person treatment?: Psychological change in two relationship skills groups. J Nerv Ment Dis 2019; 207(5): 315–319

23. Schwenk S. Ecstatic breathwork with Scott Schwenk. Available at: https://www.onecommune.com/ecstatic-breathwork-with-scott-schwenk

24. Payne P, Levine PA, Crane-Godreau MA. Somatic experiencing: using interoception and proprioception as core elements of trauma therapy. Front Psychol 2015;6:93

25. Brom D, Stokar Y, Lawi C, et al. Somatic experiencing for posttraumatic stress disorder: a randomized controlled outcome study. J Trauma Stress 2017;30(3):304–312 10.1002/jts.22189

26. Breit S, Kupferberg A, Rogler G, Hasler G. Vagus nerve as modulator of the brain-gut axis in psychiatric and inflammatory disorders. Front Psychiatry 2018;9:44

27. Kaniusas E, Szeles JC, Kampusch S, et al. Non-invasive auricular vagus nerve stimulation as a potential treatment for Covid19-originated acute respiratory distress syndrome. Front Physiol 2020;11:890

28. Rosenberg S. Accessing the Healing Power of the Vagus Nerve: Self-Help Exercises for Anxiety, Depression, Trauma, and Autism. Berkeley, CA: North Atlantic Books; 2017

29. Schwartz RC. Internal Family Systems Therapy. New York, NY: Guilford Publications; 2019

30. U.S. Department of Health & Human Services. Telehealth: delivering care safely during COVID-19. 2020. Available at: https://www.hhs.gov/coronavirus/telehealth/index.html

31. Signal Messenger. Speak freely. Available at: https://signal.org/

32. Element secure messenger—government and NGO communication. Available at: https://web.archive.org/web/20210628120240/https://element.io/pro/federation-collaboration

33. Logica: Modern Logic Programming. Available at: https://logica.dev/

34. The Clojure Programming Language. Available at: https://clojure.org/

35. Datomic. Overview. Available at: https://www.datomic.com/

36. Liu R, Rong Y, Peng Z. A review of medical artificial intelligence. Glob Health J 2020; 4(2):42–45

37. Ogidan ET, Dimililer K, Ever YK. Machine learning for expert systems in data analysis. In: 2018 2nd International Symposium on Multidisciplinary Studies and Innovative Technologies (ISMSIT). IEEE; 2018

20 Palliative Care during COVID-19

Marianne M. Holler

Introduction

Caring for patients with advanced illnesses has always been in the wheelhouse of palliative care practitioners in the American healthcare system. This challenging work took on new proportions, scope, and dimensions with the onset of the global coronavirus pandemic.[1] There was a pronounced shift in how palliative care was perceived and the skill set that could be brought to the bedside of patients and their families suddenly facing serious and, many times, unexpected illness. COVID-19 increased the need for management of the debilitating symptoms of shortness of breath, fatigue, GI complaints, and pain. It also forced patients, families, and the medical community to address end-of-life care and goals of care in a way not previously experienced.[1,2]

Having difficult conversations with patients and their loved ones was made exponentially more challenging as a result of social distancing, lack of in-person family meetings, and the inability of people to see for themselves, firsthand, the experience of being at the bedside of a loved one who may be facing the last days or hours of life. Physicians, nurse practitioners, and other providers who were not used to having these conversations found themselves in an uncomfortable space. This is no fault of the practitioner.[3,4] The medical education system does not properly equip practitioners in the art and skill of communicating bad news or how to help patients and families set goals when illness becomes advanced.[5] This lack of training leads to continued, aggressive, at times, burdensome care that does not translate into a better-quality life or change the outcome. It does impact how the patient experiences the outcome, and, potentially, how the family feels about the outcome. The default is to keep treating, keep intervening, thereby prolonging the dying process but not adding to the quality of the patient's life or allowing for conversations if things do not go well.

Many times, appropriate end-of-life care in the United States has been lacking. Defining end-of-life care not in terms of the last hours and days of life rather than the weeks, months, and sometimes years is an ongoing challenge. With emerging technology and skills, we have abilities to prolong life that we did not have in the past. What we have sacrificed in the mix is the skill of prognostication.[6] Studies have shown that physicians correctly prognosticate for seriously ill patients approximately 20% of the time. Most overestimate life expectancy and few underestimate the remaining time a patient may live.[7] This creates the perfect storm leading to overtreatment and poor communication when time may be short. The best analogy is the patient and family are left standing at the side of the road watching their house burn down. People continuously are driving by, stopping, and not talking about the house that is engulfed in flames. The patient and the family know it but no one seems to be talking about it. Instead, these well-intentioned participants talk about what they can do. The family may be thinking "gee, I think the house is burning down" and the response may be "I'm the window guy, they called me to fix the window." The next may say, "I'm the carpet guy, they called me to get a spot out of the carpet." We keep doing things "to" the patient that do not end up being "for" the patient. When the family asks, "is there anything else you can do?" We are comfortable saying, "yes, we can now try. XYZ intervention." It is difficult to communicate and to envision the end point when we are not sure ourselves where that end point actually lies. In our honest attempt to give patients and families good news we sometimes forget to provide good information. Information that will communicate the gravity of the situation, define what we can reasonably hope for, and provide a reasonable transition to the next appropriate level of care for the patient. We feel comfortable in our knowledge about what the next step is but we are unsure how to navigate care when the "next step" may be futile or burdensome to the patient without providing any clear benefit. COVID has greatly exacerbated this deficit in our system. Not only are we faced with increased numbers of patients who never thought they would be facing a potentially life-limiting illness, but our clinical workforce has been tremendously overburdened and underprepared to have discussions about the benefits and burdens and about the options for care.[8]

One big shift in the utilization of palliative care at the height of the COVID crisis happened in emergency departments.[9] At the point of entry, palliative medicine was consulted on COVID and non-COVID patients. Recognizing patients who were at risk for poor outcomes came front and center. Conversations about goals happened simultaneously with the administration of life-saving interventions. Families were given the opportunity to weigh in prior to intensive care unit (ICU) transfer or aggressive procedures. Make no mistake, these were patients who, at baseline, were debilitated, dependent on others for their care, had advanced medical problems, and were lacking documented advanced directives or POLST forms. In a perfect system, this would be the way these conversations happened on regular basis. In a utopian system, these conversations would happen outside of the hospital, in advance of a medical crisis, hopefully thereby eliminating the transfer to the emergency department.

This shift to emergency department palliative care consults highlighted another glaring hole in the system. The lack of a 24-hour palliative care practitioners present in the hospital. Our system of 11 hospitals had set up a 24-hour palliative hotline that clinicians could access to help with complex symptom management. This did not provide consult support to speak with families to determine goals of care and to weigh options for treatments being proposed. The calls to the hotline proved to be for symptom management at the end of life. Clinicians called for assistance to control shortness of breath, secretions, agitation, pain, and other distressing symptoms in the last hours to days of life.

Clinical Cases

Let's review some cases that presented during COVID-19 pandemic and strategies that may help clinicians going forward.

Case 1: We Cannot Always Fix What Is Broken

Early on in the pandemic there was a distressing amount of misinformation and false information about the virus and its spread throughout the country. None was more damaging to the situation than the notion that the virus was a hoax; it did not exist and was being blown out of proportion by political, conspiracy, and social groups for a variety of unknown purposes. Meanwhile, clinicians were experiencing the devastating destruction the virus was perpetrating on the patient. Individuals who appeared to be stable and recovering suddenly became so ill and were overwhelming critical care units. Relatives unable to see their loved ones in person were asked to rely on FaceTime meetings with medical providers and virtual visits with family members.

Mrs. R, a 68-year-old immigrant, presented to the hospital with a fever and shortness of breath. She had a history of diabetes, hypertension, heart disease, and chronic kidney disease. She tested positive for the virus upon her admission the hospital. She was from an Asian country and spoke only a specific dialect of the country's language. The language line was used to communicate with her when she was able and her illness allowed. Her husband did not speak English and requested communication take place through his two sons. Conversations with the sons had grown increasingly contentious and ended with them hanging up on the medical team who were attempting to communicate what was happening clinically with their mother. The sons clearly stated they did not "believe in the virus," that we were "lying to them" and we had all "bought into the hoax that there even was a virus." Over the course of 5 weeks she required intubation three times. After the third intubation it was clear she would not be able to sustain herself off the ventilator for any period of time. Thus, the conversations began about goals and the next steps. The family was clear the patient would not want a tracheostomy and feeding tube but refused to make the patient a do not resuscitate (DNR) and discuss the goals without these interventions. We invited them to meet, in person, with the critical care and palliative medical doctors. During the meeting, the sons became angry and hostile. At one point, one son yelled, "why are you two still insisting on this virus story?" "Who are we supposed to believe, the two of you or the government?"

My instinct was to say "the two of us." My training told me that that would be a losing position to take. At that point, he believing or not believing in the existence of the virus was secondary to the patient's immediate care needs. Arguing about how we arrived at this day would not advance the goals of the meeting and was sure to set up an "us against them" dynamic.

We let him vent for a while and then let silence overtake the room. This technique may seem like it takes valuable time away from the conversation, but it will save time and emotional energy for everyone involved. Once the silence settles, you have the opportunity to reintroduce the goals. We were able to review her clinical condition in detail discussing what was possible and what was probable. We showed them the patient's X-rays and why these test results were concerning to us and how the picture was impacting her ability to live off the ventilator. We discussed cardiopulmonary resuscitation (CPR) and the likelihood of aggressive interventions being beneficial at this stage of illness. We also discussed the burdens of those interventions. The family did agree to DNR status by the end of the meeting but not to the tracheotomy or percutaneous gastrostomy (PEG) feeding tube. They also did not consent to directing all care toward comfort.

In the coming days we had additional virtual family meetings attempting to address goals and a plan going forward. The meetings ended the same: no trach, no peg, no comfort care. The sons seemed to want another option that did not exist. I invited them to the hospital again to meet face to face. They begged to be allowed into her room to touch her and talk to her. They said they felt if they could talk to her in her own language, encourage her to get better that things would start to change. I asked what they would tell her if things were not able to change and that she truly was at the end of her life. One son looked at me and said, "we have to tell her that we are sorry." He explained that his mom was considered a peasant in their country, uneducated, unable to read, and they reminded her of this throughout their lives. They felt they treated her as a servant and did not respect as their mother as they should have all along. I left the conference room and called administration. I explained we need to let this family into the room and why it was imperative to the patient's care at this time. Permission was granted. I returned to the sons and husband. I acknowledged they did not believe the virus was real, but they would have to adhere to wearing appropriate PPE to be allowed into her room. We discussed how they should use the time with her as it would only be one at a time for ten minutes each.

One by one they entered the room, held her hand, and whispered something to her as she lay tethered to the ventilator. Each came out tearful but calm. The family gathered again in the conference room alone. We reentered the room and asked if they had any questions or thoughts. The eldest son said, "we need to let her go." Just barely above a whisper but with conviction.

There were many things broken in this family. Our interactions with them could have been better from the beginning. Their refusal to acknowledge the virus became a focal point of frustration and energy rather than the patient's needs. The emotional situation between the family and the staff deteriorated as a result. This reminded me of working with a family who was frustrated by an Alzheimer patient. A daughter once told me about a daily, frustrating encounter she had with her mother. Her mom would pick up a blanket telling her someone named Paul made it for her. The daughter would daily say, "mom, it was your niece, Mary, that made the blanket." I asked her why she did that every day. The daughter said to me, "I correct her so she will remember for the next time." I pointed out that she would not remember and you will continue to be frustrated by her inability to remember. I suggested the next she say, "Wow, Paul must really like you" and put the blanket aside. Focusing on the family's belief that the virus was a hoax gave us something other than the patient's care and goals to discuss and/or argue about. We wanted them to acknowledge the existence of the virus that we almost missed what was driving the pain, frustration, and anger in this family. They needed to heal the emotional wounds they perceived they inflected over a lifetime before we could ask them to move forward with deciding the best way to manage her care needs.

Case 2: "I Hear What You Are Saying, But Our Mom Is a Fighter"

How many times in critical care and medicine in general have we heard this response over the years? We diligently present the facts and data about why the body is failing only to be met with this particular battle cry from those closest to the patient. "We hear what you are saying but you do not know her. She is a fighter." This is a statement that

tends to stymy practitioners who then continue to move forward with care and interventions that we know or highly suspect will prove futile in hindsight. During COVID, as the onslaught of patients increased, we were faced with family members who had little to no warning that their loved ones would be facing a potentially life-limiting illness.

GW was a 73-year-old gentleman who presented with shortness of breath to the emergency department. He had been diagnosed with COVID 5 days prior to his presentation by his primary care physician and was instructed to present to the hospital, should his symptoms worsened. Initially, his respiratory failure was stabilized with the use of Hi-Flo oxygen and Bipap. As his condition worsened, Palliative Care was consulted to review goals of care and a plan going forward. During the initial consult, the patient was able to say that he was ok with being placed on a ventilator but he did not wish to be on a vent long term if he was not able to be extubated. In the early days of his hospitalization, his wife was also admitted and required intubation. She experienced multisystem organ failure requiring the use of pressers and dialysis. Eventually, she could not tolerate hemodialysis and was transitioned to continuous veno-veno hemodialysis (CVVHD).

Mr. W's brother had power of attorney for both of the patients. As each patient's condition worsened, the team had a number of phone and video conferences with the family. It became clear that code status for both would need to be discussed in detail and clarified. The conversation was detailed and family input was sought throughout. At the end of the call, the family elected to change the code status of both patients to DNR. Mrs. W's condition continued to worsen over the next 2 weeks. She was profoundly hypoxic while on ventilator settings of 100% FiO_2 with oxygen saturation's hovering in the 70s for days regardless of the interventions attempted. Despite maximizing the use of vasopressors her blood pressure remained almost incompatible with life. The family refused to consider directing all care toward comfort. The war/assault on her body continued until one day, after a number of weeks, she became bradycardic and died.

The family meetings now were completely about Mr. W following the death of his wife. He, also, required high levels of oxygen and could not be weaned from the ventilator. Over the course of the next 4 weeks, the team had a number of calls with the patient's brother to provide updates and discuss goals. We shared his brother's conversation prior to being placed on the ventilator. Despite his worsening condition, the family elected to proceed with a tracheostomy and a feeding tube. Patient appeared to be awake but was not interactive and unable to follow commands. Imaging of his head and neurological testing did clearly define what we were seeing clinically. We expressed concern about the benefits and burdens of the present level of interventions. The patient's brother invoked the all familiar battle cry, "I hear what you are saying but my brother is a fighter." Before diving into that pool to respond, I asked had they ever experienced anyone who was on a ventilator who required a tracheostomy and a feeding tube. Yes, was the response much to my surprise. Their mother had suffered a catastrophic stroke a number of years ago and required the same interventions. I asked them to share with me that experience. Once their mother was on the ventilator, the four children were split on how they should proceed. Two (including our patient) thought they should let her go peacefully and the other two thought she was a fighter and could recover. Unable to come to a consensus she remained in that condition for 4 years until she eventually died. She never regained consciousness or returned to her previous functional status. There was that phrase again, "She is a fighter...."

At times like these we are charged with helping the family reflect on what it means to be a "fighter." We discussed how it speaks to GW's spirit, his emotional, mental, and psychological state. It is what enabled him to strive, to achieve, move forward when the

odds seem against him in life. However, as the body fails the spirit cannot overcome that devastation. It is at that point that we leaned into the conversation and asked, "what is the goal if the breakdown of the physical body overcomes the will and sprit to live." It is a fact that every human must face as life comes to an end. We cannot change that as doctors or healthcare providers but can help guide patients and families on the journey. Sadly, this family pressed on for 48 days. The patient continued to deteriorate; he received the tracheostomy, the feeding tube, and was eventually transferred to a long-term acute care hospital where he died 12 days after his admission.

The lesson here is we cannot change the outcome for patients in many circumstances. The risk is how the family feels about the outcome after it is over. In 2 or 5 years they need to be able to look back on the situation and know they did what they thought was the right thing for their family member.

Case 3: "We Have Faith God Will Provide a Miracle"

Religion and the care of patients with advanced illness have shared the same space for centuries. Many practitioners have seen religion and discussions of miracles as barriers to appropriate end-of-life care in the ICU. Many years ago, in a discussion with one of my critical care colleagues, he remarked, "when they pull the Bible card on me I know to fold up my tent and move on because I will not get through to them." He clearly was in the camp that viewed faith and religion as an obstacle to be overcome before discussions could progress about the patient's poor prognosis and when to begin transition to a comfortable, peaceful, and natural end of life.

RL was a 67-year-old woman who came to the hospital with the all too familiar complaints of fever, malaise, and shortness of breath. She was an active senior citizen with a history of diabetes and obesity. She was the heart and soul of her family and a leader within her community. Within 24 hours, she required admission to the ICU and was placed on a ventilator. She tested positive for COVID-19 at the point of entry. Over the next 7 days, we were witness to the destruction the virus wrought on her body. Renal failure, strokes, and heart failure presented as the team battled to push back against what we began to see as the potential end of her life. Her four children and husband kept vigil via frequent iPad visits arranged by the ICU nurses and managers. One of the patient's sisters was a nurse and lived out of state. Another significant number of family members kept in touch from overseas. RL's sister knew early on the gravity of her sister's condition and likely outcome. As the days and weeks rolled by the patient's condition not only failed to improve but continued to worsen. Her sister began to advocate on the patient's behalf to other family members. She communicated to us and her family that this was not an existence that her sister would value or want for herself.

Early on the family identified themselves as a people of great faith. Their local parish held prayer vigils for her and the family frequently used their iPad visits to pray the rosary to her. They declared their belief that a miracle would happen and she would wake up, come off the ventilator, and return home to them. On the other side of the world a relative called to say, they had a vision during which they saw her whole and healthy and restored. They believed it was a clear message from God not to give up hope, that an intervention from God's grace was always near at hand. The critical care team began to despair along with the patient's sister that she would suffer until the end. The dynamic quietly shifted between the family and the critical care team into and "us vs. them" feeling. The gap was widening on each side of the bed. The family held onto the belief that a miracle would come regardless of how long it took to reveal itself. Meanwhile, the critical care practitioners watched as each organ system failed, the patient become unrecognizable, and the burdens of the interventions were greatly outpacing the benefits to her.

Faith appeared to become the dividing line between the two sides.

In some moments, when caring for a family such as this one, I had trouble understanding how so many people of faith have difficulty seeing the natural order of the cycle of life and death. I shared the same religion as this family. From a very young age my parents exposed us to dying relatives, being present at funerals and explaining death and loss as a natural part of our existence. Faith and religion was central to our lives. When I went to medical school I had a friend comment that the more I studied science and medicine my faith would falter and be at risk. I happened to experience the opposite. The more I studied the more it validated that something greater than us created life, the body, and the world as we experience it.

In medicine we need to stop seeing faith and religion as a barrier to good end-of-life care. It is not an obstacle to be overcome but an important addition to looking at the whole patient and their support system. Faith and religion should be seen as an opportunity, a gateway to partner with relatives to provide the best possible experience at the most devastating time in a family's life. It is important to remember that when we cannot change the outcome for the patient we can change how they experience the outcome and how the family feels about the outcome.

We arranged a virtual family meeting with all present, locally and from overseas. I outlined RLs clinical condition in detail and asked if there were questions about what was happening. We discussed the possibilities for her care along with the probabilities. I shared that I did not think it would be helpful or beneficial if I did not tell them the truth or if I beat around the bush. They all agreed that the truth was what they wanted. We discussed the benefits and burdens of what was happening and asked they place her at the center of their decision-making. We discussed how what was good for her was ultimately going to be bad for all of them. Fifteen minutes into the meeting, the conversation again turned to faith and miracles. I leaned forward closer to the screen. I told them I was happy they were a family of faith. That people who lacked faith did not always see that something greater than us is in charge of the bigger picture. We never get to decide who lives and who dies but only how they make the journey.

Having faith doesn't always mean your prayers would be answered how you imagined or how you request them to be. If that was the case, I pressed on, then people of faith would outlive those with no faith. They acknowledged this was not the case. Slowly, over the next hour, we explored what RL valued, what gave her joy, and what was meaningful to her. We discussed the importance of her faith and how she lived it every day. Her sister masterfully took over the conversation. She pointed out that taking her off the ventilator was not a sign they lacked faith. She quietly said, "if we take her off the machines and she lives, we win, we get to have her for longer in our lives. If we take her off the machines and she dies, she will be with God and she wins. Isn't that what our faith has always taught us."

I wish I could tell you the meeting ended with a plan to direct the patient's care toward comfort and less aggressive measures. The family did agree to change her code status to DNR but they decided to press on with other aggressive interventions. She died 12 days later still undergoing the full support of all modern medicine has to offer. The goal was never to change the outcome, just how the family felt about the outcome. As they look back on the 6 of 7 weeks their relative spent in ICU, on life support, dialysis, and vasopressors, they need to know they did the right thing for her and for themselves.

Case 4: She Was Fine Right before This, We Have Hope

One of the hardest things for families to wrap their head around is the concept that everyone who is not fine was fine at some point before illness or injury compromised their physical, functional, and/or cognitive condition. Never before had the sheer number of patients and families facing this devastating change in status happen than with this pandemic. Not only did we see those who were seriously compromised by other illnesses felled by COVID-19, we were also experiencing relatively young, seemingly healthy, active people end up in ICU, on life support, and battling the ravages of the virus to stay alive.

FM was a 52-year-old woman, working in an area nursing home when she woke up one morning feeling generally unwell. Out of character, she called out sick from work. Two months into the pandemic, her husband and children were immediately concerned she had contracted COVID-19. A test at the local urgent care confirmed their fears. Knowing she was healthy and active with no medical problems did little to calm their anxiety. She told them it was unlikely that she would become seriously ill and quarantined in the family basement. As the days passed she became short of breath and confused. Concerned with her obvious change in status, her husband called 911. When the rescue squad arrived at the house, her oxygen saturation was in the 70s. They intubated her in the field and transported her to the hospital. The litany of procedures and interventions began in earnest. The days and weeks became a blur of central line placements, ventilator adjustments, chest tubes, and eventually dialysis. Her once healthy body looked unrecognizable compared to the pictures the family had emailed to us. On daily video calls with her family, a familiar line was spoken and repeated "she was fine right before this" and "keep going, we have hope." The critical care team began to feel as if we were crossing that invisible yet familiar line between benefit and burden in the care we were providing. After two cardiac arrests we dove more earnestly into the discussion about code status and if further CPR would be of any clear benefit to her.

Through tears and anguish, they asked, "So are you telling us there is no hope?"

There was that word again "hope." In medicine and in general we have come to think of hope as a two-sided coin. We have hope, the patient lives. We do not have hope, the patient dies. When illness becomes advanced and there is concern about where we are going and what the destination is we must help the family redefine the meaning of hope, helping them broaden the definition from its binary constraints into a much broader concept.

We met on multiple occasions and discussed FM, what was important to her, and what she valued. We reviewed her condition and all she had been through over her 7 weeks in the ICU. I discussed how we had to talk about what they hoped for if time was short. Did they hope she knew how much she was loved, what she meant to them? Or how she was respected and loved at her job and in their church? Did they hope she felt fulfilled and accomplished? Slowly we helped them broaden their definition of hope. Through these conversations about what they were hoping for, they were able to then begin the process of letting her go more peacefully. In the coming days, the family consented to a DNR status and decided to direct her care toward comfort. She was liberated from the ventilator and died. We cried at her bedside while the family observed virtually. A nurse held her hand as she slipped away. The scars were deep for the staff, deeper for the family. Helping them redefine hope in their family and for their relatives which contributed to their acceptance of her death and letting her leave this life in a peaceful way.

Conclusion

COVID brought into sharp focus the need to train all healthcare providers in having the difficult conversations to ensure the right care is provided at the right time that is aligned with the patient and family goals. We need to understand there is a definite contrast between giving good news and providing good information. The majority of patients were provided the benefit of having many specialists care for them throughout their illness. We want so badly to provide the family with good news about a desperately ill patient that we forget to provide good information. Sometimes, good information is not always good news. For example, if a patient on a vent for an extended period of time, requiring 100% FiO$_2$, continuous dialysis, the aide of four vasopressor agents, and poor cognitive response off sedation but has a normal ejection fraction focusing on the heart muscle function may provide good news but not necessarily convey to the family the gravity of the overall clinical situation. It is the equivalent of driving by a house that is burning down and stopping to offer to fix a window that is broken on the third floor of the home. The house will continue to burn if you cannot put out the fire but it will have a new window as it goes down. The family may think, "gee, I thought the house was actually burning down but if someone is here to fix a window, may be the house isn't going to be a complete loss." Words matter.

At the start of a family meeting it is always best to fire a warning shot. I will start and tell them it is better if we talk about the truth. If I beat around the bush it may not be helpful to you or your family member. Most time people want the truth and they appreciate an honest conversation. I ask what they have been told by the various members of the team. This will allow for correction of misinformation and to explain terms that they find unfamiliar. During normal times (i.e., non-COVID times) when I read a chart and examine a patient, I ask myself, "is this patient experiencing sentinel event; something that robbed them quickly of their previous functional status or is this a culminating event; part of a long slow decline over time?" While caring for extremely ill patients with COVID-19, we saw a mixture of both categories. Asking this question of yourself as a clinician can help guide discussions about prognosis and goals.

Families need help in setting goals and translating those goals into a plan of care. We cannot be afraid to speak the truth. I once cared for an 88-year-old woman who suffered a catastrophic middle cerebral artery cerebral vascular accident. During a family meeting to discuss goals, her son told me that she rode her bicycle around the neighborhood daily and his goal was to have her return to that level of functioning. That was not a goal we could realistically hope to attain. Knowing the family goals for the patient and aligning that with care can help guide them in their decision-making. Mutually decide with the team and patient/family the steps that would be needed to achieve the goals as outlined.

The first goal stated is often: "she wants to live and we want the same." The best response is, "we want that for her also. However, we need to talk about a plan if things do not go how we hope." In serious, debilitating illness there may be a difference between being alive and living. What level of existence would be acceptable to this person? Emotional, vocal conflicts are common during these decision-making sessions. It is a time of emotional turmoil, uncertainty, and fear. Conflicts may exist between family members or between the family and the healthcare team. It is best, not to take anything personally. It is also not a time to dive into family conflicts that may have existed for years. When you see and hear conflict, think emotion. Remember communication is not always about what you say but what the other side hears. In conflict, there is often anger. Family members need to be heard, to be understood. It also may be a way to get the dialogue to go in a different direction. When patients and family start arguing and yelling, healthcare providers often run the other way. Many say, "I'll come back when you are calmer so we can talk." This accomplishes nothing. The message is, "I do not want to deal with this." This may reinforce the family's behavior. They know if they get angry when the subject arises about prognosis or discussing a plan, they can deflect and not have the conversation. Conflict make us uncomfortable, we may feel under attack. It may be the message and not the messenger. It is a time to examine your approach. How could you have done it better? Is there someone else on the team who is better equipped and more skilled at these conversations? Be attentive, be patient, and be sincere. Acknowledge the anger and ask if everyone can come to the table to help plan for the most appropriate care for their family member.

Lastly, it is important to acknowledge the power of silence. As palliative fellowship director this was the hardest skill for the fellows to master. I used to tell them, "He who speaks first loses." After reviewing the patient's clinical condition and answering questions, it is important to sit in silence. Let the patient and/or family speak first. There have been many studies about how soon practitioners interrupt patients or fill the silence with more talking.[10-12] Great things can come from silence.[11] It allows patients and families time to reflect on all that has been discussed, gather their emotions, and articulate fears, hopes, and concerns. Silence can be uncomfortable for everyone in the room. It is from this discomfort that a plan for how to go forward can emerge. Interrupting this process can easily redirect a family away from what needs to be said and explored.

There are many things we learned from working with patients and families during the pandemic. We kept pace as the science changed and as treatments emerged and we lost friends and colleagues. We fought alongside each other as we lost patients we felt we should have saved and were left bereft and overwhelmed with the sheer number of patients for whom we were caring.[13] I felt a shift in the healthcare landscape and a new appreciation of what palliative care could bring to the bedside. The importance of having goals of care conversations early on in serious illness continues to challenge many in the healthcare arena. Everyone does not have to be good at these conversations but we all need to know who among us possesses this skill set. Palliative care can help both at the bedside and with training everyone to understand how to have the conversation and how to navigate the obstacles that patients and families may present as illness becomes advanced.

References

1. Davies A, Hayes J. Palliative care in the context of a pandemic: similar but different. Clin Med (Lond) 2020;20(3):274–277

2. Powell VD, Silveira MJ. What should palliative care's response be to the COVID-19 pandemic? J Pain Symptom Manage 2020; 60(1):e1–e3

3. Romanò M. Between intensive care and palliative care at the time of CoViD-19. Recenti Prog Med 2020;111(4):223–230

4. Dujardin J, Schuurmans J, Westerduin D, Wichmann AB, Engels Y. The COVID-19 pandemic: a tipping point for advance care planning? Experiences of general practitioners. Palliat Med 2021;35(7): 1238–1248

5. Fitzpatrick D, Heah R, Patten S, Ward H. Palliative care in undergraduate medical education: how far have we come? Am J Hosp Palliat Care 2017;34(8):762–773

6. The SUPPORT Principal Investigators. A controlled trial to improve care for seriously ill hospitalized patients. The study to understand prognoses and preferences for outcomes and risks of treatments (SUPPORT). JAMA 1995;274(20):1591–1598

7. Christakis NA, Lamont EB. Extent and determinants of error in doctors' prognoses in terminally ill patients: prospective cohort study. BMJ 2000;320(7233):469–472

8. Goh KJ, Choong MC, Cheong EH, et al. Rapid progression to acute respiratory distress syndrome: review of current understanding of critical illness from coronavirus disease 2019 (COVID-19) infection. Ann Acad Med Singap 2020;49(3):108–118

9. Eygnor JK, Rosenau AM, Burmeister DB, et al. Palliative care in the emergency department during a COVID-19 pandemic. Am J Emerg Med 2021;45:516–518

10. Marvel MK, Epstein RM, Flowers K, Beckman HB. Soliciting the patient's agenda: have we improved? JAMA 1999;281(3):283–287

11. Back AL, Bauer-Wu SM, Rushton CH, Halifax J. Compassionate silence in the patient-clinician encounter: a contemplative approach. J Palliat Med 2009;12(12):1113–1117

12. Beckman HB, Frankel RM. The effect of physician behavior on the collection of data. Ann Intern Med 1984;101(5):692–696

13. Arya A, Buchman S, Gagnon B, Downar J. Pandemic palliative care: beyond ventilators and saving lives. CMAJ 2020;192(15): E400–E404

21 Comorbidities and COVID-19 Perspectives and Challenges

Jose Iglesias and Joseph Varon

Introduction

Since the earliest days of the pandemic, it became obvious that patients with pre-existing comorbidities were at high risk for developing severe COVID-19 disease, prolonged hospitalization, respiratory failure, and death. The major comorbidities included obesity, diabetes mellitus (DM), cancer patients hypertension (HTN), chronic kidney disease (CKD), chronic obstructive pulmonary disease (COPD), and cardiovascular disease (CVD).[1-3] Up to 25 to 60% of patients with severe COVID-19 have multiple pre-existing comorbidities.[1-3] Guan and coworkers observed that the greater the amount of comorbidities the higher the risk for poorer clinical outcomes.[3] Although somewhat of an oversimplification, an underlying common pathophysiologic finding in patients with these comorbidities is either a downregulation of angiotensin converting enzyme 2 (ACE2) or increase in ACE/ACE2 ratio (**Fig. 21.1**).[4-6] In addition, patients on immunosuppression, such as solid organ transplant (SOT) and bone marrow transplant (BMT) recipients, present another spectrum of patients at increased risk of adverse outcomes and a poor response to vaccination.[1-3,7-13] Patients with COPD, HTN, DM, and CVD have been noted to have a higher incidence of the acute respiratory distress syndrome (ARDS), acute kidney injury, shock, and multiorgan dysfunction syndrome (MODS).[1,2,9,10,12-16] Both the pre-COVID therapy of the disease and therapeutic management of these patients pose specific challenges.[2] In this chapter, we present a brief overview of the challenges in managing patients with comorbidities afflicted with COVID-19 and provide some representative cases illustrating the challenges these patients face (with some of the most common comorbidities present).

Obesity

In most clinical studies of individuals with COVID-19, obesity has been highly associated with increased hospitalizations, morbidity, and mortality.[17,18] A meta-analysis by Poly et al evaluated 17 studies and over 500,000 patients observed obesity to be associated with a 42% increased risk of mortality.[18] In addition, obese individuals 65 years and older demonstrated a markedly (higher 150%) increased risk of death.[19] Obesity increases the necessity of mechanical ventilation, and from a general respiratory standpoint, obesity poses significant challenges in management due to changes in airway mechanics, such as decreased compliance, airway resistance, increased work of breathing, and reduced gas exchange. In addition, ACE2, the primary receptor, is highly expressed in visceral adipose tissue.[14,15,17,18,20-22] Obesity results in alterations in T and B lymphocytes, and obese individuals have demonstrated poor antibody responses to immunization.[21,23,24] Obese individuals have an increase in net visceral adipose tissue and thus an increased ACE2, possibly making them more prone to infection and increased viral shedding.[10,25-27] Furthermore, they have a higher ACE/ACE2 ratio at baseline, resulting in an unabated Angiotensin II (ANG II) effects.[4,5,14,17,20,25,28,29] The SARS-CoV-2 infection causes downregulation of ACE2, further increasing the ACE/ACE2 ratio. The net effect is a dysregulated increase in ANG II expression, increase in circulating reactive oxygen species, a

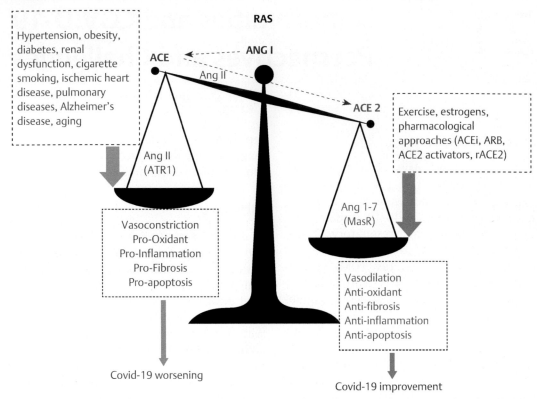

Fig. 21.1 Depiction of the critical balance between angiotensin-converting enzyme (ACE) and ACE2 products and clinical course of COVID-19. Patients with comorbidities may already have a baseline imbalance in ACE/ACE2 ratio in a proinflammatory, procoagulant vasoconstrictive state due to increased A2 which is further exacerbated by SARS-CoV-2 binding to ACE2 during infection. Pagliaro P, Penna C. ACE/ACE2 ratio: a key also in 2019 coronavirus disease (Covid-19). Front Med (Lausanne) 2020;7:335. Creative Commons Attribution License (CC BY Frontiers in Medicine).[4]

proinflammatory state, vasoconstriction, and the prothrombotic state, and increase in proinflammatory cytokine production which is characteristic of severe COVID-19 disease.[4,6,14,17,20,21,24,27] Furthermore, obesity is a chronic proinflammatory state and coupled with increases in dysregulated ANG II production may enhance cytokine production and the development of the cytokine storm, cardiovascular dysfunction, and ARDS in infected individuals.[14,17,20,25,29]

Diabetes

Diabetes mellitus (DM) and poor glycemic control are independent risk factors of mortality in patients with COVID-19 disease.[2,9,30] Furthermore, infection results marked insulin resistance and worsening glycemic control. A large percentage of type 2 diabetics afflicted with infection develop diabetic keto acidosis (DKA).[31–34] Hyperglycemia contributes to the dysregulated immune response and increases viral replication.[30] Interestingly, Zhou reported in an observational study that 10% of type II diabetics developed at last one episode of hypoglycemia.[35] Hypoglycemia also increases morbidity during the clinical course of infection by increasing proinflammatory monocytes phenotypes and inducing platelet dysfunction.[30,35–37] Similar to obesity, both type I and type II DMs are states of increase in ANG II expression which is further exacerbated in COVID-19, resulting in a marked prothrombotic, proinflammatory state, and endothelial injury which are harbingers of multiorgan failure.[4,30,32,37,38] Hyperglycemia has been known to decrease the efficacy of tocilizumab in patients with severe COVID-19 disease.[39]

A variety of therapeutic agents used in the management of COVID-19 have variable effects on blood glucose. Glucocorticoids and protease inhibitors, such as lopinavir/ritonavir, increase blood glucose levels.[2,30,32,38] Tocilizumab and remdesivir have been reported to decrease insulin resistance. Both chloroquine and hydroxychloroquine demonstrate the ability to induce hypoglycemia.[2,30,32,38] Thus, potential drug–drug interactions between therapeutic agents used during the clinical course of COVID-19 infection and those used to treat DM need to be considered.[2,30,32,38]

Therapeutic agents that can be employed with reasonable safety in the management of DM during infection include insulin, metformin, and dipeptidylpeptidase-4 (DPP-4) inhibitors such as sitigliptin.[2,30,32,38] In terms of metformin use, this agent should be discontinued if patients develop acute kidney injury or lactic acidosis. DPP-4 inhibitors have the potential to inhibit viral cell entry due to blockade of the DPP-4 receptor, a known SARS-CoV-2 receptor protein.[30,32,40–44] Furthermore, DPP-4 inhibitors possess immunomodulatory properties and thus may attenuate the dysregulated immune response commonly observed in severe infection.[30,45,46] A recent case-control observational study showed that the use of sitigliptin was associated with a decrease in mortality and an improvement in clinical outcomes.[47] Glucagon-like peptide-1 (GLP-1) agonists in combination with insulin have the potential of improving glucose control and decreasing proinflammatory cytokine expression.[30,48–50] The effects of GLP-1 agonists such as nausea, vomiting, and diarrhea result in volume depletion.[30,32,38,50] Thus, caution must be taken when employing GLP-1 agonists in patients with worsening disease. Sodium glucose transporter-1 (SGLPT2) inhibitors, such as empagliflozin, possess natriuretic and diuretic properties which can lead to volume depletion. A noted side effect of SGLPT2 inhibitors is diabetic ketoacidosis; thus, the use of these agents in COVID-19 should be avoided.[30,38]

The sulfanylurea class of oral hypoglycemics should be used with caution in patients with poor oral intake as profound hypoglycemia may occur. Pioglitazone use may result in significant fluid retention, and cardiac compromise that can commonly occur in COVID-19 disease may result in congestive heart failure (CHF). Concurrent use of angiotensin receptor blockade (A2RB) or angiotensin-converting enzyme inhibitors (ACEIs) should not be discontinued unless hemodynamic instability, hyperkalemia, or acute kidney injury develops.[2,30,38]

Chronic Obstructive Pulmonary Disease

Multiple studies have observed that patients with COPD have an increased risk of hospitalization, intensive care unit (ICU) admission, and mortality.[16,51–53] Clearly, COPD patients have less pulmonary reserve; thus, any insult during infection such as COVID-19 tracheobronchitis or pneumonia will lead to severe decompensation in a shorter time period. Many patients with COPD are chronically on inhaled corticosteroids (ICS) and initially it was presumed that these agents would predispose patients to a higher risk of infection and worse outcomes.[52,54,55] However, to date there has been no evidence to support that ICS leads to increase in infection rates and outcomes.[52,54,55] COPD patients have a higher expression of ACE2 and transmembrane protease (TMPRS) in bronchial epithelial and lung tissue allowing for the potential increased viral entry into respiratory epithelial cells that results in a more rapid progression of infection into the lower respiratory tract.[55,56] Patients with COPD have demonstrated an abnormal innate immune response to viral infection, possibly predisposing them to development of severe disease.[57,58]

Cardiovascular Disease and Hypertension

Throughout the period of the current pandemic, many observational studies have demonstrated an increased prevalence of hypertension (HTN) and cardiovascular disease (CVD) in individuals afflicted with COVID-19 disease.[59-67] Although many of the original studies were not adjusted for confounders, there is abundant data to suggest that individuals with HTN and CVD are at higher risk for the development of COVID-19 complications and death.[59-67] In a large meta-analysis involving over 15,000 patients, Barrera and collaborators demonstrated that HTN, even when adjusted for confounding risks, was associated with ICU admission and death.[68] Initially, due to the mechanism of viral cellular entry involving interactions with the viral S protein and ACE2, it was thought that the employment of ACEIs or angiotensin 2 receptor blockers (ARBs) would place individuals treated with these agents at higher risk of infection and disease complications.[66] Large observational studies by Rezel-Potts and coinvestigators, and others, have demonstrated that none of the use of ARBs, ACEI, or any of the major classes of antihypertensive agents commonly employed were associated with adverse outcomes or increased rate of infection.[69] Thus, unless hemodynamic compromise exists, hyperkalemia develops, or acute renal failure occurs, recommendations are to continue ACEI or ARB use.

A myriad of observational studies have demonstrated that CVD can be associated with poor clinical outcomes and mortality.[59-67] This is perhaps due to SARS-CoV-2 S protein interaction with ACE2 during infection, which results in a proinflammatory and prothrombotic state, potentially leading to acute myocardial infarction, myocarditis, cardiac arrhythmias, and thromboembolic events.[4,6,66] As myocarditis, elevated troponin I, and acute myocardial infarction are not uncommon, CVD complications such as CHF may occur.[60,62,66] Thiazolidinediones used to treat DM have been known to precipitate CHF and should be discontinued. Many therapeutic agents that have been employed in the therapeutic arsenal against SARS-CoV-2 such as chloroquine, hydroxychloroquine, azithromycin, lopinavir/ritonavir have cardiotoxic effects such as prolongation of the QTc interval (as is the case with hydroxychloroquine and chloroquine and azithromycin). Lopinavir/ritonavir have been reported to cause bundle branch block and prolonged QTc interval. The presumptive mechanism of these agents is that they block the human ether-a-go-go-related gene (hERG) potassium channel resulting in a risk for arrhythmogenesis.[66,70,71] Therefore, therapy with these prodysrhythmic agents in the setting viral-induced myocardial injury, cytokine-mediated myocardial dysfunction, and electrolyte abnormalities poses a significant risk for the potential development of lethal dysrhythmias.

Chronic Liver Disease

The impact of chronic liver disease (CLD) regarding the risk of infection and clinical outcomes is poorly understood. Previous experience in patients with liver disease developing acute-on chronic hepatitis and ARDS resulting in clinical decompensation has been observed during infection with influenza.[72] A small observational study demonstrated that in patients receiving corticosteroids, chronic hepatitis B was independently associated with delay in SARS-CoV-2 viral clearance.[73] In an observational study including over a thousand patients, 2.1% of the patients had chronic hepatitis B.[3] Investigators demonstrated no increased risk of decompensation in patients with chronic hepatitis B.[3,74] Patients with chronic hepatitis C have an increased risk of hospitalization; however, there does not seem to be an increased risk of ICU admission or mortality.[75] In patients with hepatitis C, hospitalization rates are higher in patients with a higher fibrosis score.[75] Although the risk of mortality and morbidity associated with CLD was initially unclear, as we learn more about this disease it has become clear that the presence of CLD is associated with poor clinical outcomes particularly as the severity of CLD increases with patients with nonalcoholic hepatic steatosis, cirrhosis, hepatocellular carcinoma, and alcoholic liver disease.[74,76–82]

Therapeutic agents used in the management of the COVID-19 disease have significant hepatotoxic side effect potential including tocilizumab, remdesivir, lopinavir/ritonavir, and azithromycin.[83,84] Tocilizumab has been observed to cause elevated transaminases which are usually mild; however, when employed with other drugs it may become more pronounced. In most cases, elevated transaminases have not resulted in terminating therapy.[83,84] Although tocilizumab has the potential to cause reactivation of hepatitis B, there appears to be very little risk of reactivation occurring during treatment for COVID-19.[85] Remdesivir has been demonstrated to cause an elevation in transaminases, and in some studies, transaminitis is the most commonly cited side effects of treatment.[83,86,87] The elevation of transaminases can be severe; however, discontinuation of therapy is usually not necessary. Generally, the current thinking is that most of the elevations in transaminases observed with remdesivir is related to the superimposed infection with SARS-CoV-2.[81,86,87] It is currently not recommended to start therapy with this agent if transaminases are greater than five times normal.[87] Elevated transaminase levels have occurred in patients with HIV treated with lopinavir/ritonavir which can also occur in patients with COVID-19 treated with these agents.[88–90] The potential hepatotoxicity of this agent is possibly due to its activation of caspases, oxidant stress, and toxic metabolites resulting in hepatocyte injury. The clinician should be constantly vigilant of drug–drug interactions, because many of these agents are inhibitors of the cytochrome p-450 system.[88–90]

Chronic Kidney Disease

Patients with chronic kidney disease (CKD) usually have multiple superimposed comorbidities such as diabetes, CVD, and HTN. Thus, it is understandable from an epidemiological and pathophysiological standpoint that individuals with CKD would represent a group at high risk for increased morbidity and mortality in the setting of COVID-19. Large observational studies have demonstrated that patients with CKD and COVID-19 have a significantly worse prognosis and mortality than those individuals with and without CKD.[91,92] Henry and Lippi performed a small unadjusted meta-analysis involving over 1,000 patients and observed an almost threefold risk for the development of severe COVID-19 in individuals with CKD.[93] Pakhchania et al employing a large electronic medical record database observed that individuals with CKD demonstrated a significant increase in hospitalization, need for mechanical ventilation, requirement for dialysis, and mortality.[92] When individuals were propensity matched for comorbidities, these significant differences in morbidity and mortality remained in patients with moderate to severe CKD.[92] After propensity matching patients with mild disease, a significant difference in need for hospitalization remained.[92] Drug dosing in the setting of impaired renal dysfunction needs to be considered. Although there is a paucity of information, attention should be paid to the timing and dosing of medications in patients requiring renal replacement therapy. Interestingly, patients with CKD in contrast to patients with SOTs demonstrate a better response to mRNA vaccines employed during the pandemic.[94–96] However, hemodialysis patients demonstrate a blunted response to vaccination.[94–96]

Organ Transplant and Patients with Cancer

Due to immunosuppressive therapy, patients with SOT and BMT are a particularly challenging group of individuals who may be at risk for SARS-CoV-2 infection and worse clinical outcomes during COVID-19 disease.[8,97–100] However, reports on the bone marrow transplant patients have been mixed.[101] In addition, potential drug–drug interactions with immunosuppressants may pose additional challenges.[8,97,99–101] Antiproliferative agents may also worsen leukopenia and neutropenia in these patients. Recent experience has demonstrated that individuals with SOT have worse disease and clinical outcomes.[97–101] Older patients and those with superimposed comorbidities and other infections seem to have the highest risk of poor clinical outcomes.[97–101] Periera et al reported that when compared with COVID-19 patients without SOT, SOT patients had more severe disease (39 vs. 6%) and increased mortality.[99] In a small observational study, Fernandez-Ruiz and coinvestigators, reported worse clinical disease and clinical course in SOT patients.[102] In early and long-term liver transplant survivors, Lee et al reported a high mortality rate.[103] The approach to care in these high-risk patients includes early diagnosis and tapering of immunosuppression and possible administration of monoclonal antibodies.[99,104] Of note, many patients with SOT demonstrate a diminished response to current vaccines directed against COVID-19 S protein. In contrast to individuals with SOT, those with BMT, at least in early reports, generate an adequate vaccine response.[95,96,105]

Patients with cancer represent another subset of immunosuppressed populations that are at increased risk for increased severity of disease and poor clinical outcomes.[12,100,106–108] However, many cancer patients are older and have superimposed comorbidities which heighten their risk for worse outcomes. Miyashita reporting on a large cohort of patients observed that age played a major factor on mortality among individuals with cancer, and risk of poor outcomes did not reach statistical significance when adjusted for age.[107] Others evaluating clinical outcomes in cancer patients with history of thoracic malignancies, and those undergoing active treatment for these neoplasms observed an increase in mortality among groups studied.[109] Thus, the overall evidence supports that cancer patients, whether diagnosed or undergoing treatment, demonstrate a high-risk group for infection, severe disease, intensive care admission, and mortality. Although patients with cancer do mount a serological response to vaccination, it is comparably less than healthy controls.[110] Those undergoing lymphocyte-depleting strategies may have a blunted or no response to current vaccines.[7] Patients with solid tumors seem to have a reasonable response after the second vaccine.[7]

Although cancer patients represent a high-risk group for poor clinical outcomes, in some cases treatment should not be delayed and therapy in cancer patients should be risk stratified and treatment should be individualized.[111]

Case Studies

Case 1

A 67-year-old gentleman with a past medical history of nonalcoholic hepatic steatosis (NASH), type 2 DM managed with metformin and sitagliptin, presented to the hospital with 3 days of upper respiratory tract symptoms, dyspnea, and diarrhea. As the patient received full vaccination series with the Moderna vaccine, his primary physician did not initially test for SARS-CoV-2 and he treated the patient symptomatically.

On admission, the patient was in marked respiratory distress with a respiratory rate of 35/min, temperature 38°C, blood pressure 90/40 torr, BMI 38, and pulse 116/min, and oximetry revealed an oxygen saturation of 80% on 100% non-rebreathing mask. On initial physical exam, he was in marked distress using accessory muscles of respiration. Pulmonary examination was significant for diffuse bilateral rales. The remaining physical examination was unremarkable. His laboratory values revealed a serum creatinine of 6.6 mg/dL, urea 100 mg/dL, serum potassium 7.2 mEq/dL, serum glucose 350 mg/dL, plasma IL-6 level 2,300 pcg/mL, serum bicarbonate (CO_2) 13 mEq/dL. Arterial blood gas analysis (ABG) with the patient being administered oxygen employing a 100% non-rebreathing mask and supplemental HFNC at 60 L/min revealed a pH 6.92, $PaCO_2$ 42 mmHg, PaO_2 100 mmHg, and HCO_3 8. Computed tomographic scan (**Fig. 21.2**) revealed severe bilateral airspace disease with peripheral ground-glass opacities and areas of organizing pneumonia. The patient rapidly deteriorated and was endotracheally intubated and was managed employing proning, lung protective strategies, and PEEP. He required 12 µg/min of norepinephrine in order to maintain a mean arterial pressure (MAP) of 65 mmHg. Due to refractory hyperkalemia he was placed on continuous renal replacement therapy and required heparinization in order to prevent dialyzer clotting. Therapeutic management was initiated with remdesivir, tocilizumab, and intravenous dexamethasone. The patient survived to discharge from the acute hospitalization at day 24. However, he failed to be liberated from mechanical ventilation; he was transitioned to intermittent hemodialysis and currently is in a long-term acute care/ventilator unit and remains dialysis- and ventilator-dependent.

Case 2

In March of 2020, a 52-year-old Hispanic gentleman with a history of HTN and coronary artery disease and DM presented to the outpatient clinic with upper respiratory tract symptoms associated with 2 days of low-grade fever and malaise. The patient's nasopharyngeal swab was positive for SARS-CoV-2. As at that time the Centers for Disease Control and Prevention stated there were no specific treatment for COVID-19, he was discharged home with a prescription of azithromycin and advised to immediately go to the emergency room if he developed respiratory distress. The patient returned to the emergency room 5 days after the onset of symptoms with a fever of 39°C, a heart rate of 130 beats/min, and low blood pressure. Hypotension (70/50 mmHg) was refractory to volume expansion and vasopressors. The patient was profoundly hypoxemic on 100% non-rebreathing mask with a pulse oximeter reading of 85%. Laboratory values were significant for a d-Dimer of 4,000 ng/mL, Troponin I of 50 ng/mL. Imaging (chest X-ray, **Fig. 21.2a**) revealed severe alveolar airspace disease. Echocardiogram revealed an ejection fraction of 15% with severe anterior wall hypokinesis, and a large right ventricular thrombus was also observed (**Fig. 21.2b**). CT scan revealed severe organizing pneumonia and peripheral airspace disease (**Fig 21.2c**). The patient expired with 8 hours of admission due to refractory shock.

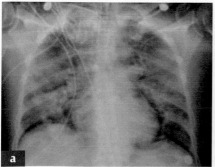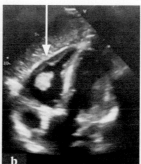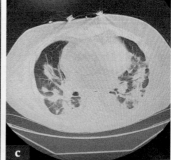

Fig. 21.2 (a) Chest X-ray demonstrating severe alveolar airspace disease. (b) Echocardiogram demonstrating large right ventricular thrombus (*white arrow*). (c) CT scan revealing organizing pneumonia and peripheral airspace disease.

Case 3

A 55-year-old Caucasian lady with stage 4 CKD and HTN called her nephrologist with a 1-day history of diarrhea, chills, fever, and severe body aches. She was advised to go to the emergency for SARS-CoV-2 by naso-pharyngeal polymerase chain reaction (PCR) testing. A rapid PCR test was positive for the SARS-CoV-2. Her chest X-ray revealed patchy peripheral ground-glass opacities. The patient was not hypoxic, and other than a temperature of 39°C, her exam and vital signs were unremarkable. The patient was admin-istered intravenous REGN-COV2 monoclonal antibody cocktail and was discharged home on aspirin 325-mg daily, doxycycline 100 mg two times per day and ivermectin 18 mg (200 µg/kg) daily for 5 days. She was educated on home pulse oximetry monitoring every 2 hours while awake and advised to go imme-diately to the emergency room should her saturation drop below 94% or she develops dyspnea. Although her fever resolved, on day 6 she developed a dry cough and wheezing. Inhaled albuterol 2.5 mg four times a day and budesonide dry powder was delivered using a turbohaler at a dose of 400 µg per actua-tion. She was asked to take two inhalations twice a day for 7 days. The patient gradually improved and did not require hospitalization.

Conclusion

Patients with comorbidities present a signifi-cant challenge in management and are at a higher risk for poor outcome. Many of these individuals have more than one comorbidity, they may have a blunted response to vaccines and therapy of comorbidities may compli-cate management. In many cases, individu-als may have a baseline ACE/ACE2 imbalance due to comorbidities favoring a proinflamma-tory, vasoconstrictive, and profibrotic state leading to poor outcomes when infection occurs. Vaccination, nontherapeutic (wear-ing masks, social distancing) prompt diagno-sis, and implementation of and adjustments to therapy of comorbidities are essential in potentially improving outcomes.

References

1. Dong G, Du Z, Zhu J, et al. The clinical characteristics and prognosis of COVID-19 patients with comorbidities: a retrospective analysis of the infection peak in Wuhan. Ann Transl Med 2021;9(4):280
2. Callender LA, Curran M, Bates SM, Mairesse M, Weigandt J, Betts CJ. The impact of pre-existing comorbidities and therapeutic inter-ventions on COVID-19. Front Immunol 2020; 11:1991
3. Guan WJ, Ni ZY, Hu Y, et al; China Medical Treatment Expert Group for Covid-19. Clinical characteristics of coronavirus disease 2019 in China. N Engl J Med 2020; 382(18):1708–1720
4. Pagliaro P, Penna C. ACE/ACE2 ratio: a key also in 2019 coronavirus disease (Covid-19). Front Med (Lausanne) 2020;7:335
5. Iwasaki M, Saito J, Zhao H, Sakamoto A, Hirota K, Ma D. Inflammation triggered by SARS-CoV-2 and ACE2 augment drives multiple organ failure of severe COVID-19: molecular mechanisms and implications. Inflammation 2021;44(1):13–34
6. Verdecchia P, Cavallini C, Spanevello A, Angeli F. The pivotal link between ACE2 deficiency and SARS-CoV-2 infection. Eur J Intern Med 2020;76:14–20
7. Addeo A, Shah PK, Bordry N, et al. Immu-nogenicity of SARS-CoV-2 messenger RNA vaccines in patients with cancer. Cancer Cell 2021;39(8):1091–1098.e2
8. Aziz H, Lashkari N, Yoon YC, et al. Effects of coronavirus disease 2019 on solid organ transplantation. Transplant Proc 2020;52(9): 2642–2653
9. Emami A, Javanmardi F, Pirbonyeh N, Akbari A. Prevalence of underlying diseases in hospitalized patients with COVID-19: a systematic review and meta-analysis. Arch Acad Emerg Med 2020;8(1):e35
10. Fadl N, Ali E, Salem TZ. COVID-19: risk factors associated with infectivity and severity. Scand J Immunol 2021;93(6):e13039
11. Grupper A, Rabinowich L, Schwartz D, et al. Reduced humoral response to mRNA SARS-CoV-2 BNT162b2 vaccine in

kidney transplant recipients without prior exposure to the virus. Am J Transplant 2021; 21(8):2719–2726

12. Höllein A, Bojko P, Schulz S, et al. Characteristics and outcomes of patients with cancer and COVID-19: results from a cohort study. Acta Oncol 2021;60(1):24–27

13. Jiang Y, Abudurexiti S, An M-M, Cao D, Wei J, Gong P. Risk factors associated with 28-day all-cause mortality in older severe COVID-19 patients in Wuhan, China: a retrospective observational study. Sci Rep 2020;10(1):22369

14. Kwok S, Adam S, Ho JH, et al. Obesity: a critical risk factor in the COVID-19 pandemic. Clin Obes 2020;10(6):e12403

15. Mahmudpour M, Roozbeh J, Keshavarz M, Farrokhi S, Nabipour I. COVID-19 cytokine storm: the anger of inflammation. Cytokine 2020;133:155151

16. Richardson S, Hirsch JS, Narasimhan M, et al; the Northwell COVID-19 Research Consortium. Presenting characteristics, comorbidities, and outcomes among 5700 patients hospitalized with COVID-19 in the New York City Area. JAMA 2020;323(20): 2052–2059

17. Aghili SMM, Ebrahimpur M, Arjmand B, et al. Obesity in COVID-19 era, implications for mechanisms, comorbidities, and prognosis: a review and meta-analysis. Int J Obes 2021; 45(5):998–1016

18. Poly TN, Islam MM, Yang HC, et al. Obesity and mortality among patients diagnosed with COVID-19: a systematic review and meta-analysis. Front Med (Lausanne) 2021; 8:620044

19. Stefan N, Birkenfeld AL, Schulze MB. Global pandemics interconnected: obesity, impaired metabolic health and COVID-19. Nat Rev Endocrinol 2021;17(3):135–149

20. Pasquarelli-do-Nascimento G, Braz-de-Melo HA, Faria SS, Santos IO, Kobinger GP, Magalhães KG. Hypercoagulopathy and adipose tissue exacerbated inflammation may explain higher mortality in COVID-19 patients with obesity. Front Endocrinol (Lausanne) 2020;11:530

21. Popkin BM, Du S, Green WD, et al. Individuals with obesity and COVID-19: a global perspective on the epidemiology and biological relationships. Obes Rev 2020;21(11):e13128

22. Valerio A, Nisoli E, Rossi AP, Pellegrini M, Todesco T, El Ghoch M. Obesity and higher risk for severe complications of Covid-19: what to do when the two pandemics meet. J Popul Ther Clin Pharmacol 2020;27(S Pt 1): e31–e36

23. Frasca D, Diaz A, Romero M, Blomberg BB. Ageing and obesity similarly impair antibody responses. Clin Exp Immunol 2017;187(1):64–70

24. Pérez-Galarza J, Prócel C, Cañadas C, et al. Immune response to SARS-CoV-2 infection in obesity and T2D: literature review. Vaccines (Basel) 2021;9(2):102

25. Gammone MA, D'Orazio N. Review: obesity and COVID-19: a detrimental intersection. Front Endocrinol (Lausanne) 2021;12:652639

26. Mohammad S, Aziz R, Al Mahri S, et al. Obesity and COVID-19: what makes obese host so vulnerable? Immun Ageing 2021;18(1):1

27. Ryan PM, Caplice NM. Is adipose tissue a reservoir for viral spread, immune activation, and cytokine amplification in coronavirus disease 2019? Obesity (Silver Spring) 2020; 28(7):1191–1194

28. Bank S, De SK, Bankura B, Maiti S, Das M, A Khan G. ACE/ACE2 balance might be instrumental to explain the certain comorbidities leading to severe COVID-19 cases. Biosci Rep 2021;41(2):BSR20202014

29. de Leeuw AJM, Oude Luttikhuis MAM, Wellen AC, Müller C, Calkhoven CF. Obesity and its impact on COVID-19. J Mol Med (Berl) 2021;99(7):899–915

30. Lim S, Bae JH, Kwon H-S, Nauck MA. COVID-19 and diabetes mellitus: from pathophysiology to clinical management. Nat Rev Endocrinol 2021;17(1):11–30

31. Chee YJ, Ng SJH, Yeoh E. Diabetic ketoacidosis precipitated by Covid-19 in a patient with newly diagnosed diabetes mellitus. Diabetes Res Clin Pract 2020;164:108166

32. Chee YJ, Tan SK, Yeoh E. Dissecting the interaction between COVID-19 and diabetes mellitus. J Diabetes Investig 2020;11(5): 1104–1114

33. Pal R, Banerjee M, Yadav U, Bhattacharjee S. Clinical profile and outcomes in COVID-19 patients with diabetic ketoacidosis: a systematic review of literature. Diabetes Metab Syndr 2020;14(6):1563–1569

34. Palermo NE, Sadhu AR, McDonnell ME. Diabetic ketoacidosis in COVID-19: unique

concerns and considerations. J Clin Endocrinol Metab 2020;105(8):2819–2829

35. Zhou J, Tan J. Diabetes patients with COVID-19 need better blood glucose management in Wuhan, China. Metabolism 2020;107:154216

36. Iqbal A, Prince LR, Novodvorsky P, et al. Effect of hypoglycemia on inflammatory responses and the response to low-dose endotoxemia in humans. J Clin Endocrinol Metab 2019;104(4):1187–1199

37. Zhu L, She Z-G, Cheng X, et al. Association of blood glucose control and outcomes in patients with COVID-19 and pre-existing type 2 diabetes. Cell Metab 2020;31(6):1068–1077.e3

38. Bornstein SR, Rubino F, Khunti K, et al. Practical recommendations for the management of diabetes in patients with COVID-19. Lancet Diabetes Endocrinol 2020;8(6):546–550

39. Marfella R, Paolisso P, Sardu C, et al. Negative impact of hyperglycaemia on tocilizumab therapy in Covid-19 patients. Diabetes Metab 2020;46(5):403–405

40. Raj VS, Mou H, Smits SL, et al. Dipeptidyl peptidase 4 is a functional receptor for the emerging human coronavirus-EMC. Nature 2013;495(7440):251–254

41. Solerte SB, Di Sabatino A, Galli M, Fiorina P. Dipeptidyl peptidase-4 (DPP4) inhibition in COVID-19. Acta Diabetol 2020;57(7):779–783

42. Valencia I, Peiró C, Lorenzo Ó, Sánchez-Ferrer CF, Eckel J, Romacho T. DPP4 and ACE2 in diabetes and COVID-19: therapeutic targets for cardiovascular complications? Front Pharmacol 2020;11:1161

43. Yang Y, Cai Z, Zhang J. DPP-4 inhibitors may improve the mortality of coronavirus disease 2019: A meta-analysis. PLoS One 2021;16(5):e0251916

44. Du H, Wang DW, Chen C. The potential effects of DPP-4 inhibitors on cardiovascular system in COVID-19 patients. J Cell Mol Med 2020;24(18):10274–10278

45. Pinheiro MM, Fabbri A, Infante M. Cytokine storm modulation in COVID-19: a proposed role for vitamin D and DPP-4 inhibitor combination therapy (VIDPP-4i). Immunotherapy 2021;13(9):753–765

46. Shao S, Xu Q, Yu X, Pan R, Chen Y. Dipeptidyl peptidase 4 inhibitors and their potential immune modulatory functions. Pharmacol Ther 2020;209:107503

47. Solerte SB, D'Addio F, Trevisan R, et al. Sitagliptin treatment at the time of hospitalization was associated with reduced mortality in patients with type 2 diabetes and COVID-19: a multicenter, case-control, retrospective, observational study. Diabetes Care 2020;43(12):2999–3006

48. Lee S, Lee DY. Glucagon-like peptide-1 and glucagon-like peptide-1 receptor agonists in the treatment of type 2 diabetes. Ann Pediatr Endocrinol Metab 2017;22(1):15–26

49. Lee Y-S, Jun H-S. Anti-inflammatory effects of GLP-1-based therapies beyond glucose control. Mediators Inflamm. 2016:3094642. doi:10.1155/2016/3094642

50. Landstra CP, de Koning EJP. COVID-19 and diabetes: understanding the interrelationship and risks for a severe course. Front Endocrinol (Lausanne) 2021;12:649525

51. Gerayeli FV, Milne S, Cheung C, et al. COPD and the risk of poor outcomes in COVID-19: a systematic review and meta-analysis. EClinicalMedicine 2021;33:100789

52. Lee SC, Son KJ, Han CH, Park SC, Jung JY. Impact of COPD on COVID-19 prognosis: a nationwide population-based study in South Korea. Sci Rep 2021;11(1):3735

53. Paranjpe I, Russak AJ, De Freitas JK, et al. Clinical characteristics of hospitalized Covid-19 patients in New York City. *medRxiv*. Published online 2020. doi:10.1101/2020.04.19.20062117

54. Choi JC, Jung S-Y, Yoon UA, et al. Inhaled corticosteroids and COVID-19 risk and mortality: a nationwide cohort study. J Clin Med 2020;9(11):E3406

55. Leung JM, Niikura M, Yang CWT, Sin DD. COVID-19 and COPD. Eur Respir J 2020;56(2):2002108

56. Leung JM, Yang CX, Tam A, et al. ACE-2 expression in the small airway epithelia of smokers and COPD patients: implications for COVID-19. Eur Respir J 2020;55(5):2000688

57. Shaykhiev R, Crystal RG. Innate immunity and chronic obstructive pulmonary disease: a mini-review. Gerontology 2013;59(6):481–489

58. Polverino F, Kheradmand F. COVID-19, COPD, and AECOPD: immunological, epidemiological, and clinical aspects. Front Med (Lausanne) 2021;7:627278

59. Sun Y, Guan X, Jia L, et al. Independent and combined effects of hypertension and diabetes on clinical outcomes in patients with COVID-19: a retrospective cohort study of Huoshen Mountain Hospital and Guanggu Fangcang Shelter Hospital. J Clin Hypertens (Greenwich) 2021;23(2):218–231

60. Guo T, Fan Y, Chen M, et al. Cardiovascular implications of fatal outcomes of patients with coronavirus disease 2019 (COVID-19). JAMA Cardiol 2020;5(7):811–818

61. Leiva Sisnieguez CE, Espeche WG, Salazar MR. Arterial hypertension and the risk of severity and mortality of COVID-19. Eur Respir J 2020;55(6):2001148

62. Li B, Yang J, Zhao F, et al. Prevalence and impact of cardiovascular metabolic diseases on COVID-19 in China. Clin Res Cardiol 2020; 109(5):531–538

63. Liang X, Shi L, Wang Y, et al. The association of hypertension with the severity and mortality of COVID-19 patients: evidence based on adjusted effect estimates. J Infect 2020;81(3):e44–e47

64. Luo L, Fu M, Li Y, et al. The potential association between common comorbidities and severity and mortality of coronavirus disease 2019: a pooled analysis. Clin Cardiol 2020;43(12):1478–1493

65. Matsushita K, Ding N, Kou M, et al. The relationship of COVID-19 severity with cardiovascular disease and its traditional risk factors: A systematic review and meta-analysis. *medRxiv*. Published online 2020. doi:10.1101/2020.04.05.20054155

66. Nishiga M, Wang DW, Han Y, Lewis DB, Wu JC. COVID-19 and cardiovascular disease: from basic mechanisms to clinical perspectives. Nat Rev Cardiol 2020;17(9):543–558

67. Salazar MR. Is hypertension without any other comorbidities an independent predictor for COVID-19 severity and mortality? J Clin Hypertens (Greenwich) 2021;23(2):232–234

68. Barrera FJ, Shekhar S, Wurth R, et al. Prevalence of diabetes and hypertension and their associated risks for poor outcomes in Covid-19 patients. J Endocr Soc 2020; 4(9):a102

69. Rezel-Potts E, Douiri A, Chowienczyk PJ, Gulliford MC. Antihypertensive medications and COVID-19 diagnosis and mortality: population-based case-control analysis in the United Kingdom. Br J Clin Pharmacol 2021;n/a(n/a). doi:https://doi.org/10.1111/bcp.14873

70. Charbit B, Rosier A, Bollens D, et al. Relationship between HIV protease inhibitors and QTc interval duration in HIV-infected patients: a cross-sectional study. Br J Clin Pharmacol 2009;67(1):76–82

71. Roden DM, Harrington RA, Poppas A, Russo AM. Considerations for drug interactions on QTc in exploratory COVID-19 treatment. Circulation 2020;141(24):e906–e907

72. Bal CK, Bhatia V, Kumar S, et al. Influenza A/H1/N1/09 infection in patients with cirrhosis has a poor outcome: a case series. Indian J Gastroenterol 2014;33(2):178–182

73. Zha L, Li S, Pan L, et al. Corticosteroid treatment of patients with coronavirus disease 2019 (COVID-19). Med J Aust 2020; 212(9):416–420

74. Xiang T-D, Zheng X. Interaction between hepatitis B virus and SARS-CoV-2 infections. World J Gastroenterol 2021;27(9):782–793

75. Butt AA, Yan P, Chotani RA, Shaikh OS. Mortality is not increased in SARS-CoV-2 infected persons with hepatitis C virus infection. Liver Int 2021;41(8):1824–1831

76. Alqahtani SA, Buti M. COVID-19 and hepatitis B infection. Antivir Ther 2020;25(8):389–397

77. Chen X, Jiang Q, Ma Z, et al. Clinical characteristics of hospitalized patients with SARS-CoV-2 and hepatitis B virus co-infection. *medRxiv*. Published online 2020. doi:10.1101/2020.03.23.20040733

78. Reddy KR. SARS-CoV-2 and the liver: considerations in hepatitis B and hepatitis C infections. Clin Liver Dis (Hoboken) 2020; 15(5):191–194

79. Yip TC-F, Wong VW-S, Lui GC-Y, et al. Current and past infections of HBV do not increase mortality in patients with COVID-19. Hepatology 2021; n/a(n/a). doi:https://doi.org/10.1002/hep.31890

80. Bajaj JS, Garcia-Tsao G, Biggins SW, et al. Comparison of mortality risk in patients with cirrhosis and COVID-19 compared with patients with cirrhosis alone and COVID-19 alone: multicentre matched cohort. Gut 2021;70(3):531–536

81. Garrido I, Liberal R, Macedo G. Review article: COVID-19 and liver disease. What we know on 1st May 2020. Aliment Pharmacol Ther 2020;52(2):267–275

82. Hegyi PJ, Váncsa S, Ocskay K, et al. Metabolic associated fatty liver disease is associated with an increased risk of severe COVID-19: a systematic review with meta-analysis. Front Med (Lausanne) 2021;8:626425

83. Ferron P-J, Gicquel T, Mégarbane B, Clément B, Fromenty B. Treatments in Covid-19 patients with pre-existing metabolic dysfunction-associated fatty liver disease: a potential threat for drug-induced liver injury? Biochimie 2020;179:266–274

84. Serviddio G, Villani R, Stallone G, Scioscia G, Foschino-Barbaro MP, Lacedonia D. Tocilizumab and liver injury in patients with COVID-19. Therap Adv Gastroenterol 2020; 13:1756284820959183

85. Rodríguez-Tajes S, Miralpeix A, Costa J, et al. Low risk of hepatitis B reactivation in patients with severe COVID-19 who receive immunosuppressive therapy. J Viral Hepat 2021;28(1):89–94

86. Bertolini A, van de Peppel IP, Bodewes FAJA, et al. Abnormal liver function tests in patients with COVID-19: relevance and potential pathogenesis. Hepatology 2020; 72(5):1864–1872

87. Aleem A, Mahadevaiah G, Shariff N, Kothadia JP. Hepatic manifestations of COVID-19 and effect of remdesivir on liver function in patients with COVID-19 illness. Proc Bayl Univ Med Cent 2021;34(4):473–477

88. Heil EL, Townsend ML, Shipp K, Clarke A, Johnson MD. Incidence of severe hepatotoxicity related to antiretroviral therapy in HIV/HCV coinfected patients. AIDS research and treatment. 2010:856542. doi:10.1155/2010/856542

89. Cvetkovic RS, Goa KL. Lopinavir/ritonavir: a review of its use in the management of HIV infection. Drugs 2003;63(8):769–802

90. Gruevska A, Moragrega ÁB, Cossarizza A, Esplugues JV, Blas-García A, Apostolova N. Apoptosis of hepatocytes: relevance for HIV-infected patients under treatment. Cells 2021;10(2):410

91. Gibertoni D, Reno C, Rucci P, et al. COVID-19 incidence and mortality in non-dialysis chronic kidney disease patients. PLoS One 2021;16(7):e0254525

92. Pakhchanian H, Raiker R, Mukherjee A, Khan A, Singh S, Chatterjee A. Outcomes of COVID-19 in CKD patients: a multicenter electronic medical record cohort study. Clin J Am Soc Nephrol 2021;16(5):785–786

93. Henry BM, Lippi G. Chronic kidney disease is associated with severe coronavirus disease 2019 (COVID-19) infection. Int Urol Nephrol 2020;52(6):1193–1194

94. Grupper A, Sharon N, Finn T, et al. Humoral response to the Pfizer BNT162b2 vaccine in patients undergoing maintenance hemodialysis. Clin J Am Soc Nephrol. 2021;16(7):1037-1042. doi:10.2215/CJN.03500321

95. Danthu C, Hantz S, Dahlem A, et al. Humoral response after SARS-CoV-2 mRNA vaccination in a cohort of hemodialysis patients and kidney transplant recipients. J Am Soc Nephrol 2021;32(9):2153–2158

96. Hou Y-C, Lu K-C, Kuo K-L. The efficacy of COVID-19 vaccines in chronic kidney disease and kidney transplantation patients: a narrative review. Vaccines (Basel) 2021; 9(8):885

97. Azzi Y, Bartash R, Scalea J, Loarte-Campos P, Akalin E. COVID-19 and solid organ transplantation: a review article. Transplantation 2021;105(1):37–55

98. Mastroianni F, Leisman DE, Fisler G, Narasimhan M. General and intensive care outcomes for hospitalized patients with solid organ transplants with COVID-19. J Intensive Care Med 2021;36(4):494–499

99. Pereira MR, Mohan S, Cohen DJ, et al. COVID-19 in solid organ transplant recipients: initial report from the US epicenter. Am J Transplant 2020;20(7):1800–1808

100. Sharma A, Bhatt NS, St Martin A, et al. Clinical characteristics and outcomes of COVID-19 in haematopoietic stem-cell transplantation recipients: an observational cohort study. Lancet Haematol 2021;8(3):e185–e193

101. Hilbrands LB, Duivenvoorden R, Vart P, et al; ERACODA Collaborators. COVID-19-related mortality in kidney transplant and dialysis patients: results of the ERACODA collaboration. Nephrol Dial Transplant 2020;35(11):1973–1983

102. Fernández-Ruiz M, Andrés A, Loinaz C, et al. COVID-19 in solid organ transplant recipients: a single-center case series from Spain. Am J Transplant 2020;20(7):1849–1858

103. Lee BT, Perumalswami PV, Im GY, Florman S, Schiano TD; COBE Study Group. COVID-19 in liver transplant recipients: an initial experience from the US epicenter. Gastroenterology 2020;159(3):1176–1178.e2

104. Dhand A, Lobo SA, Wolfe K, et al. Casirivimab-imdevimab for treatment of COVID-19 in solid organ transplant recipients: an early experience. Transplantation 2021;105(7): e68–e69

105. Redjoul R, Le Bouter A, Beckerich F, Fourati S, Maury S. Antibody response after second BNT162b2 dose in allogeneic HSCT recipients. Lancet 2021;398(10297): 298–299

106. Gosain R, Abdou Y, Singh A, Rana N, Puzanov I, Ernstoff MS. COVID-19 and cancer: a comprehensive review. Curr Oncol Rep 2020;22(5):53

107. Miyashita H, Mikami T, Chopra N, et al. Do patients with cancer have a poorer prognosis of COVID-19? An experience in New York City. Ann Oncol 2020;31(8):1088–1089

108. Yang F, Shi S, Zhu J, Shi J, Dai K, Chen X. Clinical characteristics and outcomes of cancer patients with COVID-19. J Med Virol 2020;92(10):2067–2073

109. Garassino MC, Whisenant JG, Huang L-C, et al; TERAVOLT investigators. COVID-19 in patients with thoracic malignancies (TERAVOLT): first results of an international, registry-based, cohort study. Lancet Oncol 2020;21(7):914–922

110. Massarweh A, Eliakim-Raz N, Stemmer A, et al. Evaluation of seropositivity following BNT162b2 messenger RNA vaccination for SARS-CoV-2 in patients undergoing treatment for cancer. JAMA Oncol 2021;7(8): 1133–1140

111. Fox TA, Troy-Barnes E, Kirkwood AA, et al. Clinical outcomes and risk factors for severe COVID-19 in patients with haematological disorders receiving chemo- or immunotherapy. Br J Haematol 2020; 191(2):194–206

Index